W1 529 SCH
(ORD)

CHALLENGES IN
Colorectal Cancer

CHALLENGES IN

Colorectal Cancer

EDITED BY

John H. Scholefield
Professor of Surgery
University Hospital
Nottingham, UK

Axel Grothey
Professor
Division of Medical Oncology
Mayo Clinic
Rochester, Minnesota, USA

Herand Abcarian
Turi Josefsen Professor and Chairman
Department of Surgery
University of Illinois College of Medicine
Chicago, Illinois, USA

Tim Maughan
Professor of Cancer Studies
University of Cardiff
Cardiff, UK

SECOND EDITION

Blackwell
Publishing

Blackwell Publishing, Inc., 350 Main Street, Malden, Massachusetts 02148-5020, USA
Blackwell Publishing Ltd, 9600 Garsington Road, Oxford OX4 2DQ, UK
Blackwell Publishing Asia Pty Ltd, 550 Swanston Street, Carlton, Victoria 3053, Australia

First published 2000
Second edition 2006

1   2006

Library of Congress Cataloging-in-publication Data

Challenges in colorectal cancer/edited by
    John H. Schofield. . .[et al.]. – 2nd ed.
    p. ; cm.
Includes index.
ISBN-13: 978-1-4051-2706-6 (alk. paper)
ISBN-10: 1-4051-2706-6 (alk. paper)
    1. Colon (Anatomy)—Cancer.
    2. Rectum—Cancer. I. Scholefield, John H.
    [DNLM: 1. Colorectal neoplasms—therpay. 2. Colorectal Surgery.
WI 529 C437 2006]
RC280.C6C47 2006
616.99′4347—dc22

                                                                        2006000979

ISBN-13: 978-1-4051-2706-6
ISBN-10: 1-4051-2706-6

A catalogue record for this title is available from the British Library

Set in 10/13.5 Sabon by Newgen Imaging Systems (P) Ltd., Chennai, India
Printed and bound in India by Replika Press PVT Ltd

Commissioning Editor: Alison Brown
Editorial Assistant: Jennifer Seward
Development Editor: Elisabeth Dodds
Production Controller: Kate Charman

For further information on Blackwell Publishing, visit our website:
http://www.blackwellpublishing.com

Contents

List of contributors

EDITORS

John H. Scholefield ChM, FRCS, *Professor of Surgery, Division of Gastrointestinal Surgery, Floor E, West Block, University Hospital, Queen's Medical Centre, Nottingham NG7 2UH, UK*

Herand Abcarian MD, *Turi Josefsen Professor and Chairman, Department of Surgery, University of Illinois College of Medicine, 30 N Michigan Ave, #1118 Chicago, IL 60602, USA*

Axel Grothey MD, *Professor, Division of Medical Oncology, Mayo Clinic, 200 First Street SW, Rochester, MN 55905, USA*

Tim Maughan BA, MB BS, MA, FRCP, FRCR, MD, *Honorary Professor of Cancer Studies, School of Medicine, University of Cardiff and Consultant in Clinical Oncology, Velindre Hospital, Whitchurch, Cardiff, CF14 2TL, Wales, UK*

CONTRIBUTORS

Chris Byrne MB BS, BSc(Med), MS, FRACS, *Colorectal Surgeon, Royal Prince Alfred Hospital, Missenden Road, Camperdown, New South Wales 2050, Australia*

David Chessin MD, *Clinical Research Fellow, Department of Surgery, Memorial Sloan-Kettering Cancer Center, New York, NY 10021, USA*

Rachel Cooper MRCP, FRCR, MD, *Department of Oncology, Cookridge Hospital, Leeds Teaching Hospital NHS Trust, Leeds LS16 6QB, UK*

Ian Daniels FRCS, *Surgeon, Pelican Cancer Foundation, Aldermaston Road, Basingstoke, Hampshire RG24 9NA, UK*

Jill Dean MMedSci, BSc(hons), RGN, *Nurse Consultant, Sheffield Teaching Hospitals NHS Foundation Trust, Northern General Hospital, Herries Road, Sheffield S5 7AU, UK*

Anthony El-Khoueiry MD, *Assistant Professor of Medicine, Division of Medical Oncology, Department of Oncology, School of Medicine, University of Southern California, 1441 Eastlake Ave, Suite 3440, Los Angeles, CA 90033, USA*

Ilora Finlay FRCP, FRCGP, *Professor of Palliative Medicine, Cardiff University and Velindre NHS Trust, Cardiff, Wales CF14 2TL, UK*

José G. Guillem MD, MPH, FACS, FASCRS, *Surgeon, Department of Surgery, Memorial Sloan-Kettering Cancer Center, New York, NY 10021, USA*

Pierre J. Guillou BSc, MD, FRCS, FRCPS, FMedSci, *Department of Surgery, St James University Hospital, Beckett Street, Leeds LS9 7TF, UK*

Melanie Jefferson MB ChB, BSc, FRCP, *Department of Palliative Medicine, University Hospital of Wales, Heath Park, Cardiff & Vale NHS Trust, Cardiff CF14 4XW, UK*

Seung-Yong Jeong MD, PhD, *Visiting Surgical Scientist, Department of Surgery, Memorial Sloan-Kettering Cancer Center, New York, NY 10021, USA*

Julia Jessop BSc(Hons), DCR(T), *Training Director, Pelican Cancer Foundation, North Hampshire Hospital, Aldermaston Road, Basingstoke RG24 9NA, UK*

Timothy G. John MBBCh, MD, FRCSEd(Gen), *Consultant Hepatobiliary Surgeon, North Hampshire Hospital NHS Trust, Aldermaston Road, Basingstoke RG24 9NA, UK*

George P. Kim MD, *Chief, Gastrointestinal Cancer Section, Assistant Professor, Mayo Clinic Jacksonville, 4500 San Pablo Road, Jacksonville, Florida, 32224, USA*

Heinz-Josef Lenz MD, *Associate Professor of Medicine and Preventive Medicine, Department of Oncology, School of Medicine, University of Southern California, 1441 Eastlake Ave., Suite 3440, Los Angeles, CA 90033, USA*

Brendan Moran MCh, FRCS, FRCSI(Gen), *Consultant Colorectal Surgeon, North Hampshire Hospital, Aldermaston Road, Basingstoke, Hampshire RG24 9NA, UK*

Richard Nelson BA, MD, FACS, FASCRS, *Professor and Head, Division of Colon and Rectal Surgery, Department of Surgery and School of Public Health, University of Illinois at Chicago, Rm. 2204 M/C 957, 1740 West Taylor Street, Chicago, IL 60612, USA*

John Northover MS, FRCS, *Professor of Intestinal and Colorectal Disorders, Cancer Research UK Colorectal Cancer Unit, Imperial College of Science, Technology and Medicine, St Mark's Hospital, Northwick Park, Watford Road, Harrow, Middlesex HA1 3UJ, UK*

Phil Quirke BM, PhD, FRCPath, *Pathology and Tumor Biology, Leeds Institute for Molecular Medicine, School of Medicine, Leeds University, Leeds, UK*

Myrddin Rees MS, FRCS, FRCSEd, *Consultant Surgeon, North Hampshire Hospital NHS Trust, Aldermaston Road, Basingstoke RG24 9NA, UK*

Susan Ritchie MBChB, *Division of Gastrointestinal Surgery, Nottingham City Hospital, Hucknall Road, Nottingham NG5 1PB, UK*

Theodore J. Saclarides MD, *Professor of Surgery and Head of the Section of Colon and Rectal Surgery, Rush University Medical Center, 1725 W. Harrison, Suite 810, Chicago, IL 60612, USA*

David Sebag-Montefiore FRCP, FRCR, *Department of Oncology, Cookridge Hospital, Leeds Teaching Hospital NHS Trust, Leeds LS16 6QB, UK*

Robert Steele BSc, MBChB, MD, FRCS(Ed), FRCS(Eng), FCS(HK), *Professor of Surgery, Department of Surgery and Molecular Oncology, Ninewells Hospital, University of Dundee, Dundee DD1 9SY, UK*

Foreword

Challenges in Colorectal Cancer provides a unique perspective in the management of this difficult problem. This book is aimed at the entire medical team rather than a specific specialty or subspecialty. Gastroenterologists, surgeons, oncologists, gastroenterology specialty nurses, radiotherapists, and other health care professionals involved in the management of patients with colorectal cancer can find the latest guidance for the most challenging and controversial aspects of this disease. The book features leading international editors and contributors. It provides the latest guidelines on the epidemiology and prevention of colorectal cancer, the application of molecular genetics, and new strategies for screening. It provides a synopsis of surgical management including new laparoscopic and endoscopic techniques, and the emerging role of genetic and pathologic staging. It is an up-to-date record of the rapidly evolving alternatives in the oncologic management of this disease, including the new chemotherapeutic alternatives and evolving radiotherapeutic techniques.

I am excited about this book, and particularly about this group of editors and well-recognized contributors. This should be a significant contribution to the library of anyone managing this disease.

Robert W. Beart, Jr, 2006

1: Does lifestyle cause colorectal cancer?

Richard Nelson

Introduction

Can lifestyle cause colorectal cancer (CRC)? To answer this it is best first to get an idea of the magnitude of the risk.

Suppose you wanted to get CRC, not by rechoosing your parents and therefore opting to be born with a genetic defect that might make the likelihood of getting cancer as high as 50%, but exclusively through diet/lifestyle alteration or toxic exposure after birth. Could you do it? Not with very much reliability, not even by moving to the highest risk locale, with a population with habits that maximize the chances of getting CRC, whatever they might be. This would only result in a probability of getting the disease of maybe 5–7% and even that in your dotage [1]. These are not very good odds if you are a betting man.

Well, perhaps there is a bit more that you could do, such as burdening yourself with a few chronic illnesses, like inflammatory bowel disease. The risk of cancer is certainly increased here but mostly at a younger age. But no one knows how to contract ulcerative colitis or Crohn's disease, and chronic infectious enteritides have not been reliably connected with cancer risk [2].

The risk of anal cancer can certainly be augmented by lifestyle decisions. Neglected chronic perianal disease, such as hemorrhoids, fissure, and fistula, and acquisition of sexually transmitted disease, especially related to human papilloma virus, can greatly increase the risk of anal cancer over the general population, perhaps as much as 10-fold for some factors [3]. But this type of cancer is much rarer than more proximal colon and rectal cancer, so even this great augmentation would not have a large overall effect on the chances of getting combined colorectal and anal cancer. No matter what you do, the chances are quite strong that you will never get CRC in your lifetime – better than 90%.

Okay, let's be a bit more realistic. You've seen enough CRC in your life and you want to minimize the risk of ever getting it, or of any of your loved ones ever getting it. First of all, how early is the die cast – again limiting our discussion to average risk individuals? Modification of risk in people with obvious familial syndromes has little to do with lifestyle – except for the role screening has in one's style of life. But more about that later. And, since inflammatory bowel disease tends to cluster in families, for whatever reason, screening may have an enhanced role here as well. But when you can or should do something about your life is an important point. For instance, it seems that risk is determined at quite an early age for breast cancer. This adds a new facet to parental responsibility, with the uncertainty of effect decades away. If there is going to be any good news in this discussion, it is that CRC risk seems to be determined at a much older age than with breast cancer or gastric cancer. So it may be possible to change one's ways at an age when motivation is there to do so, compared with an adolescent [4].

So, more fiber, less fat, and don't get constipated, right? Well, maybe. But the trouble is that, though there is some experimental evidence that these factors might diminish risk, what is needed to achieve a material change in the incidence of CRC through public health intervention is evidence that these or other recommendations actually work in the real world. And that is where things get interesting.

Since the establishment of the SEER (Surveillance, Epidemiology and End Results) program in 1973 by the National Cancer Institute in the United States, there has been a continual decline in CRC *mortality* in the United States. During much of the same period, however, CRC *incidence* rose rapidly [1]. In addition, underdeveloped countries, which once had vanishingly small rates of CRC, and whose lifestyles we hoped, in some degree, to emulate in order to reduce CRC incidence, were playing a rapid game of catch-up in CRC. Whereas there was in 1978 a 50-fold difference between mortality in high-risk and lowest-risk countries, by 1992 this had narrowed to only a 12-fold difference [5,6].

Numerous case/control and cohort studies generated apparently useful hypotheses for CRC prevention [7]. But, what had been conspicuous in its absence was any natural population in which CRC incidence had declined. It seemed that only social cataclysm could create such a population; that is, a rising risk of CRC was an inevitable result of peace and prosperity. Yet such a population did appear where it was least expected, in the United States. SEER reported that the rapidly rising incidence of CRC in the United

States suddenly reversed in 1986 and incidence has declined since then at a rate greater than 1% per year up to 2002 [1].

It seems reasonable to suppose that this sudden reversal of incidence, after a long period of rising risk, was preceded by a change in exposure to one or more environmental factors. Investigation of the evolution of suspected risk factors for CRC before and during this period of declining incidence offers a very different and unique perspective in the determination of causation and prevention of CRC. The precise time period of greatest interest in this investigation is uncertain, since there is considerable lag time between exposure to a risk modifier and clinical onset of CRC, but it might be assumed to be anywhere from 5 to 15 years before 1986. Fortunately it is in this period, from 1970 to 1980, in which data became available to allow trending of most risk factors in the United States.

Presented herein first is therefore an analysis of the pattern of change in CRC incidence by anatomic subsite, gender, and race, then a time-trend analysis of exposure to all suspected risk factors for CRC in the United States from 1970 to 1986. This broad focus is necessary because no proven paradigm of CRC prevention yet exists despite 50 years of intensive research. Therefore it would be premature to exclude any risk factor from consideration for being responsible for the declining incidence of CRC in the United States. Finally a summary of the randomized trials of diet interventions will be presented – the natural and necessary next steps to establish the effectiveness of a change in lifestyle in CRC prevention. Some of these trials investigated only single components and others attempted to diminish risk by a more global dietary change.

Incidence and dietary trends

The incidence of CRC is shown over the period from 1973 to 1994 in Figs 1.1 and 1.2. The colorectum is divided anatomically in those graphs into proximal (cecum, ascending, transverse, and descending) and distal (sigmoid and rectum) colorectum. This anatomic division of the colorectum was as a result of an analysis of race, gender, and age issues in CRC subsite location [8]. In that work, it became apparent that grouping the sigmoid, rectosigmoid, and rectum together as distal and all tumors proximal to that as proximal was a more rational point of division than the traditional division of the large bowel into colon and rectum (with further subdivision into the right and left colon). Pathologic misclassification became less likely than when for instance tumors had to be classified as either rectal or recto-sigmoid (a left

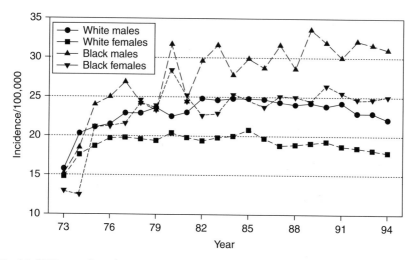

Fig. 1.1 SEER age adjusted proximal colon cancer incidence: 1973–94. Proximal colon extends from the cecum to the junction of the descending and sigmoid colon. (Reproduced from Nelson RL *et al*. *Dis Colon Rectum* 1999; 42: 741–52, with permission from Springer-Verlag.)

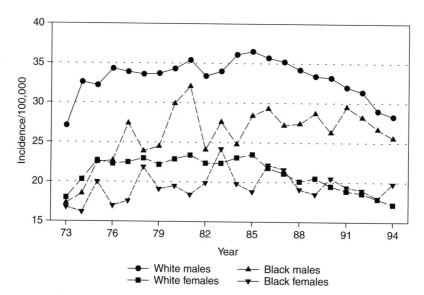

Fig. 1.2 SEER age adjusted distal CRC incidence: 1973–94. Distal colorectum includes the sigmoid, rectosigmoid, and rectum above the anorectal ring. (Reproduced from Nelson RL *et al*. *Dis Colon Rectum* 1999; 42: 741–52, with permission from Springer-Verlag.)

colon subsite) [9]. The division is more rational on embryologic (division is made at the border of the midgut and hindgut), physiologic, and anatomic grounds.

As mentioned earlier, the incidence of CRC began to decline in 1986 and has continued to drop ever since. The decline in age adjusted incidence of cancer is 24% in the distal colorectum in white men, 26% in the distal colorectum in white women, 12% in the proximal colon in white men and 14% in the proximal colon in white women. Rates among blacks are more variable from year to year but show no consistent pattern of decline in SEER, with an increase in the proximal colon in both genders, but especially in men, since 1986. Thus the decline in incidence is most apparent in both white men and white women in the distal colorectum. The lifestyle factor that had changed the most but was also gender neutral and race specific was therefore the one most likely to be associated with the sudden decline in CRC incidence.

Energy related factors. Though dietary fat has long been suspected to be the major risk factor for CRC, the time-trend data do not support this association in any aspect of energy measurement: fat intake, energy intake, obesity, physical activity, or serum cholesterol. Americans eat about the same amount of fat, exercise less, and weigh more than they did in 1970 [4].

Alcoholic beverages. National Health and Nutrition Examination Survey (NHANES) data show a decrease in ethanol intake in men. World Health Organization data show however an increase in all forms of alcoholic beverage intake [10], including the form most associated with distal CRC, beer [4]. It is interesting to note that the method of manufacture of beer in many breweries generated very high concentrations of nitrosamines, up to 50 times that found in smoked meats. The discovery of this and the delineation of the specific step in the brewing process responsible for these nitrosamines resulted in an industry-wide modification of their procedures in 1980 and the subsequent near disappearance of nitrosamines from all commercial beers [11]. But this is not a gender neutral and race-specific risk factor.

Dietary fiber and related measures. Changes in definition of fiber and instruments that measure fiber intake have made this among the most difficult dietary items to trend over time. Quantitative estimates of changes in fiber intake therefore may not be very precise but the trend appears to be upward in consumption in NHANES, though less so in the National Food Consumption Survey (see Table 1.1). Surrogates of fiber intake

Table 1.1 Time trends of non-energy related risk factors for CRC.

Risk factor	Time period	Data source	Direction + or −
Alcoholic beverages	1960–85	World Health Organization: US Consumption	+54% +61% beer +43% spirits +426% wine
	1971–88	NHANES	−10% men +28% women
Iron intake	1971–88	NHANES	+22% men +27% women
Body iron stores	1971–88	NHANES	−7.8%
Calcium intake	1971–88	NHANES	+0.5%
Constipation	1958–86	NDTI	−33%
Dietary fiber	1976–88	NHANES	+29%
Cholecystectomy	1972–90	US Hospital Discharge Survey	−1.5%
Vitamin A	1971–88	NHANES	+8%
Vitamin C	1971–88	NHANES	+18%
Parity	1960–88	NSFG	−33%
Oral contraception	1971–80	NHANES	−2%
Postmenopausal estrogen	1980–85	Ambulatory Care Survey	+22%
Cigarettes	1950–91	National Cancer Inst.	−60%
Polypectomy	1970–93	HCFA & Wisc. Hospital Assoc.	+ from negligible to >830,000 indiv.
Aspirin	1985–90	Minnesota Heart	+300%
General diet score	1965–90	National Food Consumption Survey	−10.5% (improved) (see text)

NHANES, National Health and Nutrition Examination Survey; NDTI, National Disease and Therapeutic Index; NSFG, National Survey of Family Growth; HCFA, Health Cost Finance Administration. (Reproduced from Nelson RL *et al. Dis Colon Rectum* 1999; 42: 741–52, with permission from Springer-Verlag.)

described below may more accurately reflect the trend in fiber consumption. These include constipation, vitamin A and C intake, and a combination of iron intake and body iron stores (which if diminished, imply chelation of oral iron by fiber-related phytic acid). Each of these suggest an increase in fiber ingestion from 1970 to 1985. On the other hand, data from the National Food Consumption Surveys, which report specific food groups, show an increase in these foods only in higher socioeconomic classes of both blacks and whites from 1965 to 1991. In addition there is little difference between blacks and whites in the trend for the foods, though throughout the study period whites had slightly higher fruit and vegetable (but not fiber) consumption. Neither fiber nor anti-oxidant vitamins have been associated previously with protection against specific CRC subsites.

Calcium. There seems to have been little change in dietary calcium intake over the study period. The number of people ingesting calcium supplements is however large, though skewed towards female gender. The randomized trials of calcium (see below) are more informative.

Estrogen. Parity has declined, oral contraception use has changed very little, and the use of postmenopausal estrogen has increased and then recently again declined. Again, the randomized trials described below have been more informative for this factor, which is hardly gender neutral.

Aspirin. Chronic aspirin use for the disease prophylaxis, either coronary or neoplastic, has been difficult to track before 1985, though it is unlikely to have been prominent before that date. Aspirin use may, therefore, be a cause for further decline in CRC incidence in the future, though mostly in men, since they are the principal consumers of aspirin for prophylaxis. Even if aspirin-induced bleeding resulted in polypectomy, the effect on CRC incidence should only become apparent about now (see below).

Cigarettes. Cigarette use has been consistently associated with benign colorectal adenoma risk and only recently in a study for CRC risk as well. The use of cigarettes has declined progressively in all age/race/gender cohorts in the United States since 1951.

Cholecystectomy. Cholecystectomy has been extensively investigated as a risk factor for CRC and may increase risk of proximal CRC many years after the operation [12]. The rate of cholecystectomy in the United States dropped less than 1% between 1972 (212/100,000) and 1980 (211/100,000) in data from the Hospital Discharge Survey of the National Center for Health Statistics (NCHS). From 1972 to 1990 (209/100,000) the rate dropped 1.5% [13]. In Sweden, from 1970 to 1980 the rate of cholecystectomy dropped by 25% [14].

Polypectomy. Polypectomy has grown from an occasional procedure in 1970, performed either through a rigid proctoscope or through colectomy (a huge intervention when the adenoma–carcinoma sequence was still controversial) to one performed upon almost one million individuals in the United States in 1993. It has been estimated that risk of CRC could be reduced by 70% by polypectomy [15]. If there is a 10-year lag time from polyp detection to cancer formation, which is a broadly accepted conservative estimate [16], then the rapid growth of polypectomy would be first seen in reduced CRC incidence around the mid-1980s. The National Polyp Study demonstrated that colonoscopy was most effective in preventing distal

CRC [17], which fits with SEER data (Figs 1.1 and 1.2). If population-based data could show that both white genders have had equal exposure to colonoscopy and blacks have had less access than whites to polypectomy, and even if the 70% risk reduction for CRC is wildly optimistic, polypectomy may be the most likely explanation for the declining incidence of CRC.

Indirect evidence in support of less access to polypectomy among blacks and equal access in white genders can be found in SEER CRC stage data in which whites of both genders had discovery of CRC at an earlier stage than blacks. This implies that discovery was more likely to have been made during screening of asymptomatic individuals, the same type of individuals who would be getting polypectomy.

Summary of observational epidemiology

Because this time trend review does not contain a specific experiment in a defined cohort, it might seem that the findings carry less weight than would such an experiment. However the individual findings of this report in most cases carry the weight of being derived from populations and data weightings that make them more representative of the entire American population than any other available data. Any degree of direction of change in exposure over time is therefore significant. Time trending also is a powerful tool in the determination of disease causation, especially when the trending covers a disease that has undergone such an abrupt change in incidence as CRC has in the mid-1980s. These analyses therefore have important implications related to screening for CRC. The apparent success of polypectomy in reducing CRC incidence in the general population suggests that cancer control might be more effectively achieved if the emphasis in screening would shift towards technologies that are effective in detecting adenomas [18].

Most importantly, the feasibility of incidence reduction has also been established and should encourage further attempts to accelerate this through primary prevention. Increased fiber consumption and changes in alcoholic beverages may already have played a role in this reduction and current trends in the use of estrogen, aspirin, and calcium and may accelerate this decline in CRC risk over the next decade. Altered caloric balance (eating less fat and more exercise), so heavily emphasized in recent reports, is apparently more difficult to achieve in this society than CRC reduction [4].

Randomized clinical trials in risk modification and prevention

Vegetable *fiber* has been assessed in at least four randomized clinical trials [19–23]. Amongst these trials, none so far have shown a diminished risk of adenoma recurrence with increased fiber consumption. Indeed one large trial actually showed an increased risk in the high fiber group that quite alarmed its investigators [23]. Does this translate into increased cancer risk with dietary fiber? There is statistical evidence presented below which would argue against this, and decades of observational epidemiology would be negated by such a conclusion.

Dietary *calcium* was also hoped to be a significant contributor to risk reduction and has been looked at in two relatively large trials and two much smaller cancer-prone groups, that is, individuals either with familial adenomatous polyposis or hereditary non-polyposis CRC. Similar to the results regarding dietary fiber, none of these intervention trials has shown a protective effect related to calcium [19,23–26].

Two trials, one in Australia and one in the United States, assessed more *global dietary change*, feeling that no single dietary component would obtain significant protection [19,20]. Both of these trials have unfortunately shown no benefit to a program that increased fiber, fruits, vegetable, and beta carotene and decreased fat intake. The resolution of these disappointing results with prior descriptive epidemiology, which had suggested significant dietary modification of colon cancer risk, has not been achieved.

On the other hand, several items have emerged as significant, though modest, risk modifiers in randomized trials. One is *selenium* status in the Polyp Prevention Trial [27]. Another pharmacologic intervention that appears to provide benefit in randomized controlled trials is supplementation or ingestion of non-steroidal anti-inflammatory drugs (NSAIDs) [28]. This has been demonstrated both in cancer-prone individuals, that is, individuals with hereditary polyposis, and in the randomized trials amongst intermediate-risk individuals with prior histories of either cancer or adenoma, looking at adenoma recurrence. Unlike hormone replacement therapy (HRT) in women, in whom significant harmful effects of HRT may have been found, there seems to be little risk of harm in low-dose NSAID ingestion.

These trials did not use CRC as an end point of effect, but adenoma recurrence. This was chosen for several reasons. First is that it occurs soon enough and frequently enough to make these randomized trials economically feasible. It also, being a non-lethal surrogate for CRC, allays the ethical conundrum of allocation of study participants into a research arm that one may feel could be deleterious, whether it is the intervention or the control. There is however no perfect correlation between either adenoma risk or adenoma recurrence risk and subsequent incidence of or mortality from CRC. Many patients with adenomas never get cancer. Yet, there is no other intermediate end point or usable study outcome measure that correlates as well with cancer risk as this. The suitability of this as a surrogate for population-wide reduction in CRC risk must be called into question because of the failure of these trials. Cogent statistical arguments against the use of even more perfect surrogate end points have been raised [29]. Also, the use of high-risk groups in dietary intervention trials as economic surrogates for the general population has been shown to be unwise [30].

Hormone replacement therapy, that is, postmenopausal estrogen either opposed or unopposed by progestin [31], is unique amongst these randomized intervention trials, using colon cancer as an end point. Despite some of the alarming effects noted in the Women's Health Initiative related to estrogen supplementation, there still remains one significant health benefit to HRT in addition to reduction of osteoporosis and postmenopausal symptoms, and that is the diminished risk of CRC.

Analyses of more recent novel risk factors in non-randomized trials

Novel risk factors have also been sought with interesting though preliminary data. None of these have yet achieved significant enough evidence to rationalize their assessment in randomized trials. One of the most thoroughly investigated is *iron* status, either measured as dietary iron intake, body iron stores, or as genetic carriers of a disease known to increase iron exposure, hereditary hemochromatosis. The *hemochromatosis* population is the most interesting of these because it is, first of all, the most prevalent genetic disease in the United States. Second, evidence of increased risk of cancer or adenoma in this population bypasses some of the biases inherent to etiologic studies in observational epidemiology, almost giving the strength of randomized trials. Several trials have shown a positive association even in hemochromatosis heterozygosity and colorectal neoplastic risk [32,33].

Dietary *magnesium* has recently been found to be a significant protective factor in women for colon tumors [34] and *black tea* has not [35]. No relation has been found in a meta-analysis of prior *gastric surgery* and CRC risk [36]. Looking at what is perhaps this country's most prevalent disease, *obesity*, there is also a significant risk for CRC amongst these individuals, especially in men [37]. In a loosely related vein, cholesterol lowering with *statins* may have the added advantage of diminishing CRC incidence as well [38]. This comes from a case/control study; no randomized trials of statin use have reported this as yet. *C reactive protein* has received much recent publicity as a marker of heart disease risk and it has similarly been found to correlate with colon cancer risk [39].

So, in summary, what is the most important lifestyle decision one can make to avoid getting CRC?

Get screened. There is no dietary practice that comes close to the effectiveness of this measure in disease prevention [4]. Eating healthy, being active, staying slim may help and will certainly make each day more enjoyable. Adding aspirin, a statin, or estrogen if you dare may have an incremental effect but always at some cost [40].

References

1 NCI SEER data, http://canques.seer.cancer.gov.

2 Eaden J. Review article: colorectal carcinoma and inflammatory bowel disease. *Aliment Pharmacol Ther* 2004; 20: 24–30.

3 Nelson RL, Abcarian H. Do hemorrhoids cause cancer? *Semin Colon Rectal Surg* 1995; 6: 178–81.

4 Nelson RL, Persky V, Turyk M. Determination of factors responsible for the declining incidence of colorectal cancer. *Dis Colon Rectum* 1999; 42: 741–52.

5 Segi M. Age adjusted death rates for cancer for selected sites in 46 countries. *Segi Institute of Cancer Epidemiology*, Nagoya, Japan, 1984.

6 Landis SH, Murray T, Bolden S, Wingo PA. Cancer statistics 1998. *CA* 1998; 48: 6–29.

7 Norat T, Bingham S, Ferrari P *et al.* Meat, fish, and colorectal cancer risk: the European prospective investigation into Cancer and Nutrition. *J Natl Can Inst* 2005; 97: 906–16.

8 Nelson RL, Dollear T, Freels S, Persky V. The effect of age, gender and race on colorectal cancer subsite location. *Cancer* 1997; 80: 193–7.

9 Nelson RL, Dollear T, Freels S, Persky V. The relation of age, race, and gender to the subsite location of colorectal carcinoma. *Cancer* 1997; 80: 193–7.

10 National Center for Health Statistics Health Promotion and Disease supplement of the National Health Interview Survey, 1991. Ezzati TM, Massey JT, Waksburg J *et al.* Sample design: third national health and nutrition examination survey. *Vital Health Statistics 2* 1992; 113: 2–4.

11 Scanlon RÅ, Barbour JF. N-nitrosodimethylamine content of US and Canadian beers. *IARC Sci Publ* 1991; 105: 242–3.

12 Giovannucci E, Colditz GA, Stampfer MJ. A meta-analysis of cholecystectomy and risk of colorectal cancer. *Gastroenterology* 1993; 105: 130–41.

13 Detailed Diagnoses and Procedures; National Hospital Discharge Survey. *Vital and Health Statistics.* Series 10, no. 107, series 13, nos. 37, 60, 99, 130. 1972, 1976, 1979, 1989, 1995.

14 Kullman E, Dahlin LG, Hallhagen S *et al.* Trends in incidence, clinical findings and outcome of acute and

elective cholecystectomy, 1970–86. *Eur J Surg* 1994; 160: 605–11.

15 Lieberman DA. Cost-effectiveness model for colon cancer screening. *Gastroenterology* 1995; 109: 1781–90.

16 Winawer SJ, Fletcher RH, Miller L *et al.* Colorectal cancer screening: clinical guidelines and rationale. *Gastroenterology* 1997; 112: 594–642.

17 Winawer SJ, Zauber AG, Ho MN *et al.* Prevention of colorectal cancer by colonoscopic polypectomy. *N Engl J Med* 1993; 329: 1977–81.

18 Nelson RL. Screening for colorectal cancer. *J Surg Oncol* 1997; 64: 249–58.

19 Schatzkin A, Lanza E, Corle D *et al.* Lack of effect of a low-fat, high fiber diet on the recurrence of colorectal adenomas. *N Engl J Med* 2000; 342: 1149–55.

20 MacLennan R, Macrae F, Bain C *et al.* Randomized trial of intake of faat fiber and beta-carotene to prevent colorectal adenomas. The Australian Polyp Prevention Project. *J Natl Cancer Inst* 1995; 87: 1760–6.

21 Jacobs ET, Guiliano AR, Roe DJ *et al.* Dietary change in an intervention trial of wheat bran fiber and colorectal adenoma recurrence. *Ann Epidemiol* 2004; 14: 280–6.

22 Alberts DS, Martinez ME, Roe DJ *et al.* Lack of effect of a high fiber cereal supplement on the recurrence of colorectal adenomas. Phoenix Colon Cancer Prevention Physicians Network. *N Engl J Med* 2000; 342: 1156–62.

23 Bonithon-Koop C, Kronborg O, Giacosa A *et al.* Calcium and fibre supplementation in prevention of colorectal adenoma recurrence: a randomized intervention trial. *Lancet* 2000; 356: 1300–6.

24 Hartman TJ, Albert PS, Snyder K *et al.* The association of calcium and vitamin D with risk of colorectal adenomas. *J Nutr* 2005; 135: 252–9.

25 Wallace K, Baron JA, Cole BF, Sandler RS. Effect of calcium supplementation on the risk of large bowel polyps. *J Natl Cancer Inst* 2004; 96: 921–5.

26 Cats A, Kleibueker JH, van der Meer R *et al.* Randomized double blinded placebo controlled intervention study with supplemental calcium in families with hereditary nonpolyposis colorectal cancer. *J Natl Cancer Inst* 1995; 87: 598–603.

27 Jacobs ET, Jiang R, Alberts DS *et al.* Selenium and colorectal adenoma: results of a pooled analysis. *J Natl Cancer Inst* 2004; 96: 1669–75.

28 Huls G, Koornstra JJ, Kleibeuker JH. Non-steroidal anti-inflammatory drugs and molecular carcinogenesis of colorectal carcinomas. *Lancet* 2003; 362: 230–2.

29 Baker SG, Kramer BS. A perfect correlate does not a surrogate make. *BMC Med Res Methodol* 2003; 3: 16.

30 Baker SG, Kramer BS, Corle D. The fallacy of enrolling only high risk subjects in cancer prevention trials: is there a "free lunch"? Biomedcentral.com 2004; 4: 24.

31 Chlebowski RT, Wactawski-Wende J, Ritenbaugh C *et al.* Estrogen plus progestin and colorectal cancer in postmenopausal women. *N Engl J Med* 2004; 350: 991–1004.

32 Nelson RL. Iron and colorectal cancer risk; human studies. *Nutr Rev* 2001; 59: 140–8.

33 Shaheen NJ, Silverman LM, Keku T *et al.* Association between hemochromatosis (HFE) gene mutation carrier status and the risk of colon cancer. *J Natl Cancer Inst* 2003; 95: 154–9.

34 Larsson SC, Bergkvist L, Wolk A. Magnesium intake in relation to risk of colorectal cancer in women. *JAMA* 2005; 293: 86–9.

35 Goldbohm RA, Hertog MGL, Brants HAM *et al.* Consumption of black tea and cancer risk: a prospective cohort study. *J Natl Cancer Inst* 1996; 88: 93–100.

36 Munnangi S, Sonnenberg A. Colorectal cancer after gastric surgery: a meta-analysis. *Am J Gastroent* 1997; 92: 109–13.

37 Calle EE, Rodriguez C, Walker-Thurmond K, Thun MJ.

Overweight, obesity and mortality from cancer in a prospectively studied cohort of U.S. adults. *N Engl J Med* 2003; 348: 1625–38.

38 Poynter JN, Gruber SB, Higgins PDR *et al.* Statins and the risk of colorectal cancer. *N Engl J Med* 2005; 352: 2184–92.

39 Erlinger TP, Platz EA, Rifai N, Helzlsouer KJ. C-reactive protein and risk of incident colorectal cancer. *JAMA* 2004; 291: 585–90.

40 Material on randomized trials reproduced from Nelson RL, New Developments in Colon and Rectal Cancer. In: *Business Briefing: US Gastroenterology Review 2005*. London: Touch Briefings, 2005: 86–8, with permission.

2: Screening for colorectal cancer – who, when, and how?

Robert Steele

Introduction

In Europe, the incidence of colorectal cancer is currently very similar to that of lung and breast cancer (about 135,000 cases per year), and in the developed countries there are some 250,000 deaths attributable to the disease each year [1]. The main symptoms consist of rectal bleeding, change of bowel habit, abdominal pain, and anemia, but a tumor giving rise to these symptoms is likely to be locally advanced. As a result symptomatic cancers are rarely early and, in the United Kingdom, only about 8% of colorectal cancers present at Dukes' stage A, with 25% having distant metastases at the time of diagnosis [2]. It is well established that early-stage colorectal cancer carries a much better prognosis than does late-stage disease [3] but relying purely on symptomatic presentation is unlikely to ever increase substantially the proportion of cancers treated early and thus with curative intent. It follows that the only successful strategy for detecting early disease is screening, and the purpose of this chapter is to examine current evidence relating to colorectal cancer screening and to try to answer the questions posed in its title.

Principles of screening

The main aim of screening is to identify a disease process in asymptomatic individuals but many who accept an invitation to be screened do have relevant symptoms, and, indeed, screening may be more readily accepted when symptoms are present. For example, in colorectal cancer, a recent study found that about 50% of subjects undergoing fecal occult blood test (FOBt) screening had colorectal symptoms, although these were unrelated to the findings on subsequent colonoscopy [4]. This underlines the unreliability of

Table 2.1 Principles of screening.

1. The condition should be an important health problem
2. There should be an accepted treatment for patients with recognized disease
3. Facilities for diagnosis and treatment should be available
4. There should be a recognizable latent or early symptomatic stage
5. There should be a suitable test or examination
6. The test should be acceptable to the population
7. The natural history of the condition, including development for latent to declared disease, should be adequately understood
8. There should be an agreed policy on whom to treat as patients
9. The cost of case-finding (including diagnosis and treatment of patients diagnosed) should be economically balanced in relation to possible expenditure on medical care as a whole
10. Case finding should be a continuing process and not a "once and for all" project

Source: Wilson JM, Jungner F. *Public Health Papers No. 34. 1968.*

symptoms as a pointer to early disease and emphasizes the need for reliable screening methodology.

In 1968 Wilson and Jungner [5] published principles underlying effective screening that have stood the test of time and these are summarized in Table 2.1. Despite the seemingly obvious advantages of screening, it is associated with inherent biases that appear to confer a better prognosis on screen-detected disease when compared to symptomatic disease *whether or not* the screening process has had any effect on the outcome. Thus, to be sure that screening is delivering real benefit, it is essential to carry out population-based randomized trials in which a group is offered screening and is compared with a group that is not in terms of disease-specific mortality. In this way, cancers that arise in those who decline screening and interval cancers are analyzed along with screen-detected disease and the biases are eliminated. In the sections that follow, the main modalities that have been used to screen for colorectal cancer will be examined, with emphasis on the results of randomized trials where these are available.

Fecal occult blood screening

Blood can be detected in the feces by means of a number of methods but all the published population-based screening trials used a guaiac-based test (Fig. 2.1). Guaiac tests detect peroxidases associated with heme that enters the gastrointestinal tract as hemoglobin or myoglobin in food or as red cells from bleeding pathology. In the colon, however, the heme loses its

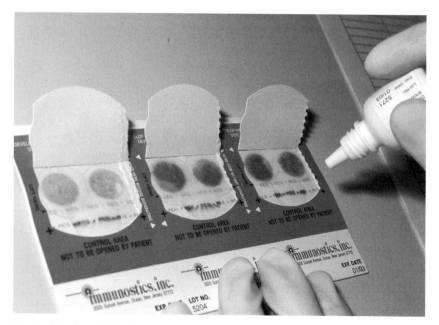

Fig. 2.1 A fecal occult blood testing kit.

peroxidase activity by the action of the microflora so that guaiac tests are more likely to pick up distal than proximal sources of bleeding [6]. Thus, a positive guaiac test is more likely to indicate colonic rather than gastric pathology.

When an unrehydrated guaiac test is used in population screening, its clinical sensitivity for colorectal cancer is probably in the region of 50% as evidenced by the interval cancer rate in randomized trials; this low sensitivity is thought to be related to the fact that cancers display an intermittent pattern of bleeding. The specificity is about 98% but, as most subjects do not have colorectal cancer, this leads to a fairly high false positive rate. Rehydration of the feces before testing can improve the sensitivity but at the expense of a decrease in specificity.

Specificity is a difficult issue with FOB testing, and although dietary restriction to eliminate peroxidases and heme can be used, a recent meta-analysis suggests that this is ineffective [7]. Immunological FOBts, which are specific for human hemoglobin, provide part of the solution to this problem. These tests, which are based on a variety of methods including reverse passive hemagglutination and immunochromatography, can be designed to have thresholds at a wide range of analytical and thus clinical sensitivities [6].

Thus, immunological FOBts can be made to be highly sensitive for colorectal cancer but, despite eliminating dietary false positives, increasing analytical sensitivity will decrease specificity by allowing the detection of trivial bleeding [8].

All the randomized and population-based trials reported to date employed Hemoccult II – a guiaic-based test – and were carried out in Minnesota (USA) [9], Nottingham (England) [10], Funen (Denmark) [11], Burgundy (France) [12], and Goteborg (Sweden) [13]. In the Minnesota study, randomization was to no screening, biennial screening or annual screening. The test was rehydrated and dietary restriction was not used. Colonoscopy was offered to all positive individuals and, after 18 years of follow-up, statistically significant reductions in colorectal cancer mortality were observed in both biennial (21%) and annual groups (33%) [14]. It is important to point out, however, that all the participants in this study were volunteers, 10% of all tests were positive, and 38% of the group screened annually underwent colonoscopy on at least one occasion. The main conclusion to be drawn from this study is that screening does reduce mortality from colorectal cancer, but it also demonstrates that unrehydrated hemoccult results in a high colonoscopy rate. Furthermore, it is difficult to extrapolate the results of this study to a non-volunteer population. One important feature of this study relates to long term follow-up; after 18 years the incidence of colorectal cancer in the groups offered screening was significantly less than in the control group [15]. The reason for this cannot be proven, but, as the rate of colonoscopy was so high, it is reasonable to conclude that polypectomy may have been at least partially responsible.

In the UK study, conducted in Nottingham [10], about 150,000 unselected subjects were randomized, and the group allocated to the screening arm was offered biennial non-rehydrated Hemoccult II testing. If an individual returned a test that was weakly positive (1–4 spots positive) they were offered further testing after dietary restriction. This algorithm resulted in 2% of those undergoing testing going on to further investigation following the first (prevalence) round and 1.2% in subsequent (incidence) rounds. Thus, the colonoscopy rate was much lower than that in the Minnesota study, and in over five screening rounds only 4% of those offered screening underwent colonoscopy. Uptake was variable but overall 60% of the group offered screening completed at least one test. The cancers detected by screening tended to be in the early stage (57% Dukes' stage A), but the interval cancer rate was high, and about 50% of cancers diagnosed in the group offered screening were not screen detected, suggesting that, in a population screening context, Hemoccult II is only about 50% sensitive. Nevertheless, despite the shortcomings of uptake and test sensitivity, when the group offered screening was compared to the control group, a statistically significant 15% reduction of colorectal cancer mortality was seen after a median of 7.8 years of follow-up [10], and at a median of 11 years this was maintained at 13% [16].

One significant effect of the Nottingham screening study was that in the *control group* the percentage of patients presenting with early stage rectal cancer (Dukes' stage A) increased from 9% in the first half of the recruitment to 28% in the second half [17]. Thus the screening program had an effect on the control group, and although the reason for this is not clear, it is reasonable to hypothesize that increased awareness of the significance of rectal bleeding may have been responsible. It is also interesting to note that during the study there were significantly fewer emergency admissions for colorectal cancer in the group offered screening [18], suggesting that screening had led to a reduction in the emergency workload.

In the Danish study, which was very similar in design to the Nottingham trial, 61,933 individuals were randomized to a control group or to a group offered biennial screening with Hemoccult II [11]. The acceptance rate was higher than in the Nottingham study with 67% completing the first screening round and with more than 90% accepting repeated screenings. Positivity was lower, however, at 1.4% following the first round and dropping to 0.8% in the second round, although it increased with subsequent rounds so that by the fifth round it was 1.8%. Again, the stage at diagnosis of the screen-detected cancers was favorable, with 48% at stage A and only 8% with distant metastases. Interval cancers were common, making up approximately 30% of all the cancers diagnosed in the group offered screening. The mortality reduction was also similar, with a statistically significant reduction of 18% after five rounds and rising to 30% after seven rounds [19].

Recently, the results of a French population-based study using non-rehydrated Hemoccult has been published [12]. In this study small geographical areas were allocated either to screening or to no screening, leading to the invitation of 1199 subjects between the ages of 50 and 74 years. The acceptance rate in the first round was 52.8% with slight increases in subsequent rounds; the positivity rate was 1.2% in the first round and 1.4% on an average thereafter; and the overall reduction in disease-specific mortality was 16%.

Finally, in Sweden all 68,308 residents of Goteborg born between 1918 and 1931 were randomized into a control group and a group offered screening using the Hemoccult II test [13]. In the first round uptake was 63%, but dropped to 60% in later rounds. Positivity was 4.4% in the first round and, as expected, screen-detected cancers were found to be at a much more favorable stage than those arising in the control group. Unfortunately, no mortality data are available from this study.

In summary, there are five large studies investigating the role of the guaiac-based Hemoccult II FOBt as a primary screening modality; four were randomized, four were truly population based, and four have reported mortality data. It is remarkable how uniform the results from these studies are, and a meta-analysis utilizing the data from all five studies has indicated that an overall 16% reduction in colorectal cancer mortality can be expected in a population offered this type of screening and, when adjusted for compliance, this reduction can be as much as 23% [20].

In the United Kingdom, to ensure that the results of the randomized trials could be reproduced in the National Health Service, a demonstration pilot was conducted [21]. This took place in two geographical areas, one in Scotland and one in England, where a total of 478,250 subjects between the ages of 50 and 69 were invited to take part in a guaiac-based FOBt screening program over a two-year period to simulate the first round of a biennial screening program. The acceptance rate was 56.8%, positivity was 1.9%, and 48% of all screen-detected cancers were at Dukes' stage A with only 1% having metastases at the time of diagnosis [22]. An independent evaluation group examined the results using the Nottingham study to provide benchmarks [23], and as a result the UK health departments have made a commitment to roll out a nationwide colorectal cancer screening program [24,25].

Flexible sigmoidoscopy

It has been proposed that a single flexible sigmoidoscopy at around the age of 60 with removal of all small adenomas at the time of initial examination and proceeding to colonoscopy in those with high-risk lesions would be effective in reducing both mortality from colorectal cancer by early detection and disease incidence by polypectomy [26].

To test this hypothesis two multicenter randomized controlled trials of identical design have been carried out, one in the United Kingdom [27] and the other in Italy [28]. In the United Kingdom, 14 centers participated and subjects aged 60–64 years were mailed a questionnaire to ask if they would attend a flexible sigmoidoscopy screening if invited. Of 354,262 people sent this questionnaire 194,726 (55%) responded in the affirmative and of these 170,432 were randomized using a 2:1 ratio of controls to those invited for screening. Those participating in the screening process underwent a flexible sigmoidoscopy with immediate removal of all small polyps and colonoscopy for those with high-risk polyps or invasive cancers. Of the 57,254 individuals invited for screening 40,674 (71%) attended, but as the study was essentially a volunteer study, the population compliance cannot be estimated with accuracy. If extrapolated, however, it is unlikely to be more than 30%.

In this UK flexible sigmoidoscopy study, distal adenomas were found in 12.1% and distal cancer in 0.3%, and in those going on to colonoscopy, proximal adenomas were found in 18.8% and proximal cancers in 0.4%. The stage at diagnosis of the cancers was particularly favorable, with 62% at Dukes' stage A. In the Italian arm of the study (the SCORE trial), 236,568 people aged between 55 and 64 were sent letters of invitation but in this case only 56,532 (23.9%) indicated that they would be prepared to be screened, and of the 17,148 assigned to screening 9999 (58%) attended. Fifty-four individuals were found to have colorectal cancer and 54% of these were diagnosed at Dukes' stage A.

Another randomized trial, carried out in the United States, has utilized flexible sigmoidoscopy as a screening modality [29]. So far no data on uptake, compliance, or pathology yield have been published, although it has been reported that repeat flexible sigmoidoscopy 3 years after an initial examination revealed advanced adenoma or cancer in the distal colon. As a result, it has been suggested that repeated flexible sigmoidoscopy is needed rather than the once only approach advocated by the UK and Italian studies.

It would therefore appear that flexible sigmoidoscopy screening is an effective means of detecting early disease and adenomas, but it does tend to miss proximal disease and currently compliance rates are modest. This raises a question mark over its use as a population-screening tool, and although the randomized trials will almost certainly show mortality reductions the issue of uptake requires attention.

Colonoscopy

In many parts of the world, colonoscopy is used as a primary screening tool on a case-finding basis (Fig. 2.2). It is, of course, highly accurate with a specificity of 100% and a very high sensitivity, although it should be emphasized that sensitivity is not 100% as back-to-back colonoscopy studies have shown that adenomas and occasionally carcinomas can be overlooked even by

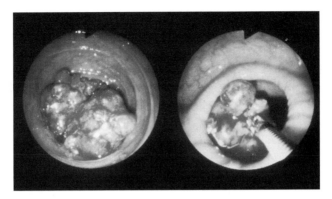

Fig. 2.2 Colonoscopy.

experienced colonoscopists [30]. There are no randomized trials of screening colonoscopy, but perhaps the most widely quoted study in this field is the US National Polyp Study [31]. This was an observational study in which 1418 patients who had undergone colonoscopy and removal of adenomas had subsequent colonoscopies during an average follow-up period of 6 years. Throughout the study period, five asymptomatic early-stage colorectal cancers were detected by colonoscopy in the study group and no symptomatic cancers were diagnosed. When compared to three reference groups, this was a much lower rate of diagnosis of colorectal cancer than expected and it was concluded that colonoscopic surveillance in adenoma patients reduces the incidence of and subsequent death rate from colorectal cancer. Although this study is of some importance, these conclusions must be interpreted with caution as the comparison group was not derived from the same population as the cases and may have led to an overestimate of the efficacy of colonoscopy. More importantly, it is not possible to extrapolate directly from polyp surveillance to the screening of asymptomatic populations.

As far as estimating the efficacy of screening colonoscopy is concerned, the best available study is a case-control study conducted amongst US military veterans [32]. Here 4411 veterans dying of colorectal cancer between 1988 and 1992 were studied and the controls were obtained from living and dead patients without colorectal cancer, matched by age, sex, and race to each case. The results indicated that colonoscopy was associated with reduced death rates from colorectal cancer with an odds ratios of 0.41 (range 0.33–0.50). Unfortunately, this study also has its limitations, not least because the reasons for colonoscopy in the study group were varied and included investigation of symptoms.

Uncontrolled data on screening colonoscopy are widely available, and one of the most useful studies estimated the ability of colonoscopy to detect colorectal neoplasia in asymptomatic males aged 50–75 years [33]. Of 17,732 potential subjects 3196 were included and 3121, with a mean age of 63 years, underwent screening colonoscopy. Invasive cancer was diagnosed in 1% and 7.5% were found to have an adenoma of 10 mm or more in diameter. Thus, extrapolating these results, if colonoscopy was used as a screening tool in men aged between 50 and 75 years the uptake would only be 20% and cancer would be detected in only 1%. Despite the widespread use of colonoscopy for screening asymptomatic individuals on demand, therefore, it could not be recommended as a population screening test on the available evidence to date.

Radiology

The use of barium enema as a screening tool has no basis in evidence, but the relatively new technology of computed tomography (CT) colography may have a role. In the most promising study so far, which used a final, unblinded colonoscopy to estimate sensitivity and specificity, the sensitivity of CT colography was found to be 93.8% for large adenomas compared to 87.5% for colonoscopy. The specificity of CT colography was 96% for adenomas [34]. However, not all researchers in this area have come to the same conclusions. A study from the Netherlands has suggested that CT colography and colonoscopy have the same ability to detect large polyps [35], but two further studies have found the radiological approach to be inferior to endoscopy [36,37]. It is interesting to note that the workers who found CT colography to be equivalent or superior used the "fly-through" technique in which the CT data are reconstructed to create a luminal view similar to that seen at colonoscopy. It would seem therefore that the accuracy of CT colography is operator and technique dependent and, given optimal conditions, there is probably little to choose between CT and colonoscopy for diagnostic purposes. There are, however, no data as yet with which to assess the performance or cost effectiveness of CT colography in population screening.

Comparative studies

The few studies that directly compare different screening methods all address FOB testing and flexible sigmoidoscopy. Researchers from Nottingham have compared FOB testing alone with combined flexible sigmoidoscopy and FOB testing [38], and while the neoplasia yield in those actually undergoing the combined approach was four times greater than in those doing the FOB test alone and the uptake of FOB testing was 50% in those offered both tests, only 20% went on to have flexible sigmoidoscopy. In a Swedish study in which 6367 individuals aged between 55 and 56 years were randomized to be offered screening with Hemoccult II or flexible sigmoidoscopy [39], uptake of the FOB test was 59% compared to 49% for flexible sigmoidoscopy. The positivity rate for the FOBt screening was 4%, and, of these, 13% were found to have had a neoplastic lesion greater than 1 cm in the rectum or sigmoid colon; in all those undergoing flexible sigmoidoscopy the neoplasia rate was 2.3%. Overall, 10 individuals were diagnosed with a neoplastic lesion in the FOBt group compared with 31 in the flexible sigmoidoscopy group. In the Norwegian Colorectal Cancer Prevention (NORCCAP) Screening Study [40], 20,780 individuals aged between 50 and 64 years were randomized to be invited for flexible sigmoidoscopy only or for a combination of flexible sigmoidoscopy and FOB testing. Uptake was high at 65%, and in total 41 (0.3%) cancers and 2208 (17%) adenomas were found. The two groups were identical in terms of the diagnosis of colorectal cancer or high-risk adenomas suggesting that there was very little benefit in adding a FOBt to a flexible sigmoidoscopy.

Thus, although uptake of flexible sigmoidoscopy tends to be less than that for FOB testing, there is little doubt that the sensitivity of flexible sigmoidoscopy is higher. On the other hand, all the evidence that FOBt screening reduces colorectal cancer mortality is based on repeated testing and in a non-randomized study from Denmark comparing once only flexible sigmoidoscopy plus FOB testing with FOB testing alone over 16 years demonstrated that the FOBt screening program had a diagnostic yield at least as high as a single flexible sigmoidoscopy [41]. It has to be concluded, therefore, that the evidence relating to the relative merits of a FOBt program and once only flexible sigmoidoscopy is insufficient to make a direct comparison, and this issue can only be resolved by an appropriate randomized trial.

The cost of screening

The cost of screening may be considered in two ways: the financial cost and the morbidity and mortality occasioned by a screening intervention. These will be dealt with in turn.

Morbidity and mortality

Although both FOB testing and flexible sigmoidoscopy are safe, the subsequent colonoscopy for those with a positive test and the surgery for those who are diagnosed with cancer both carry the risk of complications and even death. Furthermore, false negative results, inevitable owing to the low sensitivity of both FOB testing and flexible sigmoidoscopy, might persuade an individual with colorectal cancer to ignore symptoms and therefore present with advanced disease ("certificate of health effect").

Both of these issues have been examined by the Nottingham group who have studied both investigation- and treatment-related mortality and the stage at presentation of interval cancers [42]. In those with screen-detected cancers, no colonoscopy-related deaths were observed, and there were five postoperative deaths, representing a 2% operative mortality at a time when mortality after elective colorectal cancer surgery in the United Kingdom could be expected to be 5% [43]. As far as the interval cancers were concerned, the stage distribution of cancers that were diagnosed after a negative FOBt or colonoscopy was identical to that of the cancers in the control group, and the survival was significantly better. These findings suggest that any certificate of health effect must be very small.

One of the major concerns voiced about colorectal cancer screening is the finding that all-cause mortality is not reduced and indeed, in the Nottingham study, it was found to be increased in the group offered screening [44]. However, as colorectal cancer only accounts for around 2% of all deaths, a 15% reduction in disease-specific mortality could only be expected to reduce all-cause mortality by 0.3%. A randomized trial powered to demonstrate an effect of this magnitude would not be feasible, and, in any case, the excess of all-cause deaths observed in the group offered screening did not reach statistical significance.

Psychological morbidity is another potential disadvantage of screening. There has been relatively little work done in this field relating to colorectal cancer screening, but there are two studies worthy of consideration. In Sweden, a questionnaire study demonstrated that 4.7% experienced sufficient worry to influence daily life from the invitation letter, and this figure increased to 15% after receipt of a positive test [45]. However, this worry declined rapidly after the screening process was complete and after 1 year 96% reported that they were happy to have had the opportunity to be screened. A similar study carried out within the Nottingham trial showed anxiety to be highest in those with a positive test result, but in those with false positive tests it fell the day after colonoscopy and remained low when testing was repeated 1 month later [46]. It seems, therefore, that psychological morbidity associated with screening certainly exists but is relatively short lived.

Financial implications of screening

Cost effectiveness is an important consideration before introducing a screening program. Unfortunately, cost-effectiveness data are not available from the randomized controlled trials and the only available approach at present is to use information provided by health economic models. In a recent study 17 relevant papers were identified, and although none assessed biennial FOB testing or once only flexible sigmoidoscopy, data were available for the yearly FOB testing, sigmoidoscopy done every 5 years, or colonoscopy done every 10 years, or a combination of these strategies [47].

Using an advanced technique that took uncertainties into account, the data suggested that FOB screening costs €8900 per life year saved. When uncertainty was incorporated it was still 95% certain that an annual FOB test is cost effective provided society is willing to pay €30,000 per life year saved. As this is below the threshold that most countries are prepared to pay it is possible to say with a high degree of certainty that FOBt screening is cost effective. Based on this first model, sigmoidoscopy and colonoscopy were compared with FOBt screening. Sigmoidoscopy was estimated to cost €8000 per life year saved, but when uncertainty was incorporated into the model it was not even possible to be 80% certain that sigmoidoscopy is cost effective compared with FOBt screening no matter how much is paid for each life year saved. This uncertainty is caused by the lack of data on mortality reduction brought about by flexible sigmoidoscopy and will be resolved when the results of the randomized trials are available. As far as colonoscopy is concerned when the 10-yearly examination was compared with the annual FOB testing it was estimated that each life year saved would cost €28,500, and when uncertainty was taken into account it became clear that to be 95% certain of cost effectiveness it would be necessary to pay €90,000 per life year saved. Thus what can be said at present is that FOBt screening is cost effective, flexible sigmoidoscopy screening might be cost effective but further data is required to make a definitive statement, and colonoscopy is unlikely to be cost effective for population screening.

New approaches to screening

Research into improving screening methods has focused largely on stool tests; transferrin [48], albumin [49], α-1 antitrypsin [50], and the neutrophil-associated calcium binding protein calprotectin [51] have all received attention, but none have been found to be sufficiently sensitive or specific. Stool cytology, aided by the immunohistochemical detection of MCM2, a protein expressed strongly by neoplastic epithelium, has also been advocated, but never developed as a feasible screening test [52]. Most recently, however, interest has focused on the development of tests that can detect genetic abnormalities in deoxyribonucleic acid (DNA) extracted from the stool, but because colorectal cancer is heterogeneous in terms of genetic mutations, it is essential to use a panel of tests for screening purposes. The most commonly studied markers in this context are mutations of K-ras, APC, and P53; the BAT26 marker of microsatellite instability; and, because of their propensity to be shed by tumors, long fragments of DNA [53,54].

Various groups have explored this approach [54–56] and recently a study from Indianapolis, which employed a fecal DNA panel of 21 mutations, reported a 51.6% sensitivity for invasive cancer compared with a sensitivity of 12.9% for Hemoccult II testing [57]. The sensitivity for the FOBt was very low, however, in contrast to the 50% sensitivity found in the randomized trials. It would appear, therefore, that fecal DNA testing has promise, but it has a long way to go before it could replace FOB testing, especially in view of the complex technology currently required.

Conclusions

In this chapter, evidence relating to screening for colorectal cancer has been presented in an attempt to answer the questions posed in the title. In terms of population screening, as opposed to the surveillance of high-risk groups, the only criterion that can be used to define *who* should be screened is age. The age range that should be screened is practically dependent upon the extent of a society's willingness to pay for a screening program but current thinking would favor the group aged 50–74 years. As far as *when* is concerned, it has to be accepted that the ideal screening test has yet to be found; at present, the truly non-invasive tests are neither very sensitive nor specific, and the more accurate tests are expensive and unlikely to be sufficiently acceptable to be useful as population-screening tools. However, the evidence firmly points to mortality reductions of significant proportions, certainly greater than with any known adjuvant therapy, and it is difficult to argue against immediate introduction of screening at this point in time. Finally, the issue of *how* colorectal cancer screening should be conducted raises some important philosophical questions. If the aim of screening is to inform an individual, for whatever reason, whether or not they are harboring colorectal cancer, then the sensitivity and specificity of the test are paramount, and the choice must lie between colonoscopy and CT colography. If, however, the aim is to reduce the burden of disease on a community (true population screening) a test that is both acceptable and affordable must be employed, and at present the guaiac-based FOB test is the only modality proven to be effective.

References

1 Cancer Research Campaign. Cancer in the European Community. Factsheet 5.2 1992.

2 Slaney G *et al.* Cancer of the large bowel. *Clinical Cancer Monograph* Vol 4. Macmillan Press, 1991.

3 Black RJ, Sharp L, Kendrick SW. *Trends in Cancer Survival in Scotland* 1968–90. ISD Publication, Edinburgh, 1993.

4 Ahmed S, Leslie A, Thaha M *et al.* Lower gastrointestinal symptoms do not discriminate for colorectal neoplasia in a faecal occult blood screen-positive population. *Br J Surg* 2005; 92: 478–81.

5 Wilson JM, Jungner F. Principles and practice of screening for disease. *Public Health Papers No. 34.* WHO, Geneva, 1968.

6 Young GP, Macrae FA, St John DJB. Clinical methods for early detection: basis, use and evaluation. In: Young GP, Rozen P, Levin B (eds.) *Prevention and Early Detection of Colorectal Cancer.* Philadelphia: W.B. Saunders, 1996.

7 Pignone M, Campbell MK, Carr C, Phillips C. Meta-analysis of dietary restriction during fecal occult blood testing. *Eff Clin Pract* 2001; 4: 150–6.

8 Robinson MH, Marks CG, Farrands PA *et al.* Screening for colorectal cancer with an immunological faecal occult blood test: 2-year follow-up. *Br J Surg* 1996; 83: 500–1.

9 Mandel JS, Bond JH, Church JR *et al.* Reducing mortality from colorectal cancer by screening for faecal occult blood. *N Engl J Med* 1993; 328: 1365–71.

10 Hardcastle JD, Chamberlain JO, Robinson MHE. Randomised controlled trial of faecal occult blood screening for colorectal cancer. *Lancet* 1996; 348: 1472–7.

11 Kronborg O, Fenger C, Olsen J *et al.* Randomised study of screening for colorectal cancer with faecal occult blood test. *Lancet* 1996; 348: 1467–71.

12 Faivre J, Dancourt V, Lejeune C *et al.* Reduction in colorectal cancer mortality by fecal occult blood screening in a French controlled study. *Gastroenterology* 2004; 126: 1674–80.

13 Kewenter J, Brevinge H, Engaras B *et al.* Results of screening, rescreening, and follow-up in a prospect randomized study for detection of colorectal cancer by fecal occult blood testing. Results for 68,308 subjects. *Scand J Gastroenterol* 1994; 29: 468–73.

14 Mandel JS, Church TR, Ederer F, Bond JH. Colorectal cancer mortality: effectiveness of biennial screening for fecal occult blood. *J Natl Cancer Inst* 1999; 91: 434–7.

15 Mandel JS, Church TR, Bond JH *et al.* The effect of fecal occult-blood screening on the incidence of colorectal cancer. *N Engl J Med* 2000; 343: 1603–7.

16 Scholefield JH, Moss S, Sufi F *et al.* Effect of faecal occult blood screening on

mortality from colorectal cancer: results from a randomised controlled trial. *Gut* 2002; 50: 840–4.

17 Robinson MHE, Thomas WM, Hardcastle JD *et al.* Change towards earlier stage at presentation of colorectal cancer. *Br J Surg* 1993; 80: 1610–12.

18 Scholefield JH, Robinson MH, Mangham CM, Hardcastle JD. Screening for colorectal cancer reduces emergency admissions. *Eur J Surg Oncol* 1998; 24: 47–50.

19 Jorgensen OD, Krongborg O, Fenger C. A randomised study of screening for colorectal cancer using faecal occult blood testing: results after 13 years and seven biennial screening rounds. *Gut* 2002; 50: 29–32.

20 Towler B, Irwig L, Glasziou P *et al.* A systematic review of the effects of screening for colorectal cancer using the faecal occult blood test, Hemoccult. *Br Med J* 1998; 317: 559–65.

21 Steele RJC, Parker R, Patnick J *et al.* A demonstration pilot for colorectal cancer screening in the United Kingdom: a new concept in the introduction of health care strategies. *J Med Screen* 2001; 8: 197–202.

22 Steele RJC for the UK Colorectal Cancer Screening Pilot Group. Results of the first round of a demonstration pilot of screening for colorectal cancer in the United Kingdom. *Br Med J* 2004; 329: 133–5.

23 Evaluation of the UK colorectal screening pilot. A report for the UK Department of Health. http://www.cancerscreening.nhs.uk/ colorectal/finalreport.pdf. Department of Health, June 2003.

24 Department of Health Press Release 2003/0047 (http://www.info.doh.gov.uk/doh/ intpress.nsf/page/2003-0047).

25 Cancer in Scotland. Action for Change. Bowel cancer framework for Scotland. NHS Scotland. Scottish Executive, 2004.

26 Atkin WS, Edwards R, Wardle J *et al.* Design of a multicentre randomised trial to evaluate flexible sigmoidoscopy in colorectal cancer screening. *J Med Screen* 2001; 8: 137–44.

27 UK Flexible Sigmoidoscopy Screening Trial Investigators. Single flexible sigmoidoscopy screening to prevent colorectal cancer: baseline findings of a UK multicentre randomized trial. *Lancet* 2002; 359: 1291–300.

28 Segnan N, Senore C, Andreoni B *et al.* SCORE working group. Baseline findings of the Italian multicenter randomized controlled trial of "once-only sigmoidoscopy" – SCORE. *J Natl Cancer Inst* 2002; 94: 1763–72.

29 Schoen RE, Pinsky PF, Weissfeld JL *et al.* Results of repeat sigmoidoscopy 3 years after a negative examination. *JAMA* 2003; 290: 41–8.

30 Rex DK, Cutler CS, Lemmel GT *et al.* Colonoscopic miss rates of adenomas determined by back-to-back colonoscopies. *Gastroenterology* 1997; 112: 24–8.

31 Winawer SJ, Zauber AG, Ho MN *et al.* Prevention of colorectal cancer by colonoscopic polypectomy. The National Polyp Study Working Group. *N Engl J Med* 1993; 329: 1977–81.

32 Muller AD, Sonnenberg A. Protection by endoscopy against death from colorectal cancer. A case-control study among Veterans. *Arch Intern Med* 1995; 155: 1741–8.

33 Lieberman DA, Weiss DG, Bond JH *et al.* Use of colonoscopy to screen asymptomatic adults for colorectal cancer. Veterans Affairs Cooperative Study Group 380. *N Engl J Med* 2000; 343: 162–8.

34 Pickhardt PJ, Choi JR, Hwang I *et al.* Computed tomographic virtual colonoscopy to screen for colorectal neoplasia in asymptomatic adults. *N Engl J Med* 2003; 349: 2191–200.

35 Van Gelder RE, Nio CY, Florie J *et al.* Computed tomography compared with colonoscopy in patients at increase risk for colorectal cancer. *Gastroenterology* 2004; 127: 41–8.

36 Cotton PB, Durkalski VL, Pineau BC *et al.* Computed tomographic

colonography (virtual colonoscopy): multicentre comparison with standard colonoscopy for detection of colorectal neoplasia. *JAMA* 2004; 291: 1717–19.

37 Rockey DC, Paulson E, Niedzwiecki D *et al.* Analysis of air contrast barium enema, computed tomographic colonography and colonoscopy: prospective comparison. *Lancet* 2005; 365: 305–11.

38 Berry DP, Clarke P, Hardcastle JD, Vellacott KD. Randomized trial of the addition of flexible sigmoidoscopy to faecal occult blood testing for colorectal neoplasia population screening. *Br J Surg* 1997; 84: 1274–6.

39 Brevinge H, Lindholm E, Buntzen S, Kewenter J. Screening for colorectal neoplasia with faecal occult blood testing compared with flexible sigmoidoscopy directly in a 55 years' old population. *Int J Colorectal Dis* 1997; 12: 291–5.

40 Gondal G, Grotmol T, Hofstad B *et al.* The Norwegian Colorectal Cancer Prevention (NORCCAP) screening study: baseline findings and implementations for clinical work-up in age groups 50–64 years. *Scand J Gastroenterol* 2003; 38: 635–42.

41 Rasmussen M, Fenger C, Kronborg O. Diagnostic yield in a biennial Haemoccult-II screening programme compared to a once-only screening with flexible sigmoidoscopy and Haemoccult-II. *Scand J Gastroenterol* 2003 Jan; 38: 114–18.

42 Robinson MHE, Hardcastle JD, Moss SM *et al.* The risks of screening: data from the Nottingham randomised controlled trial of faecal occult blood screening for colorectal cancer. *Gut* 1999; 45: 588–92.

43 Mella J, Biffin A, Radcliffe AG *et al.* Population-based audit of colorectal cancer management in two UK health regions. *Br J Surg* 1997; 84: 1731–6.

44 Black WC, Haggstrom DA, Welch HG. All-cause mortality in randomised trials of cancer screening. *J Natl Cancer Inst* 2002; 94: 167–73.

45 Lindholm E, Berglund B, Kewenter J, Halind E. Worry associated with screening for colorectal carcinomas. *Scand J Gastroenterol* 1997; 32: 238–45.

46 Parker MA, Robinson MH, Scholefield JH, Hardcastle JD. Psychiatric morbidity and screening for colorectal cancer. *J Med Screen* 2002; 9: 7–10.

47 Steele RJC, Gnauck R, Hrcka R *et al.* ESGE/UEGF Colorectal Cancer – Public Awareness Campaign, The Public/Professional Interface Workshop, Oslo, Norway, June 20–22, 2003. Methods and Economic Considerations: Group 1 Report. *Endoscopy* 2004; 36: 349–53.

48 Miyoshi H, Ohshiba S, Asada S *et al.* Immunological determination of fecal haemoglobin and transferrin levels: a comparison with other fecal occult blood tests. *Am J Gastroenterol* 1992; 87: 67–73.

49 Saitoh O, Matsumoto H, Sugimori K *et al.* Intestinal protein loss and bleeding assessed by fecal hemoglobin, transferrin, albumin and alpha-1-antitrypsin levels in patients with colorectal diseases. *Digestion* 1995; 56: 67–75.

50 Moran A, Robinson M, Lawson N *et al.* Fecal alpha 1-antitrypsin detection of colorectal neoplasia. An evaluation using HemoQuant. *Dig Dis Sci* 1995; 40: 2522–5.

51 Tibble J, Sigthorsson G, Foster R *et al.* Faecal calprotectin and faecal occult blood tests in the diagnosis of colorectal carcinoma and adenoma. *Gut* 2001; 49: 402–8.

52 Davies RJ, Freeman A, Morris LS *et al.* Analysis of minichromosome maintenance proteins as a novel method for detection of colorectal cancer in stool. *Lancet* 2002; 359: 1917–19.

53 Mak T, Lalloo F, Evans DGR, Hill J. Molecular stool screening for colorectal cancer. *Br J Surg* 2004; 91: 790–800.

54 Ahlquist DA, Skoletsky JE, Boynton KA *et al.* Colorectal cancer screening by detection of altered DNA in stool: feasibility of a multitarget assay panel. *Gastroenterology* 2000; 119: 1219–27.

55 Rengucci C, Maiolo P, Saragoni L *et al.*
   Multiple detection of genetic alterations
   in tumors and stool. *Clin Cancer Res*
   2001; 7: 590–3.

56 Dong SM, Traverso G, Johnson C *et al.*
   Detecting colorectal cancer in stool with
   the use of multiple genetic targets. *J Natl*
   Cancer Inst 2001; 93:
   858–65.

57 Imperiale TF, Ransohoff DF, Itzkowitz
   SH *et al.* Fecal DNA versus fecal occult
   blood for colorectal-cancer screening in
   an average-risk population. *N Engl J*
   Med 2004; 351: 2704–14.

3: What can the pathologist tell the multidisciplinary team about rectal cancer resection?

Phil Quirke

The pathologist is an essential member of the multidisciplinary team. Their skills and advice change clinical management and can improve team performance for the benefit of the patient. To do this they need the support of the team in ensuring that adequate time and resources are available to them.

Pathologists can play an important role in the prediction of prognosis, the need for further therapy, and audit of the quality of surgery and radiology. In return, the patient and team members should expect high-quality pathology.

Staging

The United Kingdom changed from reporting using Dukes' staging to TNM version 5 (Tumor, Nodal status and presence of Metastases V5) in 1997 with the publication of the Royal College of Pathologists minimum dataset for reporting colorectal cancer [1]. This was an important change, bringing UK pathologists into line with international colleagues. The minimum dataset itself also fulfills several functions. First, it sets standards, second, it is an aide mémoire, third, it is a concise summary of key features, and finally, it can be entered onto audit databases or returned to cancer registries. The first revision will appear in 2005. This document aims to use the best available evidence to guide practice and yet be simple enough to be used in all sizes of hospital.

The TNM staging is an improvement over Dukes' in that it allows different modalities of staging and these are denoted with a prefix: "c" for clinical, "u" for ultrasound, "p" for pathology, and a further prefix "y" if neoadjuvant therapy has been given. Thus pathology staging post therapy is "yp." It also includes a staging system for complete resection "R0," microscopic involvement of a margin "R1," and "R2" where macroscopic disease is left behind. The pathologist can also describe pathological features denoting high-risk states such as vascular invasion, for example, v1, if present. TNM V5 was a robust staging system that worked well in practice. TNM V6 has proved problematic. First, the R1 definition has not been revised to take account of the evidence from over 5000 patients [2–13] that 0–1 mm is the optimum definition of microscopic involvement of a surgical margin, but more importantly, major issues have arisen with its change of definition of lymph node and venous involvement, two key treatment factors. From a definition that was quantitative of tumor deposits ≥3 mm in diameter as nodal involvement and a standard definition of venous involvement, it has changed to describing lymph nodes as round structures and venous involvement as irregular nodules. The latter is an unusual approach as veins are round structures and early venous involvement will always be round. The evidence base for these changes were weak, based on retrospective single institution studies of relatively small numbers of cases. The weakness of these changes have been proven in a Cardiff study [14] where they demonstrated poor reproducibility with a kappa value of 0.36 and significant upstaging with 5/80 (6%) cases changing from N0 to N1. TNM V6 has thus undermined confidence in this system and also changed patient treatment in the absence of clinical trial evidence. In those countries adopting this version, it may also distort cancer registry data by increasing the pathological stage of TNM V6 cases vs previous years staged under TNM V5. After consultation, it has been agreed that the United Kingdom will remain on TNM V5 until further notice and likewise the national Belgium PROCARE project is also recommending TNM V5 rather than V6.

A number of features are very important for the pathologist to report. The presence of tumor deposits within lymph nodes or mesorectal deposits greater than 3 mm will lead to a tumor being designated as node positive and would be eligible for adjuvant chemotherapy. The current benefits of 5-fluorouracil (5-FU) appear to be around 7%. A combination of 5-FU and oxaliplatin [15] has been reported to increase disease-free survival in Dukes' C cases by up to 5% over 5-FU alone. Failure to find involved lymph nodes leads to an increased risk of recurrence for patients and must be avoided. A median of 12 lymph nodes for every case is possible in routine practice and has been achieved in the Yorkshire region, and higher median node counts of 15 or more are achieved by specialist gastrointestinal (GI) pathologists. It is also important to describe peritoneal involvement and extramural vascular invasion. These factors, alongside incomplete resection, are high-risk features for recurrent disease in node negative cases [16]. At a recent multidisciplinary National Cancer Research Institute in a colorectal cancer studies group 100% of the oncologists stated they would consider adjuvant therapy in such "high risk" Bs.

The pathologist needs to look carefully for an incomplete resection. This occurs most frequently in the rectum, but also occurs in the right colon. In the Conventional vs Laparoscopic Assisted Surgery in Colorectal Cancer (CLASICC) study [17] 13% of the right hemicolectomies showed involvement of the posterior cecal/ascending colon retroperitoneal surgical margin. Involvement of this margin has been reported by Warren [18] in 7% of 100 right hemicolectomies, but there are as yet no local recurrence or survival figures available. In 1072 cases of colon cancer in the Colon Carcinoma Laparoscopic or Open Resection (COLOR) study, where there was no specific pathological training or proforma asking this question, only 1.5% of cases were reported as involved [19].

Involvement of the rectal circumferential margin has now been assessed in over 5000 patients, many of them in clinical trials. These studies show a higher rate of local recurrence and a poorer survival for patients within 1 mm of the surgical margin [2–12]. It has been suggested that 2 mm should be used [13], but this study alone is recommending this and is based only on small numbers of patients in this group. Data on a further 1350 patients from MRC CR07 study and 300 patients in the MRC CLASICC study will become available in early 2006 and will confirm or refute this idea. The involvement of the circumferential resection margin (CRM) by tumor contained wholly within a lymph node but within 1 mm of the margin is also controversial. Unfortunately there are few cases reported [6]. Review of CR07 cases may help to decide this matter. At present patients with involved CRMs are being offered postoperative chemoradiotherapy or radiotherapy alone. The effect of such therapy is uncertain and CR07 should help in such decision making. By accurately reporting this margin the pathologist not only alerts the team to the possibility of local failure but also indirectly helps to provide feedback on the effectiveness of the team treatment decision.

Quality of surgery

In 1994 on a visit to Norway, I was privileged to dissect a Total Mesorectal Excision (TME) rectal cancer specimen removed by Professor Bill Heald. This specimen with its mesorectal bulk and smooth surfaces was clearly

(a)   (b)   (c)

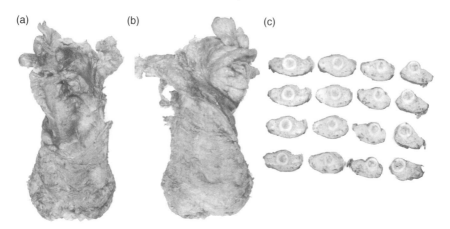

Fig. 3.1 Examples of a good mesorectal excision. (a) Anterior surface with Denovilliers fascia and (b) posterior surface with mesorectal fascia apparent. (c) Cross sections of the rectum showing a regular smooth surface covered in black ink.

superior to the specimens seen in my routine surgical pathology practice in the United Kingdom and also to many of the Norwegian specimens alongside it. Subsequently, we devised a quality grading system that was incorporated into the MRC CLASICC and MRC CR07 trials. It was also adopted into the Dutch mesorectal excision and short-course radiotherapy study [20]. This classification described the smoothness and bulk of the mesorectum and divided them into three groups. Subsequently, it was decided that the best way of describing the surgery was by the plane of the surgical dissection.

Mesorectal fascial plane. The mesorectum should be smooth with no violation of the fat, good bulk to the mesorectum anteriorly and posteriorly, and the distal margin should appear adequate with no coning near the tumor. No defect should be more than superficial or 5 mm deep (see Fig. 3.1).

Intramesorectal plane. Moderate bulk to mesorectum but irregularity of the mesorectal surface is present. Moderate coning of the specimen toward the distal margin. At no site is the muscularis propria visible with the exception of the area of insertion of levator muscles. Moderate irregularity of the CRM.

Muscularis propria plane. There will be areas of substantial loss of mesorectal tissue. Deep cuts and tears down onto the muscularis propria will be present. On cross-section there will be a very irregular CRM with

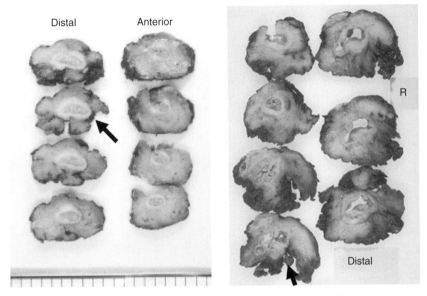

Fig. 3.2 Two resections where the dissection plane reaches onto the muscularis propria (arrows). These are poor resections.

little bulk to the mesorectal fat and the muscularis propria will form the CRM in places (see Fig. 3.2).

We are still awaiting the CR07 and CLASICC results, but a small study was performed within the Dutch trial. This showed that an involved CRM had the greatest effect but resections where the CRM reached down onto the muscularis propria had a higher rate of local recurrence and a poorer survival than resections where this did not happen [20]. So-called incomplete resections (muscularis propria plane) also had a CRM much closer to the tumor and a higher rate of CRM involvement.

Other features to note when describing the mesorectum are the anatomical variation between individuals. Some people have very small mesorectums whereas others are quite large. Thus the distance of extramural penetration of a tumor into the mesorectum may have very different implications in different people. The other feature of interest is the variation in shape of the mesorectum. Anteriorly, there is less tissue leading to a higher risk of CRM involvement. This is also the hardest area for the surgeon to dissect due to the poor visibility and difficult access in some pelvises. The distal part of the mesorectal dissection is the most arduous to undertake and frequently

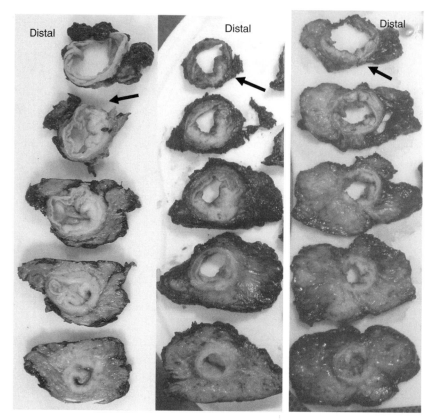

Fig. 3.3 Coning at the distal margin of three specimens leads to the tumor being very close to the CRM even though it is clear of the distal margin. The arrow shows the site of the lowest part of the tumor.

an excellent mesorectal dissection can be ruined by coning of the surgical margin as shown in two cases in Fig. 3.3.

Quality and the abdominoperineal dissection

In a recent study [12], we have demonstrated that the CRM is involved in 36.5% of abdominoperineal excisions of the rectum (APERs) compared to 22.3% of anterior resections (ARs). This was also seen in the MRC CLASICC study where 21% APERs showed margin involvement vs 10% ARs [17]. In the MERCURY study [21,22], 33% of APERs vs 13% of ARs below 6 cm showed CRM positivity; in the Dutch TME/RT [23] study, 29% APERs had margin involvement vs 13% of ARs; and in the Norwegian national audit of curative excisions of rectal cancer, 12% APERs and 5% ARs had positive margins [11]. In series with the follow-up, the increased rate of margin positivity always equated with an increased rate of local recurrence and a poorer survival. Thus when pathologically assessing, APERs always look carefully for CRM positivity in the area of the low mesorectum and sphincter.

There is also a much higher rate of tumor perforation in APERs than in ARs; in the Dutch study 13.7% of APERs were perforated vs 2.5% ARs, and in the Norwegian study 16% APERs vs 4% ARs [24].

With this data it became apparent that there was a wide variation in the quality of the APER resections and a new quality classification was derived. This was similar to the mesorectal grading system in that it describes the surgical plane of dissection.

Levator plane. The surgical plane lies external to the levators with them being removed *en bloc* with the specimen. This creates a cylindrical specimen with the levators forming an extra protective layer on the sphincters.

Sphincteric plane. Either there are no levator muscles attached to the specimen or only a very small cuff and the resection margin is on the surface of the sphincters. The specimen has a waisted/apple core appearance.

Intrasphincteric/submucosal plane. The surgeon has inadvertently entered the sphincters or even deeper into the submucosa or perforated the specimen at any point.

It has been possible to review photographs of 271 of the APERs from the Dutch TME trial with interesting results. This review showed that in one-third of the cases the surgical margin was either in the sphincter muscle, the submucosa, or into the lumen with a perforation. In the other two-thirds the CRM was on the sphincter muscle. This plane of surgical dissection explains the high frequency of CRM involvement. This study also showed that the cylindrical radical APER of Holm from the Karolinska was not performed in Holland. This operation has the theoretical advantage of approaching the tumor from below, outside of the levator plane. This avoids the difficulties of the very low pelvic floor dissection from above, removes the risk of perforation by maintaining a cylindrical package around the tumor, increases the bulk of tissue around the tumor avoiding the waist seen on standard APERs, and, importantly, increases the ease of the anterior dissection as this occurs under excellent vision. It creates a very different shaped

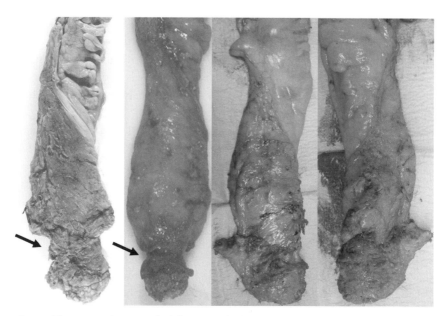

Fig. 3.4 The two specimens on the left are standard British APERs showing the typical waist (arrows) formed by the surgeon following the mesorectal fascial plane and coming down onto the sphincters. The two pictures on the right show the two sides of a Swedish APER performed by Mr T Holm from the Karolinska hospital. The projection is the coccyx that has also been removed *en bloc*.

specimen that should reduce the frequency of margin positivity at this site (see Fig. 3.4).

Reporting the tumor after neo-adjuvant therapy

Within the United Kingdom we are seeing an increasing usage of preoperative radiotherapy and chemotherapy. These are increasingly being used together and the number of chemotherapy agents used in combination is rising.

Short-course radiotherapy was popularized by the improvement in survival and reduction in local recurrence as seen in the Swedish rectal cancer studies [24–29] and the effect of halving the local recurrence was confirmed by the Dutch TME/RT trial [23]. Short-course 5×5 Gy radiotherapy is reported not to downstage tumors but is aimed at small micro-metastases within the mesorectum. There are, however, tumors that do show significant damage from such therapy, but the relative effect of this on patient outcome is not known.

Long-course radiotherapy over a period of 6 weeks can cause significant effects on the tumor, although complete response is unusual at between 0 and 8%. The addition of 5-FU to radiotherapy increases the complete response rate to 8% [30]. Combination chemotherapy of 5-FU with irinotecan or oxaliplatin has been reported to increase the complete response rate up to 10–30% but these are small phase II studies and definitive studies are awaited.

CRM and preoperative treatment

A major source of debate is the relative importance of achieving a clear CRM over a complete response. Recent results [31] on 150 patients strongly suggest that clear CRM is the key factor. After chemoradiotherapy with 5FU local recurrence occurred in 10% of negative CRM and 62% of positive CRM or R2 resections. Distant metastases occurred in 29% of negative CRM and 75% of positive CRM or R2 resections. Three-year overall survivals were 25 and 64% respectively for patients with and without a positive CRM. A multicenter audit of 650 patients confirmed these results [32] as did a study performed in Leeds [33]. This is important as the assessment of this margin is well described whereas the reporting of a complete response is highly variable. For the assessment of complete response we recommend using the criteria established for the dissection and reporting of complete response in the Capicitabine/Oxaliplatin, Radiotherapy and Excision (CORE) trial. The recommendations were to extensively sample the area of the tumor by taking a minimum of five blocks. If no tumor is found the whole of the area of the tumor should be embedded. If there is still no tumor then three levels should be cut on each block. If there is still no tumor then the case should be reported as a complete response. Since the efficacy of chemoradiotherapy regimens is frequently judged on complete response it is essential that such assessments are standardized across all trials.

It is also possible to grade the degree of regression of tumor after neoadjuvant therapy. The results from the preoperative radiochemotherapy vs postoperative radiochemotherapy study [34] support the use of regression grading. Unfortunately grading has become complicated by the reversal of the scoring system by different authors. They all use a modification of Mandard grading [35] first described in the esophagus, and for the CORE study we used the Dworak scoring [36] where grade 4 equals a complete response. This was also used in a preoperative 5-FU plus radiotherapy study by Rodel *et al.* [37] with complete loss of tumor cells and the presence of very few tumor cells (defined as difficult to find microscopically) leading to a 72% relapse-free survival vs 28% in the tumors showing less regression. Bouzourene *et al.* [38] also reported that the presence of rare tumor cells was associated with a similar disease-free survival of 75% vs 25–50% for the other groups. More recently the German group has reported regression grading to be a good predictor of outcome. However, the relative importance of the regression grade was not compared to margin positivity to see whether it was of additional value over the assessment of complete resection alone. Use of the description rather than a number should ease communication between different groups and studies.

Chemoradiotherapy response scoring

Dworak scoring used for the CORE study

Grade 0 No regression detectable.
Grade 1 Minimal regression: dominant tumor mass with obvious fibrosis and/or vasculopathy.
Grade 2 Moderate regression: dominantly fibrotic changes with few tumor cells or groups (easy to find).
Grade 3 Good regression: very few (difficult to find microscopically) tumor cells in fibrotic tissue with or without mucin.
Grade 4 Total regression: no tumor cells, only fibrotic mass or mucin.

Simplified scoring system for CORE study

Poor response – No regression to moderate regression: dominantly fibrotic changes with few tumor cells or groups (easy to find) (Dworak 0–2).

Excellent response – Good regression: very few (difficult to find microscopically) tumor cells in fibrotic tissue with or without mucin to total regression (Dworak 3–4).

High-risk rectal cancer for adjuvant chemotherapy

It is now well established that node positive colonic cancer patients benefit from adjuvant chemotherapy. The Quasar adjuvant chemotherapy study also suggests that rectal cancer patients benefit too. It is a proven fact that the higher the number of lymph nodes found by the pathologist the higher the chance of finding a positive node [9]. The average number of lymph nodes retrieved in routine practice is still too low in many countries. In the United Kingdom the numbers of nodes found has been rising with an increase in a population-based study in Yorkshire from 8 to 13 in Dukes' B and from 9 to 14 in Dukes' C from 1995 to 2000 after the introduction of a proforma. Reviews of CR07 and the MRC CLASICC [17] studies have shown a respectable harvest of lymph nodes of a median of 13. Audits in Leeds and Gloucester report an average of 15 and 17 lymph nodes respectively. In Sweden local audits have revealed an average of 8 lymph nodes and the COLOR study, 10 nodes [19]. Many rectal cancer trials do not report the average number of lymph nodes found thus we do not know the true stage of the patients. Centers should strive for an average of 15 lymph nodes; indeed TNM suggests that a case with under 12 lymph nodes should not be staged but this dictat is widely ignored even in many European and US studies. Thus it is essential for the pathologist to retrieve as many nodes as possible. If a good node yield has been obtained and there is no evidence of metastatic spread, high-risk features should be reported. The nature of these features has been reported for colonic cancer [16] but is less well investigated in rectal cancer. High-risk features that should be reported are extramural vascular invasion, peritoneal involvement, perforation, and the distance the tumor has spread from the muscularis propria. Incomplete resection is important but may need local as well as systemic treatment depending on prior therapy.

Locally advanced and metastatic cancer

In some specialist centers the pathologist will be presented with *en bloc* resections or even extenterations. These represent a major challenge. The surgeon who performed the operation should be invited to demonstrate the anatomy and highlight any areas that he/she had concerns over. The presence of residual recurrent tumor, the completeness of excision, and which organs are involved are all important. The resection of liver metastases in patients with spread to the liver is increasingly common and in selected patients relatively good outcomes are achievable. How are these specimens reported? The surgeon wants to have each lesion confirmed as adenocarcinoma and to know whether excision is complete, whether there is spread through the liver capsule, whether there is venous invasion present, and the state of the surrounding liver. Occasionally, lung resections will be performed for metastatic colorectal cancer, especially in younger patients.

The pathologist and the radiologist

The use of Magnetic Resonance Imaging (MRI) has transformed the management of rectal cancer. The early work of Blomquist [38] and Brown [39] and confirmed by Beets Tan [40] and other centers [41] demonstrated the potential for this modality. The recent MERCURY [21,22] data has confirmed the accuracy of a well-performed MRI in predicting distance of extramural spread to within 1 mm and involvement of the CRM with an accuracy of 82%. Seeing the preoperative MRI can help the pathologist to dissect complicated specimens and to look for extramural vascular invasion and peritoneal involvement. The presentation of the macroscopic pathology slices at the MDT meeting can help the radiologist to improve their accuracy for the benefit of the patient and the team. This will become increasingly important if 3 Tesla scanners become routine instruments, increasing the resolution available to radiologists.

Conclusions

Thus the pathologist is an important member of the multidisciplinary team guiding their colleagues on the accuracy of the preoperative assessment of the MRI, the completeness of excision and the presence of residual disease, the pathological stage of the tumor, the quality of the excision, and in suggesting the change to a more radical perineal approach to low rectal cancer. We identify complete resection after chemoradiotherapy and surgery and determine the degree of regression and whether there has been a complete response. In Dukes' stage B cancers (TNM Stage II) we can identify high-risk cases and guide adjuvant therapy.

References

1 Quirke P, Williams GT. The Royal College of Pathologists. Minimum dataset for colorectal cancer histopathology reports. London: The Royal College of Pathologists, 1998.
http://www.rcpath.org/ resources/pdf/ colorectal cancer.pdf

2 Quirke P, Durdey P, Dixon MF, Williams NS. Local recurrence of rectal adenocarcinoma is caused by inadequate surgical resection. Histopathological

study of lateral tumour spread and surgical excision. *Lancet* 1986; 2: 996–9.

3 Ng IO, Luk IS, Yuen ST *et al*. Surgical lateral clearance in resected rectal carcinomas. A multivariate analysis of clinicopathological features. *Cancer* 1993; 71: 1972–6.

4 Adam IJ, Mohamdee MO, Martin IG *et al*. Role of circumferential margin involvement in the local recurrence of rectal cancer. *Lancet* 1994; 344: 707–11.

5 de Haas-Koch DF, Baeten CGMI, Jager JJ *et al*. Prognostic significance of radial margins of clearance in rectal carcinoma. *Br J Surg* 1996; 83: 781–5.

6 Birbeck KF, Macklin CP, Tiffin NJ *et al*. Rates of circumferential margin involvement vary between surgeons and predict outcomes in rectal cancer surgery. *Ann Surg* 2002; 235: 449–57.

7 Wibe A, Rendedal PR, Svensson E *et al*. on behalf of the Norwegian Rectal Cancer Group. Prognostic significance of the circumferential resection margin following total mesorectal excision for rectal cancer. *Br J Surg* 2002; 89: 327–34.

8 Nagetaal ID, Marijnen CAM, Kranenbarg EK *et al*. Circumferential margin involvement is still an important predictor of local recurrence in rectal carcinoma. Not 1 mm but 2 mm is the limit. *Am J Surg Pathol* 2002; 26: 350–7.

9 Maughan NJ, Morris E, Craig SC *et al*. Analysis of Northern and Yorkshire Cancer Registry Data 1995–2001. *J Pathol* 2003; 201: 18A.

10 Martling A, Singnomklao T, Holm T *et al*. Prognostic significance of both surgical and pathological assessment of curative resection for rectal cancer. *Br J Surg* 2004; 91: 1040–5.

11 Wibe A, Syse A, Andersen E *et al*. on behalf of the Norwegian Rectal Cancer Group. Oncological outcomes after total mesorectal excision for cure for cancer of the lower rectum: anterior resection vs abdominoperineal resection. *Dis Colon Rectum* 2004; 47: 48–58.

12 Marr R, Birbeck K, Garvican J *et al*. The abdomino-perineal excision – the next

challenge after total mesorectal excision. *Ann Surg* July 2005; 242: 74–82.

13 Nagtegaal ID, van de Velde CJH, Marijnen CAM *et al*. for the pathology review committee and the cooperative clinical investigators of the Dutch ColoRectal Cancer Group. Low rectal cancer; a call for a change of approach in abdominoperineal resection. *J Clin Oncol* 2005; 23: 9257–64.

14 Howarth SM, Morgan JM, Williams GT. The new (6th edition) TNM classification of colorectal cancer – a stage too far. *Gut* 2004; 53: A21.

15 Andre T, Bonni C, Mounedjii-Boudiaf L *et al*. Oxaliplatin, fluorouracil and leucovorin as adjuvant treatment for colon cancer. *N Engl J Med* 2004; 350: 2343–51.

16 Petersen VC, Baxter KJ, Love SB, Shepherd NA. Identification of objective pathological prognostic determinants and models of prognosis in Dukes' B colon cancer. *Gut* 2002; 51: 65–9.

17 Guillou P, Quirke P, Thorpe H *et al*. for the MRC CLASSICC Trial Group. Short-term endpoints of conventional versus laparoscopic assisted surgery in patients with colorectal cancer (MRC CLASICC trial): multicentre, randomised controlled trial. *Lancet* 2005; 365: 1718–26.

18 Bateman AC, Carr NJ, Warren BF. The retroperitoneal surface in distal caecal and proximal ascending colon carcinoma: the Cinderella surgical margin? *J Clin Pathol* 2005; 58: 426–8.

19 Laparoscopic surgery versus open surgery for colon cancer: short-term outcomes of a randomized trial. The Colon Laparoscopic or Open Resection Study Group. *Lancet Oncol* 2005; 6: 477–84.

20 Nagtegaal ID, van de Velde CJH, van der Worp E *et al*. and the pathology review committee for the cooperative clinical investigators of the Dutch Colorectal Group. Macroscopic evaluation of rectal cancer resection specimen: clinical significance of the

pathologist in quality control. *J Clin Oncol* 2002; 20: 1729–1734.

21 Daniels I and the MERCURY Study Group. Magnetic resonance imaging of low rectal cancers: a multicentre, multidisciplinary European study of 285 tumours located within 6 cm of the anal verge. *Colorectal Dis* 2004; 6: 1.

22 The MERCURY study group. MRI predicts extramural tumour spread and circumferential resection margin status in patients with rectal cancer: Results of the MERCURY study. *Br Med J* submitted May 2005.

23 Kapiteijn E, Marijnen CAM, Nagtegaal ID *et al.* for the Dutch Colorectal Cancer Group. *NEJM* 2001; 345: 638–46.

24 Eriksen MT, Wibe A, Syse A *et al.* Norwegian Rectal Cancer Group; Norwegian Gastrointestinal Cancer Group. Inadvertent perforation during rectal cancer resection in Norway. *Br J Surg* 2004; 91: 779.

25 Cedermark B, Johansson H, Rutqvist LE, Wilking N. The Stockholm I trial of preoperative short term radiotherapy in operable rectal carcinoma. A prospective randomized trial. Stockholm Colorectal Cancer Study Group. *Cancer* 1995; 75: 2269–75.

26 Martling A, Holm T, Johansson H *et al.* The Stockholm II trial on preoperative radiotherapy in rectal carcinoma: long-term follow-up of a population-based study. *Cancer* 2001; 92: 896–902.

27 Stockholm Rectal Cancer Study Group. Preoperative short-term radiation therapy in operable rectal carcinoma. A prospective randomized trial. *Cancer* 1990; 60: 49–55.

28 Stockholm Colorectal Cancer Study Group. Randomised study on preoperative radiotherapy in rectal carcinoma. *Ann Surg Oncol* 1996; 3: 423–30.

29 Sauer R, Becker H, Hohenberger W *et al.* for the German Rectal Cancer Study Group. Preoperative versus postoperative chemoradiotherapy for rectal cancer. *N Engl J Med* 2004; 351: 1731–40.

30 Mawdsley S, Glynne-Jones R, Grainger J *et al.* Can the histopathological assessment of the circumferential margin following pre-operative pelvic chemo-radiotherapy for T3/4 rectal cancer predict for three year disease free survival? *Int J Radiat Oncol* 2005; 63: 745–52.

31 Sebag-Montefiore D, Glynne-Jones R, Mortensen N *et al.* Pooled analysis of outcome measures including the histopathological R0 resection rate after preoperative chemoradiation for locally advanced rectal cancer. *Colorectal Dis* 2005; 7: A20.

32 Sebag-Montefiore D, Hingorani M, Cooper R, Chesser P. Circumferential resection margin status predicts outcome after pre-operative chemoradiation for locally advanced rectal cancer. http://www.asco.org/ac/1,003,12-002636-0018-0036-00190010208.00.asp

33 CORE study: Capicitabine/Oxaliplatin, Radiotherapy and excision protocol Study No. C8601. Sanofi-Synthelabs 2002 Appendix 7, Pathological techniques (P. Quirke).

34 Mandard AM, Dalibard F, Mandard JC *et al.* Pathological assessment of tumour regression after preoperative chemoradiotherapy of esophageal carcinoma. Clinicopathological correlations. *Cancer* 1994; 73: 2680–6.

35 Dworak O, Keilholtz L, Hoffmann A. Pathological features of rectal cancer after preoperative radiochemotherapy. *Int J Colorectal Dis* 1997; 12: 19–23.

36 Rodel C, Grabenbauer GG, Papadopoulos T *et al.* Apoptosis as a cellular predictor for histopathological response to neo-adjuvant radiochemotherapy in patients with rectal cancer. *Int J Rad Oncol Biol Phys* 2002; 52: 294–303.

37 Bouzourene H, Bosman FT, Seelentag W *et al.* Importance of tumour regression assessment in predicting outcome in patients with locally advanced rectal carcinoma who are treated with

preoperative radiotherapy. *Cancer* 2002; 94: 1121–30.

38 Blomquist L, Rubio C, Holm T *et al.* Rectal adenocarcinoma:assessment of tumour involvement of the lateral resection margin by MRI of the resected specimen. *Br J Radiol* 1999; 72: 18–23.

39 Brown G, Richards CJ, Newcombe RG *et al.* Rectal carcinoma: thin-section MR imaging for staging in 28 patients. *Radiology* 1999; 211: 215–22.

40 Beets-Tan RGH, Beets GL, Vliegen RFA *et al.* Accuracy of magnetic resonance imaging in prediction of tumour-free resection margin in rectal cancer surgery. *Lancet* 2001; 357: 497–504.

41 Botterill ID, Blunt DM, Quirke P *et al.* Evaluation of the role of pre-operative magnetic resonance imaging in the management of rectal cancer. *Int J Colorectal Dis* 2001; 3: 295–304.

4: MRI-directed rectal cancer surgery

Brendan Moran and John H. Scholefield

Introduction

Rectal cancer is a common problem and accounts for approximately 30% of all colorectal malignancies. The treatment is predominantly surgical excision, with the addition of neoadjuvant therapy (preoperative radiotherapy or chemoradiotherapy) in selected cases. There is universal agreement that surgery alone can cure localized rectal cancer and now increasing evidence that neoadjuvant therapy may facilitate surgical excision in advanced disease. There is currently ongoing controversy as to whether all, or selected patients, should have neoadjuvant therapy. Major resectional rectal cancer surgery is both technically challenging and complex due to the relative inaccessibility within the confines of the bony pelvis, the difficulty in reconstruction with a high risk of leakage, and the particular problem of local recurrence within the pelvis.

Major surgery is associated with significant mortality and morbidity and is inappropriate for some cases. There is now a range of treatments, both surgical and non-surgical, for management of rectal cancer. For some patients with early tumors, local excision alone may be curative, while some elderly, unfit, or those with very advanced disease may only benefit from symptom control, for example, luminal ablation techniques. Furthermore, novel chemotherapeutic and radiotherapy regimens can result in local symptom control in patients who either refuse or are unsuitable for major surgery.

With this range of treatment options, patient assessment, cancer staging, and selection for appropriate therapy is becoming crucial to the optimal management of rectal cancer. Despite the range of treatments, and ongoing controversy as to their merits in individual situations, there is general agreement that, for the majority of patients with rectal cancer, trans-abdominal resection is the optimal treatment.

The main aims in rectal cancer surgery are to cure the patient and if possible preserve normal bowel, bladder, and sexual function. The main mechanisms available to achieve these aims encompass two key treatment modalities, namely surgical technique [1,2] and neoadjuvant therapy, both of which have been shown to reduce the local recurrence rates [3,4]. There is substantial evidence that optimal surgery, in the form of total mesorectal excision (TME), reduces local recurrence and improves survival [1–5]. With regards to preoperative radiotherapy, there is good quality evidence for a reduction in local recurrence from large randomized trials [3,6–8], though to date only one trial has reported improved survival with the addition of radiotherapy [8].

The key advances in rectal cancer have resulted from awareness of the problem of local recurrence, the risk factors influencing recurrence, and the strategies needed to reduce it. These factors when combined almost always translate to both better quality of life and improved overall survival in patients with rectal cancer.

Local recurrence of rectal cancer

Local recurrence after rectal cancer surgery is defined as disease in the pelvis, including recurrence at the site of the anastomosis and in the perineum [9]. Local recurrence is for the most part incurable and results in severe morbidity with debilitating symptoms of pelvic pain, ureteric obstruction, intestinal and urinary tract fistulation, and poor bowel and urinary function. Palliative treatment has limited success. Increasingly local recurrence is being recognized as a failure of complete removal of tumor at the primary surgical procedure. Thus, in reality, local "recurrence" may, in many cases, represent persistent and progressive disease rather than true recurrence. There are a number of predictors of risk of local recurrence following surgery for rectal cancer, including size of the primary [10] involvement of the circumferential resection margin (CRM) [11], distal location of the tumor [10–12], extramural vascular invasion [13,14], tumor differentiation [13,14], nodal status [11,13,14], extent of extramural spread [11,13,14], and peritoneal involvement by tumor [12,13,15]. Practically all of these features with a high risk of local recurrence are associated with both locally advanced tumors and frequently, in addition, metastatic disease at presentation. These risk factors for local recurrence are also highly predictive of disseminated distant recurrence following surgery. Traditionally, the majority of these risk factors came to light either at surgery or, more commonly, at histopathological assessment of the excised specimen.

Current topical issues are whether some or all of these factors can be predicted preoperatively and if so, whether there are adjunctive treatments that can improve the outcome in high-risk patients?

Reported local recurrence rates vary from 2.6 to 32% and are probably most influenced by surgical technique [16,17]. The lowest recurrence rates and best survivals have been consistently reported with TME [1,2,5,16–18]. It is now well documented that low local recurrence rates translate into better overall survival with increasing evidence that the optimal treatment of rectal cancer undoubtedly involves strategies to minimize local recurrence.

Local recurrence and the circumferential resection margin

Rectal cancer spreads by local extension, via the lymphatics and via the bloodstream. Lymphatic drainage is associated with the vascular pedicle and is generally addressed by a combination of TME and high ligation of the inferior mesenteric artery. Local spread of a rectal cancer in the confines of the narrow pelvis results in a risk of involvement of the CRM. Of all the risk factors for local recurrence of rectal cancer, involvement of the CRM appears to be the main determinant of risk. A number of reports, initially from Quirke's group, have shown that a positive CRM, defined as tumor within 1 mm of the edge of the resected specimen, and depth of extramural invasion are independent predictors of local recurrence and poor prognosis [10,11]. These observations are supported by recent reports from large studies, such as the Norwegian [19] and Dutch [20] studies.

While the CRM may be involved directly by tumor, CRM involvement may also be due to metastatic nodal disease. There is debate as to whether involved nodes, in their own right, increase local recurrence even if not directly involving the CRM. Jatzko et al. [21] reported that patients with positive lymph nodes had a higher risk of local recurrence. However, others found that lymph node involvement was not associated with higher local recurrence, attributed to the beneficial effects of TME [19,22]. Recently Cecil et al. [23] reported their experience in patients with lymph node positive rectal cancer with little impact on local recurrence rates which they attributed to optimal CRM clearance by TME.

While other risk factors, such as vascular invasion, differentiation, and so on are undoubtedly major determinants of long-term survival, the single main factor that can be manipulated by treatment is the CRM.

Surgical technique and total mesorectal excision

Total mesorectal excision involves a number of steps, which aim to maximize circumferential clearance. TME surgery has been reported to reduce the rate of local recurrence from 30–40 to 5–15% [17,24]. A paper from Stockholm has been the first report of a direct benefit in a whole population following a video-based surgical training program [4]. Local recurrence was significantly lower in the TME group compared with historical controls from the Stockholm randomized controlled trials of preoperative radiotherapy (Stockholm I and II groups) (6 vs 15% and 14% respectively) as was cancer-related death (9 vs 15% and 16% respectively) [4]. The CRM positive rate was 4% – the lowest-reported incidence so far in any published series. They have recently updated their results at 5 years with significant survival benefits in patients who had TME surgery [25].

Evidence for preoperative radiotherapy

There is ongoing debate as to the role of preoperative radiotherapy in rectal cancer. However, there is now evidence that radiotherapy, particularly in the preoperative setting results in a reduction of local recurrence. The advantages and disadvantages of preoperative vs postoperative radiotherapy have been extensively discussed in the medical literature. The main disadvantage of preoperative treatment is the risk of overtreating some patients due to staging inaccuracies and thus exposing patients to unnecessary risks. Postoperative radiotherapy can be more appropriately targeted with the benefit of histopathology but has major tolerance problems, with acute toxicity, in patients who have just undergone major surgery. Pahlman and Glimelius [26] reported the results of, until recently, the only randomized trial to address this issue. There was a significantly lower recurrence rate in the preoperative arm (12 vs 21%) which may have been partly attributable to a delay of 6 weeks or more in over 50% of the patients randomized to postoperative radiotherapy [26].

The recently reported German Rectal Cancer Study Group of a randomized trial of preoperative vs postoperative chemoradiotherapy for rectal cancer is a major addition to this ongoing debate [27]. In total, 799 patients staged preoperatively as T3 or T4 tumors were randomized. Staging' was by endorectal ultrasound and Sauer *et al.* found that 18% of the patients randomized to postoperative treatment had been overstaged compared to the pathology of the resected specimen. These 18% had been considered to have tumor penetration through the bowel wall (T3 or T4 disease) or nodal involvement but were subsequently found to have stage T1, or T2, lymph node negative disease. This is not surprising as the accuracy of endorectal ultrasonography is reported to be 67–93% for the assessment of rectal wall penetration and 62–83% for determination of nodal status [28].

The overall 5-year survival rates in the German Rectal Cancer Trial were similar (67 and 74%). The local recurrence was 6% for patients assigned to preoperative chemoradiotherapy vs 13% in the postoperative treatment group ($p = 0.006$).

Much of the background evidence in support of preoperative radiotherapy comes from the Swedish and Stockholm Rectal Cancer Trials [6–8]. The Swedish Rectal Cancer Trial showed a relative survival benefit of 21%, with an increase in the 5-year survival from 48 to 58% and a reduction in local recurrence from 27 to 11% [8]. A meta-analysis in 2000 of the then published randomized controlled trials concluded that in patients with resectable rectal cancer, preoperative radiotherapy significantly improved overall and cancer-specific survival compared with surgery alone, though these benefits were mainly attributable to the Swedish trial results [29].

It is now generally agreed that preoperative radiotherapy can reduce local recurrence rates to approximately half that in surgery alone. Therefore in situations with a high local recurrence rates, routine usage might be acceptable. However, with local recurrence rates of less than 10%, there is no data demonstrating a beneficial effect with the routine addition of radiotherapy [30]. In the Norwegian report [19], only 5% of patients with an uninvolved CRM developed local recurrence, so radiotherapy would have overtreated 97% of the patients with clear margins if all patients had routine preoperative radiotherapy.

The Dutch Colorectal Cancer Group attempted to address the role of preoperative radiotherapy when surgery was standardized to TME for rectal cancer [3]. The entry criteria included only mobile rectal cancer. With addition of radiotherapy, local recurrence was reduced from 8.2 to 2.4% after a median follow-up of 2 years in 1784 patients who underwent a macroscopically complete resection [3]. However, the surgery alone arm had high local recurrence rates for mobile tumors suggesting inadequate surgery in a significant proportion. The Dutch trial had attempted to standardize the surgery and provide quality control measures through workshops and live-video demonstrations. Despite this "standardization" of surgery, the involved margin rate in what were considered mobile tumors was 18.3%.

Nevertheless, this is an important trial which has shown a reduction in local recurrence at 2 years with the updated results confirming a similar degree of reduction of local recurrence with no difference in overall survival (unpublished results). As practically all patients with local recurrence die from the disease, it seems surprising that 5-year survival is similar. This suggests that radiotherapy may either have lethal side-effects or, more likely, that the reduction in local recurrence is offset by death from systemic metastases in a group predestined to die of disease. Nevertheless, if radiotherapy was without harm, a reduction in local recurrence would still be worthwhile. Unfortunately there are risks, as well as inconvenience and costs, associated with radiotherapy.

Complications of preoperative radiotherapy

Preoperative radiotherapy is associated with toxicity, early postoperative complications, and long-term side effects. Early complications include perineal wound breakdown, diarrhoea, proctitis, urinary tract infection, small bowel obstruction, leucopenia, and venous thrombosis.

Radiotherapy has been shown to have adverse effects on anal function with negative effects on the function and integrity of a coloanal anastomosis with, or without, formation of a colonic pouch [31].

In the recently reported German Rectal Cancer Study [27], Grade 3 or 4 acute toxicity occurred in 27% with preoperative chemoradiotherapy vs 40% in the postoperative group ($p = 0.001$); the corresponding rates of long-term toxic effects were 14 and 24%, respectively ($p = 0.01$).

Downstaging and downsizing rectal cancer with neoadjuvant therapy

Rectal cancer staging has traditionally been a histopathological analysis of the excised specimen and the "Dukes' staging" system described initially by Cuthbert Dukes [32] specifically in rectal cancer, and subsequently applied to colon cancer, is still in widespread use. However, the TNM classification system has advantages and is now considered the optimal universal staging system for colorectal cancer (Fig. 4.1).

The particular advantage of the TNM system, as applied to rectal cancer, is the "T" aspect whereby the depth of penetration within the bowel wall is a major determinant of the prognosis, particularly with regard to local recurrence in the lowest tumors. The rectum has been arbitrarily divided into three parts with the lower rectum 0–6 cm, the middle rectum 7–11 cm,

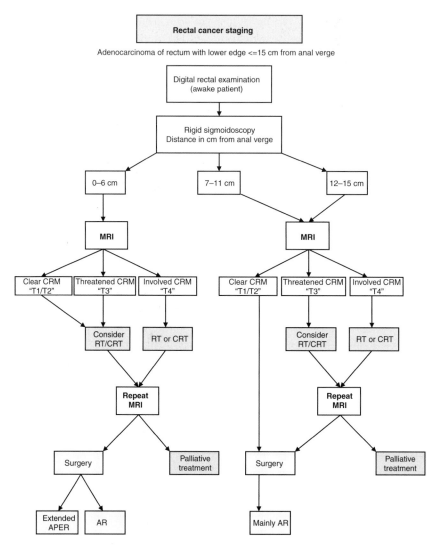

Fig. 4.1 Rectal cancer staging.

and the upper rectum 12–15 cm from the anal verge. There is a debate as to whether a T3 middle or upper rectal cancer (that is, above 7 cm) is particularly at high risk of local recurrence, providing surgery is adequate and that a TME has resulted in an intact cover of mesorectal fat and fascia.

However in the lower rectum a T3 tumor has, by definition, gone through the wall of the bowel and commonly will have an involved margin at the level of the sphincter complex unless the rectum is excised *en bloc* with the sphincter. One of the advantages of the TNM system is the ability to extrapolate this staging system to a preoperative staging system which may be helpful in planning treatment. Assessing the factors most likely to lead to local recurrence the detectable features might theoretically include the local extent of the tumor (T stage) and the nodal status (N stage). Obviously the M stage is of great prognostic importance, though local symptoms from a rectal cancer may override the presence of metastatic disease in proceeding to major resectional surgery.

Endoanal ultrasound appears to be particularly good at estimating the T stage [28]. An ultrasound staging system has been developed which is analogous to the pathological TNM system with a prefix "u" denoting that this is an ultrasound rather than a pathological staging. Correlations with pathology indicate that accuracy of ultrasound, particularly in the T staging, though less so in the N staging are accurate [28].

Endoluminal ultrasound (EUS) is particularly helpful in selecting patients who may be suitable for local excision, generally agreed to be T1 tumors. However the main determinant of local recurrence is undoubtedly a positive CRM and EUS is poor at assessment of the CRM.

In an attempt to improve the imaging of rectal cancer, endoluminal magnetic resonance imaging (MRI) has been assessed with good results from specialist centers [33]. However the very tumors most in need of accurate staging, in particular stenotic tumors, or low painful lesions, are unable to be staged by endoluminal techniques. Fortunately developments in phased-array surface coil MRI now allow accurate local assessment of most patients with rectal cancer [34,35].

While the TNM staging is important, a key aspect of the local staging of rectal cancer is the relationship of the tumor, or its metastases, to the CRM. MRI has been particularly useful in the ability to visualize the CRM and to accurately predict either involved, threatened, or clear margins and thus direct the treatment strategy [34,35]. A patient with an obviously involved margin on MRI should be considered for preoperative neoadjuvant therapy to reduce margin involvement at subsequent surgery by "downstaging" and perhaps "downsizing" the tumor. All patients with a threatened margin (which really includes most very low tumors) should also be considered for preoperative treatment, whereas patients with clear margins can be treated by optimal surgery alone.

Increasingly neoadjuvant therapy includes a combination of chemotherapy and radiotherapy. Frykholm *et al.* [36] published a small randomized controlled trial in 2001 whereby patients with fixed rectal carcinomas were randomized to preoperative radiotherapy or chemo-radiotherapy (CRT). This trial showed a significant improvement in resectability and reduction in local failure with the use of CRT [36]. With preoperative irradiation of clinically mobile lesions, pathological complete response (PCR) rates of 10–20% have been reported, and with preoperative chemoradiation, higher PCR rates of 30–35% have been reported [37].

The delay following neoadjuvant treatment may be important. The 25 cGy in five fractions (short-course radiotherapy) is usually combined with surgery within 1 week with minimal downstaging or downsizing. A trial is ongoing in Stockholm assessing whether a delay of 6–8 weeks after short-course radiotherapy might result in similar downstaging and downsizing to conventional long-course radiotherapy which has always included an interval of 6–8 weeks between completion of radiotherapy and surgery. Personal anecdotal experience of a small number of patients who had an unplanned delay suggests that a 4–6 week interval can result in effective responses, including PCR in some cases.

There has been debate as to the optimal delay even in long-course regimens. The Lyon R90-01 trial reported that long-course radiotherapy with a delay of 6–8 weeks for surgery results in a significantly better tumor response and pathological downstaging of rectal cancer compared to an interval of 3 weeks [38]. In the same trial, there was a non-significant increase in the number of sphincter preserving operations in the long-interval group compared with the short-interval group (76 vs 68% respectively) [38].

The very low rectal cancer – APER vs ultralow AR

Cancers of the distal rectum are difficult to stage, have high local recurrence rates, and exist with particular problems in sphincter preservation. Abdominoperineal excision of the rectum (APER) was long considered the standard treatment of tumors within 6 cm from the anal verge. However, it is increasingly accepted that in some low cases "ultra" low anterior resection is possible without compromising oncological safety, as pathological assessment of rectal cancer has shown that spread is mainly circumferential and not distal. Most surgeons consider a distal margin of 1–2 cm safe, as distal intramural spread rarely exceeds 1 cm [39–41].

The optimal surgical treatment of low rectal cancer remains controversial with an absence of randomized trials comparing APER and restorative resection. It is generally accepted that patients with low tumors have a high CRM positive rate, particularly in those who have an APER [2,3,17]. This may be due to the mesorectum tapering out completely below the levator sling accounting for a higher chance of the tumor spreading to perirectal tissues. Therefore, there is a higher risk of tumor involvement of the CRM. In addition, cancers of the low rectum present with more of the adverse risk factors prognostically significant for local recurrence, including lymphatic and vascular invasion, perineural invasion, and positive nodal disease [42].

In a recent report of a consecutive series of 683 rectal cancer operations, 45% of patients had cancers in the lower rectum. Of the patients who had a curative low anterior resection (LAR) for tumors below 6 cm, the 5-year local recurrence rate was 7% and systemic recurrence rate was 27%, compared with 17 and 27% in patients who had curative APER [12]. Local recurrence after APER tends to be higher than for LAR in most series comparing rectal cancers of all stages, with a range of 10–33% from a review by Dehni *et al.* [43]. This is in contrast with a local recurrence rate of 4–8% for anterior resection in all stages of rectal cancer, using TME techniques [1,2,17].

Inferior cancer cure rates with APER may be due to less precision in the excision of the surrounding tissues and thus a definable dissection plane when compared with TME for higher tumors. It may be that adjuvant radiotherapy should be considered for all low rectal tumors. To avoid involved CRM margins in an abdominoperineal excision (APE) specimen, it has recently been recommended that abdominal dissection should stop at the pelvic floor and perineal dissection should encompass the tumor with a wide resection margin, taking a wide cuff of levators above the level of puborectalis, in a "cyclindrical fashion" [44]. Additionally, the higher rates of positive margins and local recurrence with APER may be due to the alternative lymphatic drainage of low rectal cancers through the internal iliac lymphatic vessels.

MRI can predict a clear margin and histopathological T staging

There is recent data which suggests that a CRM at risk of tumor involvement can be reliably seen at the preoperative MRI scan, which correlates with the postsurgery histological specimen of the rectal tumor [33–35]. Recent unpublished data from the prospective, multicentered MRI and Rectal Cancer European Equivalence Study (MERCURY) confirms accurate prediction of both the T staging and CRM clearance of 1 mm of the resection margin. When the CRM was predicted free of tumor and the patient had surgery alone a histologically clear CRM was achieved in 91%. Furthermore the extramural depth of penetration was accurately predicted to within 0.5 mm in 95% of 295 patients who had surgery alone. Thus it is possible to predict tumors preoperatively into T3a (extramural tumor extension less than 5 mm) and T3b (extramural tumor extension greater than 5 mm) subgroups and thus consider the use of neoadjuvant treatment. Vascular invasion and lymph nodes can also be documented, though sensitivity and specificity for involved nodes remains problematic.

Previous studies reported a varying accuracy for T staging between 67 and 83% with a considerable inter-observer variability [33].

However, it has been shown that the distance of tumor to the CRM is the most powerful predictor of local recurrence and not the T stage. In a large series of magnetic resonance (MR) evaluation of CRM, there was higher accuracy for predicting tumor-free resection margins (95%) than for the prediction of T stage [35].

Conclusions

Though radiotherapy may reduce local recurrence rates, its associated toxicity, early complications, long-term side effects, and costs suggest that it is best reserved for patients at high risk of recurrence. Nicholls and Hall [16] have identified two groups of tumors, locally not-extensive and locally extensive. The former group includes those tumors which are confined to the bowel wall or with less than 5 mm penetration into the extra-rectal tissues, where the survival is high and recurrence is low. This includes T1, T2, and less extensive T3, and Dukes' A and less extensive B tumors. Tumors that have extended more than this (T3 and T4) would be locally extensive with a high risk of local recurrence and poor survival. The same subdivision of T3 tumors into T3a (up to 5 mm tumor invasion outside the muscularis propria) and T3b (more than 5 mm) was made by Merkel *et al.* [45] who noted a locoregional recurrence rate at 5 years of 10.4% for pT3a and 26.3% for pT3b tumors, and a 5-year survival of 85.4% for pT3a and 54.1% for pT3b. The use of MRI is the most promising modality to select out cases where the surgical resection margin is threatened, with consideration of preoperative radiotherapy in this group.

In summary, the optimal treatment for rectal cancer is complete surgical excision with selective use of preoperative neoadjuvant therapy. The outcomes can be evaluated from local recurrence rates and overall survival. The management of rectal cancer increasingly encompasses a treatment strategy based on the CRM. Personal experience suggests that most patients presenting with rectal cancer have clear margins and can be adequately treated by surgery alone [22,23].

In patients with involved or threatened margins, downstaging by neoadjuvant therapy and TME surgery are the major factors in reduction of local recurrence. MRI can accurately assess both the CRM and the extent of extramural tumor extension, can predict areas of surgical difficulty, and can in some cases predict nodal involvement and extramural vascular invasion. This information, together with a permanent objective map of the height and extent of the tumor can direct optimal surgery with a resultant low local recurrence rate, a high rate of restoration of normal function, and good survival rates.

References

1 Enker WE. Total mesorectal excision – the new golden standard of surgery for rectal cancer. *Ann Med* 1997; 29: 127–33.

2 Heald RJ, Moran BJ, Ryall RD. *et al.* Rectal cancer: the Basingstoke experience of total mesorectal excision, 1978–97. *Arch Surg* 1998; 133: 894–9.

3 Kapiteijn E, Marijnen CAM, Nagtegaal ID *et al.* Pre-operative radiotherapy combined with total mesorectal excision for resectable rectal cancer. *N Engl J Med* 2001; 345: 638–46.

4 Martling AL, Holm T, Rutqvist LE *et al.* Effect of a surgical training programme on outcome of rectal cancer in the County of Stockholm. Stockholm Colorectal Cancer Study Group, Basingstoke Bowel Cancer Research Project. *Lancet* 2000; 356: 93–6.

5 Kapiteijn E, Putter H, van de Velde CJ. Impact of the introduction and training of total mesorectal excision on recurrence and survival in rectal cancer in The Netherlands. *Br J Surg* 2002; 89: 1142–9.

6 Cedermark B, Johansson H, Rutqvist LE, Wilking N. The Stockholm I trial of preoperative short term radiotherapy in operable rectal carcinoma. A prospective randomized trial. Stockholm Colorectal Cancer Study Group. *Cancer* 1995; 75: 2269–75.

7 Randomized study on preoperative radiotherapy in rectal carcinoma. Stockholm Colorectal Cancer Study Group. *Ann Surg Oncol* 1996; 3: 423–30.

8 Improved survival with preoperative radiotherapy in resectable rectal cancer. Swedish Rectal Cancer Trial. *N Engl J Med* 1997; 336: 980–7.

9 Marsh PJ, James RD, Schofield PF. Definition of local recurrence after surgery for rectal carcinoma. *Br J Surg* 1995; 82: 465–8.

10 Birbeck KF, Macklin CP, Tiffin NJ *et al.* Rates of circumferential resection margin involvement vary between surgeons and predict outcomes in rectal cancer surgery. *Ann Surg* 2002; 235: 449–57.

11 Quirke P, Durdey P, Dixon MF, Williams NS. Local recurrence of rectal adenocarcinoma due to inadequate surgical resection. Histopathological study of lateral tumour spread and surgical excision. *Lancet* 1986; 2: 996–9.

12 Croxford MA, Salerno G, Watson, M et al. Colorectal 23–28. *Br J Surg* 2004; 91: 63–5.

13 Hermanek P. Current aspects of a new staging classification of colorectal cancer and its clinical consequences. *Chirurg* 1989; 60: 1–7.

14 Hermanek P. International documentation system for colorectal cancer – reporting pathological findings. *Verh Dtsch Ges Pathol* 1991; 75: 386–8.

15 Shepherd NA, Baxter KJ, Love SB. Influence of local peritoneal involvement on pelvic recurrence and prognosis in rectal cancer. *J Clin Pathol* 1995; 48: 849–55.

16 Nicholls RJ, Hall C. Treatment of non-disseminated cancer of the lower rectum. *Br J Surg* 1996; 83: 15–18.

17 Abulafi AM, Williams NS. Local recurrence of colorectal cancer: the problems, mechanisms, management and adjuant therapy. *Br J Surg* 1994; 81: 7–1911.

18 Scholefield JH. How does surgical technique affect outcome in rectal cancer? *J Gastroenterol* 2000; 35: 126–9.

19 Wibe A, Rendedal PR, Svensson E et al. Prognostic significance of the circumferential resection margin following total mesorectal excision for rectal cancer. *Br J Surg* 2002; 89: 327–34.

20 Nagtegaal ID, Marijnen CA, Kranenbarg EK et al. Circumferential margin involvement is still an important predictor of local recurrence in rectal carcinoma: not 1 mm but 2 mm is the limit. *Am J Surg Pathol* 2002; 26: 350–7.

21 Jatzko GR, Jagoditsch M, Lisborg PH et al. Long-term results of radical surgery for rectal cancer: multivariate analysis of prognostic factors influencing survival and local recurrence. *Eur J Surg Oncol* 1999; 25: 284–91.

22 Simunovic M, Sexton R, Moran BJ, Heald RJ. Optimal pre-operative assessment and surgery for rectal cancer may greatly limit the need for radiotherapy. *Br J Surg* 2003; 90: 999–1003.

23 Cecil TD, Sexton R, Moran BJ, Heald RJ. Total mesorectal excision results in low local recurrence rates in lymph node positive disease. *Dis Colon Rectum* 2004; 47: 1145–9.

24 Heriot AG, Grundy A, Kumar D. Preoperative staging of rectal carcinoma. *Br J Surg* 1999; 86: 17–28.

25 Martling AL, Holm T, Rutqvist LE et al. Impact of a surgical training programme on rectal cancer outcome in Stockholm. *Br J Surg* 2004; 992: 225–9.

26 Pahlman L, Glimelius B. Pre- or postoperative radiotherapy in rectal cancer and rectosigmoid carcinoma. Report from a randomised multicenter trial. *Ann Surg* 1990; 211: 187–95.

27 Sauer R, Becker H, Hohenberger W et al. Preoperative vs postoperative chemoradiotherapy for rectal cancer. *N Engl J Med* 2004; 351: 1731–40.

28 Pijl MEJ, Chaoui AS, Wahl RL, van Oostayen JA. Radiology of colorectal cancer. *Eur J Cancer* 2002; 38: 887–98.

29 Camma C, Giunta M, Fiorica F et al. Preoperative radiotherapy for resectable rectal cancer: a meta-analysis. *JAMA* 2000; 284: 1008–15.

30 Ross A, Rusnak C, Weinerman B et al. Recurrence and survival after surgical management of rectal cancer. *Am J Surg* 1999; 177: 392–5.

31 Da Silva GM, Berho M, Wexner SD et al. Histologic analysis of the irradiated anal sphincter. *Dis Colon Rectum* 2003; 46: 1492–7.

32 Dukes CE. The classification of cancer of the rectum. *J Pathol Bacteriol* 1932; 35: 323–32.

33 Blomqvist L, Holm T, Rubio C, Hindmarsh T. Rectal tumours – MR imaging with endorectal and/or phased-array coils, and histopathological staging on giant sections. A comparative study. *Acta Radiol* 1997; 38: 437–44.

34 Brown G, Radcliffe AG, Newcombe RG et al. Preoperative assessment of prognostic factors in rectal cancer using high-resolution magnetic resonance imaging. *Br J Surg* 2003; 90: 355–64.

35 Beets-Tan RG. MRI in rectal cancer: the T stage and circumferential resection margin. *Colorectal Dis* 2003; 5: 392–5.

36 Frykholm GJ, Pahlman L, Glimelius B. Combined chemo- and radiotherapy vs radiotherapy alone in the treatment of primary, nonresectable adenocarcinoma of the rectum. *Int J Radiat Oncol Biol Phys* 2001; 50: 427–34.

37 Sebag-Montefiore D. Treatment of T4 tumours: the role of radiotherapy. *Colorectal Dis* 2003; 5: 432–5.

38 Gerard JP, Chapet O, Nemoz C *et al.* Improved sphincter preservation in low rectal cancer with high-dose preoperative radiotherapy: the Lyon R96-02 randomized trial. *J Clin Oncol* 2004; 22: 2404–9.

39 Williams NS, Dixon MF, Johnston D. Reappraisal of the 5 cm rule of distal excision for carcinoma of the rectum: a study of distal intramural spread and of patients' survival. *Br J Surg* 1983; 70: 150–4.

40 Madsen PM, Christiansen J. Distal intramural spread of rectal carcinomas. *Dis Colon Rectum* 1986; 29: 279–82.

41 Moore HG, Riedel E, Minsky BD *et al.* Adequacy of 1-cm distal margin after restorative rectal cancer resection with sharp mesorectal excision and preoperative combined-modality therapy. *Ann Surg Oncol* 2003; 10: 80–5.

42 Enker WE, Thaler HT, Cranor ML, Polyak T. Total mesorectal excision in the operative treatment of carcinoma of the rectum. *J Am Coll Surg* 1995; 181: 335–46.

43 Dehni N, McFadden N, McNamara DA *et al.* Oncologic results following abdominoperineal resection for adenocarcinoma of the low rectum. *Dis Colon Rectum* 2003; 46: 867–74; discussion 874.

44 Marr R, Birbeck K, Garvican J *et al.* The modern abdomino-perineal excision: the next challenge after total mesorectal excision. *Ann Surg* 2005; 242: 74–82.

45 Merkel S, Mansman U, Siassi M *et al.* The prognostic inhomogeneity in pT3 rectal carcinomas. *Int J Colorectal Dis* 2001; 16: 298–304.

5: Minimally invasive surgery – where are we?

Laparoscopic surgery for cancer of the colon and rectum

Pierre J. Guillou

> *In appropriately selected patients who are operated upon by experienced surgeons laparoscopic surgery for colorectal cancer may be the new gold standard.*
>
> Myriam J. Curet [1]

Introduction

The concept of successfully undertaking resection of cancer of the colon and rectum by laparoscopic techniques has been propounded for almost a decade and a half and yet laparoscopic or laparoscopically assisted resections have not been widely accepted by the surgical community. The reasons for the concerns surrounding minimal access laparoscopic techniques for colorectal cancer have been thoroughly rehearsed and are well recognized – concerns relating to adequacy of resection margins, local recurrence, survival, atypical patterns of recurrence such as port site and cerebral recurrences, and cost-effectiveness given the skill levels and time required to perform the operations. The feasibility of using laparoscopic techniques to resect potentially curable colorectal cancer was established within a few years after the advent of the laparoscopic revolution in the late eighties and a number of enthusiastic surgeons have carried the banner for laparoscopic colorectal surgery despite the absence of data from large randomized controlled trials (RCTs) [2–5].

In a systematic review published in 2001 [6] it was concluded that the evidence base in favor of laparoscopic-assisted resection of colorectal malignancies was inadequate to determine the procedure's safety and efficacy and that a randomized controlled clinical trial should be conducted.

The results of such RCTs are now beginning to emerge and it does seem an appropriate time to take stock of the current position. Interestingly those trials which have been presented have left us with new questions which will require answers in the next few years before laparoscopic surgery for colorectal cancer will, as suggested by Curet, truly be regarded as the new gold standard.

Currently available RCTs

The recent publication of the results of several large-scale RCTs has enabled some conclusions to be drawn and the ones which have provided the most information are as follows:

1 The Barcelona trial is a single-center trial of laparoscopic vs open surgery for surgically curable colon cancer only excluding the transverse colon. Between 1993 and 1998, 219 patients were randomized and the preliminary short-term end points in the first 51 were published in 1995 [7] and the survival data for the whole trial were published in 2002 [8].

2 The Milan trial is a single-center trial of laparoscopic vs open surgery for cancer of the colon and rectum which recruited 269 patients. The short-term outcomes and immunological end-points were reported in 2002 [9].

3 The COST (Clinical Outcomes of Surgical Therapy) study group is a multicenter randomized trial of laparoscopic-assisted vs conventional open surgery for colon cancer, again excluding the transverse colon, initiated by the American National Institute of Health in which 872 patients were randomized. The short-term quality of life outcomes for this trial were published in 2002 [10] and the survival and recurrence data in 2004 [11].

4 The COLOR (Colon Carcinoma Laparoscopic or Open Resection) is a multicenter RCT of laparoscopic vs open surgery for colon cancer conducted in Europe which accrued its target of 1200 patients in 2002 [12] and short-term outcomes published in 2005 [13].

5 The Hong Kong trial is a single center RCT of laparoscopic vs open resection of rectosigmoid cancers which randomized 403 patients whose probabilities of survival at 5 years was published in 2004 [14]. This trial continues to recruit patients with rectal cancer only.

6 The CLASICC (Conventional vs Laparoscopic-Assisted Surgery in Colorectal Cancer) trial is a UK Medical Research Council-sponsored trial of laparoscopic vs open surgery in patients with cancer of the colon and rectum, excluding the transverse colon. A unique attribute of this study was the fact that in each center the resection specimen was treated by an identical technique which permitted the pathologist not only to record the local stage of the tumor but also the adequacy of the resection performed by the

corresponding surgeon [15,16]. The pathology of each resection specimen was centrally reviewed by an expert colorectal pathologist and the stage and adequacy of resection confirmed. Recruitment commenced in 1996 and by 2002 had randomized 794 patients in a ratio of 2 : 1 laparoscopic-assisted to open surgery. The short-term end points of this trial were published in 2005 [17].

7 The Singapore trial is a trial of laparoscopic vs open surgery for colonic cancer randomized according to the CLASICC trial protocol but with the intention of including 200 patients into each arm of the trial. As yet, no clinical outcome results have been reported but the immunological end points were presented with 118 patients randomized to each arm [18].

Have the concerns been addressed?

Adequacy of excision

The first and perhaps most important of the concerns which have been raised against laparoscopic colorectal cancer surgery was whether or not those surgeons who practised the approach were performing resections which were as radical as those undertaken by conventional open approaches. Reports from single-center and multicenter large retrospective series [4,3,19] suggested that the pathological margins of the resected specimens were not less extensive than those removed by conventional open surgery but it could be argued that these reports were written by "enthusiasts" and the general applicability of this conclusion was questioned (Table 5.1). In general however the RCTs appear to have confirmed this conclusion that the numbers of lymph nodes and the longitudinal and circumferential resection margins appear to

Table 5.1 Resection margins and adequacy of excision.

	Barcelona	Milan	COST	COLOR	Hong Kong	CLASICC
Proximal margin (cm)						
Lap	—	—	13	—	—	11.0
Open	—	—	12	—	—	10.5
Distal margin (cm)						
Lap	—	—	10	—	4.5	8.0
Open	—	—	11	—	4.5	8.0
L. node yield (No)						
Lap	11.1	14.8	12	10	11.1	12
Open	11.1	14.5	12	10	12.1	13.5

be no different between the two arms. However, the CLASICC trial did highlight that in those patients undergoing sphincter-preserving surgery for rectal cancer, there was a higher (but statistically nonsignificant) incidence of positive circumferential resection margins in those undergoing laparoscopic surgery than in those who had open surgery, though paradoxically the frequency with which total mesorectal excision was performed for rectal cancer was significantly higher in the laparoscopic than in the open group (77 and 66% respectively). Whether the positive resection margins in the laparoscopic group has clinical implications in terms of local recurrence remains to be seen but the long-term recurrence rates in this trial are under analysis at the time of writing. For other colonic resections and abdominoperineal excisions of the rectum (APERs) for rectal cancer circumferential resection margin positivity rates were identical suggesting that the long-term outcomes should be no different. In summary, therefore, the pathological data thus far confirm that there is no difference in resection margins between the laparoscopic approach and the open operation, but pending the analysis of clinical results in terms of local recurrences and survival some caution is required before the laparoscopic approach can be widely adopted for sphincter-preserving resections of rectal cancers.

Atypical recurrence rates

The next most disturbing aspect of laparoscopic-assisted surgery for colorectal cancer which deterred many surgeons from adopting the approach relates to the possibility that it is associated with atypical patterns of recurrence such as cerebral metastases [20], peritoneal metastases [21], and port-site metastases [22]. The controversy over port-site metastases was hugely amplified by a letter to the *Lancet* in 1994 [23] which described three subcutaneous port-site metastases in 14 patients who underwent laparoscopic colon cancer resections. This worrisome complication has rather faded from the horizon in recent years, possibly because of repeated warnings from experienced laparoscopic colorectal surgeons about not grasping the segment of bowel bearing the tumor during any phase of the operation. In the Barcelona trial, at 5 years of follow-up, there was just one port site recurrence in the laparoscopic arm and no wound recurrences in the open arm. Peritoneal seedlings recurred in three of 106 patients in the laparoscopic arm and in five of 102 patients in the open arm. No port site or wound recurrences were observed in the Hong Kong trial and local or peritoneal recurrences were recorded in 6.6 and 4.4% of the laparoscopic and open arms respectively. In the Milan trial, at 1 year of follow-up, there were no port site recurrences and only one wound recurrence in the open group. Patterns of recurrence have not yet been reported for the COST trial but they are in the process of being analyzed for the CLASICC trial. Of data reported from randomized trials at this stage therefore there has been one port site metastasis in 409 patients randomized to laparoscopic resection and one wound recurrence in 405 patients randomized to open surgery. At this stage therefore it would appear that the issue of port site metastases has been resolved but this does not absolve laparoscopic surgeons from their responsibility to be vigilant in their surgical technique. There are precautions which should be taken such as the use of retrieval bags in order to avoid implantation of tumor cells within the extraction site. At present there are few, if any, surgeons who would accomplish totally laparoscopic left-sided resection for large tumors by transanal retrieval of the specimen.

Are the proposed advantages of laparoscopic surgery actually realized?

All the reported trials identify that the operative complication rates are statistically identical between the laparoscopic and open arms of the trials (2 vs 4% in the COST trial, 7 vs 8% in the CLASICC trial, and 7 vs 2% in the Barcelona trial) (Table 5.2). The difficulty in relating to these data revolves around the interpretation of what constitutes an intraoperative complication but on balance there appears to be no statistically significant difference between laparoscopic surgery and open surgery, despite the fact that in many of the trials there is a small (statistically nonsignificant) incidence of complications which are specific to laparoscopic surgery such as bowel perforation or vascular injury which occur during induction of the pneumoperitoneum. Modern methods of pneumoperitoneum induction such as use of the Hasson technique of introducing the first laparoscopic port, followed by insertion of the remaining ports under direct internal vision, have diminished these complications. In all the trials the 30-day mortality is very low with a trend toward a slightly lower mortality in the laparoscopic arm.

All the nominated randomized clinical trials which have reported their short-term results appear to agree that with regard to the recovery of bowel function and length of hospital stay, the laparoscopic resection group enjoy statistically significant advantages over their counterparts who undergo open surgery. The magnitude of this advantage varies between the trials where such parameters as length of hospital stay may be influenced by local

Table 5.2 Short-term end points (colon cancers only – intention to treat).

	Barcelona	Milan	COST	COLOR	Hong Kong	CLASICC
Operative complication rates (%)						
Lap	2	N/A	4	N/A	N/A	7
Open	7	N/A	2	N/A	N/A	8
30-day complication (%)						
Lap	8	20.6	19	21	22	26
Open	30.8	38.3	19	20	8	27
30-day mortality (%)						
Lap	1	1	<1	1	2.0	4
Open	3	0	1	2	2.4	5
Time to recovery of bowel function (days)						
Lap	1.5	2.1	N/A	3.6	4	5
Open	3	3.3	N/A	4.6	4.6	6
Hospital stay (days)						
Lap	5.2	10.4	5	8.2	8.2	9
Open	7.9	12.5	6	9.3	8.7	9

factors. What is impressive about the data in these trials is the remarkable consistency between them with regard to the magnitude of the differences. For example, hospital stay is always lower in the laparoscopic group by the order of only 1 to 2 days. Whilst this may have global implications for overall healthcare economics, when considering the total number of patients undergoing surgery for colorectal cancer within any healthcare system, it is difficult to imagine that this has a huge impact on the individual patient's impression of their hospital journey. Similarly the lower pain-scores and lower consumption of analgesia may impress statistically minded clinicians but the magnitude of the difference to an individual patient may not be so obvious. Nevertheless, that these differences exist cannot be denied, but increasingly the question is being raised as to whether the same effects cannot be achieved by alternative means such as the multimodal fast track procedures pioneered by Henrik Kehlet and his colleagues [24]. In a recently reported randomized double-blinded trial of laparoscopic (30 patients) and open (30 patients) colonic resection in which both groups received fast track rehabilitation (optimized pain relief, early oral feeding, and mobilization with a view to hospital discharge at 48 h), there was no difference between the laparoscopic and open groups in terms of their short-term functional recovery [25]. If this finding is verified in larger trials then at least one rationale for laparoscopic surgery (i.e. benefits for the patient) is considerably undermined and the future of laparoscopic colorectal surgery may be determined by the potential differences in major morbidity and mortality and the economic considerations. However, multimodal postoperative rehabilitation programs are quite labor-intensive and the economic question will reside between the costs of laparoscopic-assisted surgery and that of such intensive programs.

As far as the important 1- and 3-month postoperative complications are concerned the majority of the randomized trials are universal in their findings that the laparoscopic approach results in either fewer or similar postoperative complication rates for events such as wound infections, other infections, deep venous thrombosis, pulmonary embolism, and anastomotic dehiscence. In the Barcelona, the Hong Kong, and the Madrid trial, the incidence of wound infection was lower in the laparoscopic arm, whereas it was identical in the CLASICC trial and was not reported in detail in the COST trial. The analysis of the CLASICC trial data suggested that chest infections were more common after the laparoscopic operation. This is under further analysis but it may be related to the prolonged operative times which has been universally recorded for laparoscopic surgery in all the trials in which short-term results have been reported. The magnitude of the difference in complication rates is therefore small or negligible and certainly should not in itself deter those who wish to undertake laparoscopic surgery for colorectal cancer.

Last but certainly not the least, the randomized trials have reported that the operative mortality in the laparoscopic arm is not greater than that in the open surgical group. Indeed, overall the 30-day mortality may even be lower in the laparoscopic arm.

In summary there is little to choose between laparoscopic and open surgery for colorectal cancer with regard to the intraoperative and immediate postoperative complications. However the CLASICC trial has identified a difference in postoperative complication rates in the group of patients who undergo attempted laparoscopic surgery but have to be converted to open surgery, irrespective of the reason for the conversion.

Does the laparoscopic approach provide healthcare economic and quality of life benefits?

This is perhaps the single most difficult question to answer from the available data. The reasons for this are that healthcare economic assessments are notoriously difficult to conduct and subsequently to compare between different countries. In the United States, assessment is complicated by the fact that the

Table 5.3 Surgical details and estimated costs.

	Barcelona	Milan	COST	COLOR	Hong Kong	CLASICC
Operative time (min)						
Lap	118	222	150	202	189.9	180
Open	142	177	95	170	144.2	135
Length of incision (cm)						
Lap	—	—	6	—	—	10
Open	—	—	18	—	—	22
Conversion rates (%)						
Lap	16	5.1	21.0	17	23.2	25
Estimated costs						
Lap	—	$931 higher than open surgery	—	—	$2100 higher than open surgery	—
Open	—	—	—	—	—	—

analyses are based on health insurance charges rather than the actual costs (Table 5.3). A further complication has been the assessment of the costs of readmissions after the primary surgery, the costs of visits by community healthcare resources and General Practitioners. Perhaps the simplest assessments are the easiest to conduct and to accept as measures of the immediate comparative healthcare costs. Naturally these relate to the immediate costs of the operative procedure and the duration of hospital stay, but difficulties are encountered in determining the impact of complications and readmissions. Furthermore, the effects of transferring the costs of postoperative care from the hospital setting to the community currently do not benefit from models which can be employed to compare the overall cost effectiveness of laparoscopic surgery compared with open surgery and the value of any cost benefit which may accrue from this.

In the Hong Kong trial, the direct costs of the operations were determined from operative time, costs of disposable instruments, and standardized cost of hospital in-patient services. This calculation led to the conclusion that the laparoscopic procedures cost, on average, US$2100 more than the open group. Comparison of the healthcare costs of the subsequent complications and readmissions could not be quantified, but because these appeared to be equivalent across the two arms it is assumed that they were approximately equal. In the Madrid study the hospital costs of the laparoscopic operation were US$931 greater than that of the open procedure but this was offset by a saving of $840 per patient for their reduced hospital stay. The health-care cost analyses for the COLOR, COST, and CLASICC trials are being analyzed and there are no data reported for the Barcelona trial. A detailed methodology for assessing the healthcare economic analyses of laparoscopic trials has been published and the data from these trials will require analysis along these lines [26].

As far as quality of life is concerned, analyses so far have been only for the short-term data from the COST [10] and CLASICC trials [17] and in essence there is no difference between laparoscopic and open surgery in the short term.

Oncological outcomes

Three- to five-year survival data have been published for the Barcelona, COST, and Hong Kong trials. For patients undergoing curative resection of colon cancer overall survival and disease-free survival are identical between the open and laparoscopic arms of the trials. Only in the Barcelona trial [8] was there a suggestion that laparoscopic surgery was independently asso-ciated with a reduced risk of tumor relapse and this was almost entirely due to the majority of the overall benefit being in patients with stage III disease. A similar effect in these patients was not observed in the COST or Hong Kong trials. This effect has been attributed to improved preservation of immunological responses as shown by some authors [27,28] but not by others [18,29]. The CLASICC and COLOR trials have already analyzed the 3-year survival data but these are as yet unpublished, as is a meta-analysis of the 3-year follow-up of all patients with colon cancer randomized in the COST, COLOR, and CLASICC trials. The published data so far, however, would seem to indicate that laparoscopic surgery is at least as effective from the oncological standpoint as conventional surgery for colon cancer.

New issues raised by data from randomized clinical trials

The RCTs published so far have posed several new questions for which answers are needed. These are given below.

Is the laparoscopic approach suitable for treating rectal cancer?

The evidence is now becoming firm that laparoscopic-assisted resections for colon cancer are at least as effective as conventional open surgery.

The question as to whether or not the same is true for rectal cancer remains to be answered from randomized data despite enthusiastic single-series reports of its efficacy [30,31]. Moreover, there were initial claims that because it was easier to perform APER laparoscopically than anterior resection, the frequency with which sphincter-saving laparoscopic resection was performed was less than was acceptable in some of the earlier series. The only trials to systematically address rectal cancer are the CLASICC trial and the ongoing Hong Kong trial. In the CLASICC trial the APER rate was 25% in both arms and there were no differences in circumferential resection margins positivity (which was itself very low for all rectal cancers in the trial) in patients undergoing APER. For those undergoing laparoscopic anterior resection, however, 12% of resection specimens had positive resection margins compared with only 6% in the open group (not statistically significant). This was despite the fact that the laparoscopic group had a higher rate of total mesorectal excision (TME) than the open group. Time will tell whether or not this pathological finding translates into a clinical consequence in terms of local recurrence but at present until the long-term results are reported, laparoscopic assisted anterior resection should be employed with caution.

This observation that TME was performed more readily in the laparoscopic arm than in the open group may have other consequences. In 2002 the Singapore Group [32] raised the concern that bladder and sexual function might be more often impaired after laparoscopic resection of rectal cancers than it was after open resection. This was investigated using postal questionnaires delivered to patients with rectal cancer who participated in the CLASICC trial. This study did indeed identify that male sexual function tended to be worse after the laparoscopic approach [33]. This was independently related to the performance of TME. This may underline the difficulties involved in the low dissection around the autonomic nerves in the region of the anterolateral mesorectal fascia which is difficult to identify clearly and laparoscopically.

What are the effects of conversion?

Conversion rates from laparoscopic to open surgery vary between the trials and range from 17% in the COLOR trial, 21% for COST, 23.2% in Hong Kong, 25% for colon resections in CLASICC, and 34% for rectal resections. In 1995 Slim *et al.* [34] suggested that the morbidity may be higher after converted laparoscopic colorectal surgery. Therefore the outcomes for the converted patients in CLASICC were systematically examined and although not statistically significant, the mortality and postoperative complications in these patients were higher than for the successful laparoscopic group and randomized open group. This suggests either that the reasons for conversion were related to tumor and/or patient characteristics, which rendered the patient unsuitable for laparoscopic surgery, or that the laparoscopic surgery followed by open surgery compromised patient recovery (e.g. by excessively prolonging the operative time). If the former then it should be possible to identify the unsuitable patient preoperatively and further analysis of this group of patients is currently under way.

Implications for training

Both the COST and the CLASICC trials required that participating surgeons should have performed at least 20 laparoscopic-colorectal resections before they were allowed to participate [35]. In the United States only 48 institutions contributed patients with a corresponding figure of 32 surgeons in the CLA-SICC trial. The number of surgeons able to train in laparoscopic colorectal surgery is therefore limited on both sides of the Atlantic. This is not a trivial issue because it is clear in retrospect that defining the learning curve as 20 cases was a singular underestimation [36]. Analysis of conversion rates year-on-year for the CLASICC trial identified a fall in the conversion rate from 38% overall in the first year of the trial to 16% in the sixth year. The fact that complications and mortality tend to be higher after conversion under-scores the need not only for appropriate preoperative selection but also for adequate training for these technically demanding laparoscopic procedures. Initiatives such as the Laparoscopic Colorectal Fellowship Scheme in the United Kingdom are clearly very much to be welcomed.

Conclusions

The answers to questions about laparoscopic surgery for colorectal cancer posed over a decade ago [37] are now beginning to emerge. At present it seems appropriate to say that laparoscopic-assisted surgery for colonic cancer possesses some short-term advantages and produces long-term onco-logical results which are at least as good as conventional open surgery. There seems no reason therefore not to recommend its use by appropri-ately trained surgeons. As far as rectal cancer is concerned the current data requires some amplification before its routine use can be unequivocally rec-ommended. It is also worth noting that things have moved on technically since the current trials were designed and initiated, and the introduction of ultrasonic dissection and improved videolaparoscopic imaging are contributing to the ease with which laparoscopic colorectal surgery may be conducted. The experience and results generated in the current RCTs represent proof of principle and with further refinement it may not be too many years before laparoscopic surgery does become the new gold standard.

References

1 Curet MJ. Laparoscopic-assisted resection of colorectal carcinoma. *Lancet* 2005; 365: 1666–8.
2 Phillips EH, Franklin M, Carroll BJ *et al.* Laparoscopic colectomy. *Ann Surg* 1992; 216: 703–7.
3 Falk PM, Beart RW, Wexner SD, Thorson AG. Laparoscopic colectomy: a critical appraisal. *Dis Colon Rectum* 1993; 36: 28–34.
4 Monson JRT, Darzi A, Carey PD, Guillou PJ. Prospective evaluation of laparoscopic-assisted colectomy in an unselected group of patients. *Lancet* 1992; 340: 831–3.
5 Milsom JW, Bohm B, Hammerhofer KA *et al.* A randomized trial comparing laparoscopic vs conventional techniques in colorectal cancer surgery: a preliminary report. *J Am Coll Surg* 1998; 187: 46–54.
6 Chapman AE, Levitt MD, Hewett P *et al.* Laparoscopic-assisted resection of colorectal malignancies. A systematic review. *Ann Surg* 2001; 234: 590.
7 Lacy AM, Garcia-Valdecasas JC, Piqué JM *et al.* Short-term outcome analysis of a randomized study of laparoscopic vs open colectomy for colon cancer. *Surg Endosc* 1995; 9: 1101–5.
8 Lacy AM, Garcia-Valdecasas JC, Delgado S *et al.* Laparoscopic-assisted colectomy vs open colectomy for treatment of non-metastatic colon cancer: a randomised trial. *Lancet* 2002; 359: 2224–9.
9 Braga M, Vignali A, Gianotti L *et al.* Laparoscopic vs open colorectal surgery. A randomized trial on short-term outcome. *Ann Surg* 2002; 236: 759–67.
10 Weeks JC, Nelson H, Gelber S *et al.* Short-term quality of life outcomes following laparoscopic-assisted colectomy vs open colectomy for colon cancer. A randomized trial. *JAMA* 2002; 287: 321–8.
11 The COST Study Group. A comparison of laparoscopically-assisted and open colectomy for colon cancer. *N Engl J Med* 2004; 350: 2050–9.
12 COLOR, Hazebrock EJ. A randomized clinical trial comparing laparoscopic and open resection for colon cancer. *Surg Endosc* 2002; 16: 949–54.
13 COLOR Group. Laparoscopic surgery vs open surgery for colon cancer: short-term outcomes of a randomized trial. http://oncology.thelancet.com. 21st June 2005. Published online.
14 Leung KL, Kwok SPY, Lam SCW *et al.* Laparoscopic resection of rectosigmoid carcinoma: prospective randomised trial. *Lancet* 2004; 363: 1187–92.
15 Quirke P, Durdey P, Dixon MF, Williams NS. Local recurrence of rectal adenocarcinoma due to inadequate surgical resection. *Lancet* 1986; 328: 996–9.
16 Adam IJ, Mohausdee MO, Martin IG *et al.* Role of circumferential resection margin in the local recurrence of rectal cancer. *Lancet* 1994; 344: 707–11.
17 Guillou PJ, Quirke P, Thorpe H *et al.* Short-term endpoints of conventional vs laparoscopic-assisted surgery in patients with colorectal cancer (MRC CLASICC trial): multicenter randomised controlled trial. *Lancet* 2005; 365: 1718–26.
18 Tang CL, Eu KW, Tai BC *et al.* Randomized clinical trial of the effect of

open vs laparoscopically assisted colectomy on systemic immunity in patients with colorectal cancer. *Br J Surg* 2001; 88: 801–4.

19 Fleshmann JW, Nelson H, Peter WR. Early results of laparoscopic surgery for colorectal cancer: retrospective analysis of 372 patients treated by COST study group. *Dis Colon Rectum* 1996; 39: 553–8.

20 Lumley J, Stitz R, Stevenson A *et al.* Laparoscopic colorectal surgery for cancer. Intermediate to long-term outcomes. *Dis Colon Rectum* 2002; 45: 867–74.

21 Ramos JM, Gupta S, Anthone GJ *et al.* Laparoscopy and colon cancer: is the port site at risk? A preliminary report. *Arch Surg* 1994; 129: 897–900.

22 Cirrocco WC, Schwartzman A, Golub RW. Abdominal wall recurrence after laparoscopic colectomy for colon cancer. *Surgery* 1994; 116: 563–5.

23 Bereduo FJ, Kazemeier G, Bonjer HJ, Lange JF. Subcutaneous metastases after laparoscopic colectomy. *Lancet* 1994; 344: 58.

24 Kehlet H, Wilmore DW. Multimodal strategies to improve surgical outcome. *Am J Surg* 2002; 183: 630–41.

25 Basse L, Jakobsen DH, Bardram L *et al.* Functional recovery after open vs laparoscopic colonic resection. A randomized blinded study. *Ann Surg* 2005; 241: 416–23.

26 Stead ML, Brown JM, Bosanquet N *et al.* Assessing the relative costs of standard open surgery and laparoscopic surgery in colorectal cancer is a randomised controlled trial in the United Kingdom. *Crit Rev Oncol Haematol* 2000; 33: 99–104.

27 Hewitt PM, Ip Sm, Kwok SPY *et al.* Laparoscopic-assisted vs open surgery for colorectal cancer: comparative study of immune effects. *Dis Colon Rectum* 1998; 41: 901–9.

28 Ozawa A, Konishi F, Nagai H *et al.* Cytokine and hormonal responses in laparoscopic-assisted colectomy and open conventional open colectomy. *Surg Today* 2000; 30: 107–12.

29 Klava A, Windsor A, Boylston AW *et al.* Monocyte activation after open and laparoscopic surgery. *Br J Surg* 1997; 84: 1152–6.

30 Darzi A, Lewis C, Menzies-Gow N *et al.* Laparoscopic abdomino-perineal resection of the rectum. *Surg Endosc* 1995; 9: 414–17.

31 Baker RP, White EE, Titu L *et al.* Does laparoscopic abdomino-perineal resection of the rectum compromise long-term survival. *Dis Colon Rectum* 2002; 45: 1481–5.

32 Quah HM, Jayne DG, Eu KW, Seow-Choen F. Bladder and sexual dysfunction following laparoscopically assisted and conventional open mesorectal excision for cancer. *Br J Surg* 2002; 89: 1551–6.

33 Jayne DG, Brown JM, Thorpe H *et al.* Bladder and sexual function following resection for rectal cancer in a randomized trial of laparoscopic versus open technique. *Br J Surg* 2005; 92: 1124–32.

34 Slim K, Pezet D, Riff Y *et al.* High morbidity rate after converted laparoscopic colorectal surgery. *Br J Surg* 1995; 82: 1406–8.

35 Simons AJ, Anthone GJ, Ortega AE *et al.* Laparoscopic-assisted colectomy learning curve. *Dis Colon Rectum* 1995; 38: 600–3.

36 Reissman P, Cohen S, Weiss EG, Wexner SD. Laparoscopic colorectal surgery: ascending the learning curve. *World J Surg* 1996; 20: 277–82.

37 Guillou PJ. Laparoscopic surgery for disease of the colon and rectum – quo vadis? *Surg Endosc* 1994; 8: 669–71.

6: Minimally invasive surgery – where are we?

Is there a role for TEM?

Theodore J. Saclarides

Introduction

Transanal (local) excision of rectal adenomas and superficial rectal cancers is a sphincter-preserving means of addressing selected neoplasms that has less morbidity and faster recovery than transabdominal or trans-sacral approaches. Excision of adenomas is straightforward and technically easy with conventional instruments such as self-retaining or hand-held retractors. This is especially so when the lower edge of the lesion is within 5 cm of the dentate line. Exposure with these instruments can be problematic when the lesion is higher in the rectum or in obese patients and the surgeon may need to resort to a more invasive approach. Excision of recurrent adenomas may also be difficult with conventional instruments; fibrosis at the site will limit mobility of the lesion.

With respect to cancer, careful patient selection for transanal excision is essential to achieve recurrence and survival rates comparable to open resections. Transanal excision as definitive and sole treatment for cancer should be limited to lesions which, by ultrasound, are limited to the mucosa and submucosal and have moderate to well differentiation and no evidence of perineural or lymphovascular invasion. Negative lateral and deep margins are necessary in obtaining adequate locoregional control. Failure to meet these standards may predispose to higher recurrence rates because of persistent cancer within the mesorectum and the wound itself. Conventional transanal excision of rectal cancers has recently been closely scrutinized because of higher recurrence rates than might be achieved with radical surgery [1–3]. In fact, there has been skepticism that such treatment is not in the patient's best interest.

Pioneered and developed by Professor Gerhard Buess (Tubingen, Germany), transanal endoscopic microsurgery (TEM) has emerged as an accepted means of transanally removing selected neoplasms [4–7].

The highly specialized instrumentation was designed to circumvent the limitations posed by conventional transanal instruments, namely short reach and poor visibility. The experience gained in Europe, the United Kingdom, and the United States thus far has shown that TEM can be safely used and has few complications.

Transanal endoscopic microsurgery first received attention when minimally invasive surgery, specifically laparoscopy, began to stimulate interest in alternatives to open surgery. However, TEM has distinguished itself from laparoscopy in several ways. First, TEM has not changed the frequency with which local excision is performed for rectal cancer. Our institutional experience has shown that although the arrival of TEM was associated with an increase in the volume of rectal cancer referrals, the portion treated by TEM vs low anterior resection or abdominoperineal excision of the rectum (APER) has remained unchanged. Second, whereas exposure in laparoscopy can be facilitated by inserting another port to provide traction and counter-traction, this is not possible with TEM, where the instruments are inserted and manipulated only in parallel. Improved exposure can only be achieved by repositioning the scope. This adds considerably to the technical difficulty. Third, the conditions treated with TEM, namely rectal cancers and adenomas, are encountered far less often than the wide variety of disorders treated laparoscopically, where the same instruments can be used for morbid obesity surgery, colectomy, fundoplication, or splenectomy. Finally, the lack of a specific procedure code for TEM, in contrast to laparoscopy, has discouraged its wide acceptance. These factors, combined with the cost of the equipment, will render TEM the domain of but a few surgeons.

Transanal endoscopic microsurgery utilization

Currently, there are approximately 600 TEM systems in use worldwide. As expected, it is most frequently used in the United Kingdom and Europe where approximately 110 units are present in Germany and 300 are in use in England and in the remaining areas of the continent. In Japan and Southeast Asia approximately 58 units are in use. In the United States, approximately 60 systems are functional; however, usage has been slow to catch on for the reasons mentioned above.

Indications

Virtually any adenoma regardless of size, location, and degree of circumferential involvement can be removed with TEM. As long as the lesion can be reached and completely visualized with a standard rigid proctoscope, removal will likely be possible. If the lesion extends around the rectosigmoid junction and cannot be completely visualized, then perhaps TEM is not the best approach, although many lesions can be pulled downward into closer view and the procedure can still be successfully employed. Following removal of lesions which encompass 360° of the rectal circumference, intestinal continuity can be re-established with a hand-sewn end-to-end anastomosis performed through the scope.

Proper patient selection is extremely important when using TEM to remove cancers for cure. These selection criteria include superficial penetration (preoperative staging with endorectal ultrasound), well to moderately-well differentiation, lack of lymphovascular invasion, lack of perineural invasion, and perhaps no mucinous component. If these criteria are not satisfied, the risk of lymph node metastases is increased and TEM should not be considered since extramural disease cannot be addressed by any of the currently available transanal techniques [8,9]. Large size (>3–4 cm) has been considered a relative contraindication for transanal excision of rectal cancers, simply because adequate exposure has been difficult to obtain with bi-valve retractors and other conventional equipment. TEM, however, circumnavigates the size issue since visualization and exposure of the entire lesion is less of a problem and complete removal with negative margins is more likely.

There are instances where transanal excision can be considered even though cure may not be possible. Palliative excision may be performed when diffuse systemic metastases are present; however, most primary tumors in these instances are bulky or stenotic and may not be amenable to transanal excision. If the patient is medically unfit to undergo radical surgery because of co-morbid diseases, TEM may be considered. If a patient refuses radical surgery or a colostomy when indicated, then transanal excision can be considered as an alternative either before or after radiation therapy and chemotherapy [7]. A large number of patients have not been treated in this fashion, and consequently direct comparison with open procedures is not possible. Further studies are needed to determine whether the oncologic results are acceptable.

It has been our practice to proceed directly with TEM resection of uT1 tumors; however, the patient should be informed that additional treatment may be required if final pathologic assessment of the lesion reveals that it is more deeply invasive. It is important to let a month or so elapse before considering radical surgery in order to let the wound contract and heal. Otherwise, the cavity could open during laparotomy and rectal mobilization.

If the ultrasound reveals that the tumor has partially invaded the muscularis propria (uT2), *and the lesion is small,* we will still proceed with TEM and compare pathologic staging with sonographic staging. If ultrasound over-staged the lesion, TEM resection should be curative. If ultrasound showed that the tumor deeply penetrated into but not completely through the muscularis propria and, by proctoscopic examination, the tumor is large, we will proceed promptly with a radical resection of the tumor. If ultrasound reveals that the lesion is penetrating into the extrarectal fat or there are suspicious lymph nodes in the vicinity, we recommend preoperative chemoradiation over 6 weeks and then radical surgery after an additional 4–6 weeks have elapsed.

Equipment

The combined, multifunctional endosurgical unit is an essential component of the TEM setup. This unit simultaneously regulates four different functions, namely suction, irrigation, carbon dioxide (CO_2) insufflation, and monitoring of intrarectal pressure. Suction removes fluid, blood, waste, and smoke. Irrigation helps to maintain a relatively clean operative field and can rinse the end of the scope. CO_2 insufflation maintains distention of the rectum throughout the operation, since the TEM system is a closed unit. Flow can be increased to a rate of 6 L/min. Visibility is greatly enhanced by CO_2 distention, and consequently excision of the lesion and closure of the wound is greatly facilitated. Intrarectal pressure is constantly monitored and the surgeon generally tries to maintain it between 12 and 15 cm of water. When the desired pressure is set at this level, suction and rate of CO_2 insufflation are automatically adjusted to maintain that pressure. If additional suction is desired this can be manually regulated by the surgeon; however, the endo-surgical unit will compensate and increase CO_2 flow to maintain intrarectal pressure. If pressure does not rise or if the rectum does not distend, there is a leak in the system and the surgeon should systematically check his/her setup. This is probably the most frequently encountered problem that the surgeon must learn to successfully troubleshoot.

The operating rectoscopes are either beveled or straight faced and approximately 4 cm in diameter. If one is using a beveled scope, the beveled end must face down at the lesion, and consequently patients are positioned according to where the lesion is located along the anterior–posterior diameter of the rectum. For example, if a patient has an anteriorly located lesion, he or she should be placed in the prone position and the legs spread apart and secured to long arm-boards placed under the mattress. When the foot of the table is dropped, the surgeon has unhindered access to the patient's perineum and can sit immediately next to the patient. For a posteriorly located lesion, the patient is placed in the lithotomy position, and if the lesion is laterally located, the patient is placed in the appropriate lateral decubitus position with the hips flexed at 90°. A straight, non-beveled recto-scope is also available and may be preferable for distal lesions. The surgeon's end of the rectoscope is covered with a sealed locking-facepiece which has air-tight, sealed working ports through which are inserted the long-shafted instruments necessary for the dissection (Fig. 6.1). The suction catheter can be electrified; in this way a bleeding vessel can be coagulated while blood is simultaneously aspirated. Tissue graspers can also be electrified for control of a bleeding vessel. Vision is obtained either through a binocular stereo-scopic eyepiece or an accessory scope which can enable video recording

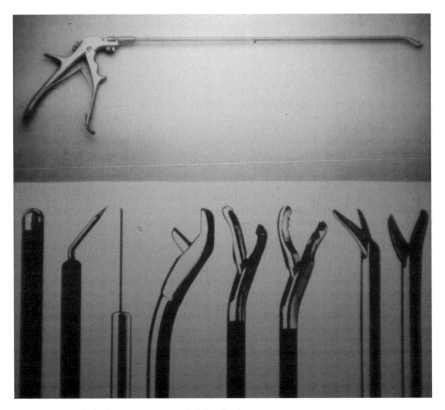

Fig. 6.1 Long-shafted instruments needed for the dissection.

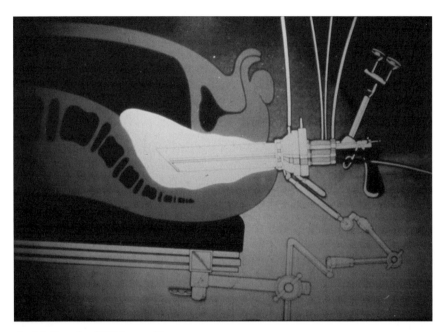

Fig. 6.2 Completed TEM assembly.

and viewing by surgical assistants, students, and residents. The binocular eyepiece provides $6\times$ magnification, has a 50° downward view and a 75° lateral field of view. In contrast, the accessory scope has a 40° downward view and a reduced lateral field of view. Because of this discrepancy, the image seen through the accessory scope and the video monitor is more narrow in its scope and it may appear as though the surgeon is going off the field. The complete assembly is shown in Fig. 6.2.

Preoperative consideration

A complete colonic evaluation with colonoscopy or air-contrast barium enema must be performed to rule out synchronous adenomas or cancer. For cancer, suitability for a transanal excision must be determined so that only those lesions with a low likelihood for nodal metastases are selected. In our practice, endorectal ultrasound is found to be excellent in providing accurate determination of depth of mucosal penetration; however, it is less so in detecting metastatic lymph nodes within the mesorectal fat. One may estimate the likelihood of nodal metastases based on the degree of mural penetration with which there is a direct correlation. For example, lesions which are confined to the mucosa and submucosa metastasize to regional nodes in less than 5% of cases. For lesions which have penetrated partially into the muscularis propria, the incidence of nodal metastases is approximately 30%, and if the lesion has penetrated into the fat, the incidence of nodal metastases is 50%. The risk of spread to lymph nodes is also influenced by degree of tumor differentiation (poor differentiation confers an increased risk) and lymphatic invasion within the tumor itself [10]. Certainly if suspicious nodes are seen by ultrasound, this overrides the risk assessment based on degree of tumor penetration. However, in the absence of identifiable nodes, tumor penetration has clear significance.

Magnetic resonance imaging (MRI) is more widely used in Europe than transanal ultrasound as a means of staging rectal cancers. In a study comparing these two imaging modalities, Bianchi *et al.* examined 49 consecutive patients with a Pentax FG36UX ultrasound scanner. The first 28 patients were then studied using a linear body coil supplied with the MRI machine, and the next 21 patients were examined with a multichannel system of four coils. Patients who received preoperative radiation and chemotherapy were excluded from the study. Radical surgery was performed a mean 7.5 days from the time of staging, operative specimens were examined, and 931 lymph nodes were retrieved. Accuracies of T-staging were 70% for ultrasound, 43% for body coil MRI, and 71% for phased-array coil MRI (PA-MRI). No significant difference was noted between the techniques. The accuracies of N-staging were 63% for ultrasound, 64% for body-coil MRI, and 76% for PA-MRI. These differences were not significantly different [11].

Kim *et al.* studied 89 patients with ultrasound (in all), pelvic computed tomography (in 69), and MRI with an endorectal coil (in 73). Results were compared with histopathologic staging. For depth of invasion, accuracies were 81% for ultrasound, 65% for computed tomography (CT), and 81% for MRI. For staging regional lymph nodes, accuracies were 64% for ultrasound, 57% for CT, and 63% for MRI. The authors concluded that ultrasound and magnetic resonance had similar accuracies and were superior to conventional computed tomograms [12].

If a candidate for transanal excision is identified and the lesion is accessible with rigid proctoscopy, no further workup is needed. A CT scan is unnecessary and is not superior to ultrasound in determining the extent of local disease. Furthermore, the risk of distant disease within the liver or lungs is sufficiently low for superficial lesions that CT scans are not required. In contrast, for locally advanced cancers, that is, those that are large, fixed, deeply penetrating, or have already spread to nodes, CT scans have a useful role; that is, if unresectable disease within the liver or lungs is identified, radical surgery for the primary tumor may not be justified.

In preparation for TEM, a bowel cleansing with lavage solutions or cathartics is needed to ensure visibility and to lower the risk of infection if penetration into the peritoneal cavity should inadvertently occur. Oral, non-absorbable antibiotics may be given and intravenous antibiotics may be added as well. Informed consent should include possible laparotomy for lesions that pose a risk of entry into the peritoneum, that is, anterior tumors in women where the location of the anterior peritoneal reflection is unpredictable and may be quite low.

We perform TEM usually under general anesthesia; however, spinal or epidural anesthesia may be considered if the patient cannot tolerate general anesthesia. Patients are released from the hospital within 3–4 h following completion of the procedure. Proper consideration to coexisting morbid conditions that place the patient at higher risk for complications should be addressed and the appropriate precautions taken. Included are an assessment of cardiac, pulmonary, and deep venous thrombosis risk.

Technique

The patient is positioned according to the location of the tumor within the rectum. The buttocks and perineum are then washed with antiseptic solution, sterile drapes are placed, and the rectoscope is inserted up to the lesion under direct vision with manual insufflation of air. The scope is then secured to the operating room table and the facepiece is locked onto the end of the scope. Rubber sleeves and caps are placed onto the working ports on the facepiece. The long-shafted instruments are inserted and the tubing necessary for CO_2 insufflation, saline irrigation, and pressure monitoring are connected. The binocular eyepiece and the accessory scope are inserted.

Dissection begins provided the bowel cleansing has been adequate, the entire lesion is visible and accessible, and intraluminal pressure can be maintained without signs of an air leak. If the entire lesion is not initially visible, one can still proceed with TEM provided it can be pulled down into view. The technique of excision will vary according to preoperative histology, suspicion that a "benign" lesion may harbor an occult cancer, and the location of the lesion within the rectum. Small adenomas may be removed by dissecting within the submucosal plane. This is especially appropriate for an anterior lesion in a woman where the anterior peritoneal reflection is unpredictable in its location and a full thickness excision may be hazardous. A 5 mm margin of normal appearing mucosa is marked around the lesion, the mucosal edge lifted up with the tissue grasper, and the lesion excised without entering the muscularis propria. Larger adenomas may contain cancer; therefore such lesions are excised with a full-thickness technique facilitating assessment of depth of penetration if cancer is present. If the peritoneum is violated, it should be promptly repaired. This does not mandate immediate conversion to laparotomy; in fact, in the instances of peritoneal entry in our experience, the peritoneum was transanally repaired as a separate layer and TEM completed as planned. In one of the patients, intra-abdominal escape of CO_2 caused a significant pneumoperitoneum which required needle decompression prior to extubation. Cancers are removed with a full thickness excision after a 1 cm margin of normal appearing mucosa has been marked around the lesion. The extrarectal fat is easy to identify and serves as a landmark to signify transmural penetration. Wounds are closed transversely with a running suture of long-lasting absorbable monofilament material with a tapered gastrointestinal needle (Fig. 6.3). After the lesion is excised, it should be fixed onto a cork board or Telfa paper to facilitate histologic examination of the deep and lateral margins.

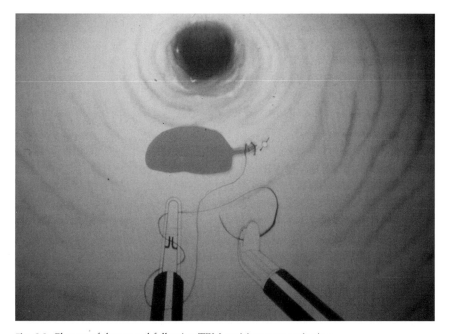

Fig. 6.3 Closure of the wound following TEM excision: surgeon's view.

The following are technical pearls:

1 Short sutures are preferable. If the suture is too long, it is cumbersome and it may be impossible to pull the stitch taut within the confines of the scope. If the wound is large, closure requires several sutures.

2 Cross over of instruments should be avoided; the surgeon should manipulate them in parallel.

3 The needle should be passed from instrument to instrument. If the needle is dropped, it may retract out of the operative field and time may be wasted in frustrating attempts at needle retrieval.

4 Lesions located in the distal 5 cm of the rectum may be better addressed with conventional instruments. If the lower lip of the beveled scope falls out of the anus, CO_2 will be lost and the operative field will collapse. Furthermore, one may encounter more bleeding just above the anus because of the hemorrhoidal veins. Alternatively, one can use the straight-ended scope that is not beveled at the end.

5 The most important aspect of the operation is patient positioning. The tumor should be located in the anterior–posterior plane during the office exam. The patient is then positioned accordingly so that the beveled end of the scope faces down at the lesion.

6 If there is an air leak, the operative field collapses and visibility is hampered. All tubing connections must be re-secured and the rubber tube and caps which seal the ports must be checked for cracks or tears which may occur secondary to normal wear and tear. The locking mechanisms which secure the scopes (accessory and main) and facepiece must be re-tightened. An adequate supply of CO_2 with unrestricted flow should be verified if the rectum remains collapsed.

7 The operating rectoscope must be repositioned several times during the course of the dissection in order to keep the lesion in the center of the operative field.

Results

Following TEM, digital rectal examination and rigid proctosigmoidoscopy are performed at 3, 6, and 9 months. A follow-up colonoscopy should be performed at 1 year. For cancers, rectal ultrasound may be combined with proctosigmoidoscopy; however, caution should be exercised in interpreting the results. Tissue plans will be altered as a result of the excision. Consequently, no definitive decision should be made based upon the first examination. With serial ultrasound examinations, however, one can find enlarging hypoechoic nodules either within the rectal wall or the rectal mesentery suggesting tumor recurrence. Such lesions can be biopsied using ultrasound-guided needle techniques.

Complications are relatively infrequent and include entry into the peritoneal cavity, conversion to laparotomy, bleeding, fecal soilage, fever, wound dehiscence, urinary dysfunction, and fistulas. In the author's experience, soilage has occurred in only 2% of patients and has usually been of short duration.

Gerhard Buess has published extensively on his experience [4–6]. Of his first 186 TEMs, 137 were performed for adenomas and 49 for cancers. With respect to location in the rectum, 25, 47, and 18% of adenomas were located in the distal, mid, and upper rectum, respectively. Five percent recurred and were treated with endoscopic snare or cautery in the majority. Of the cancers, 18, 45, and 31% were located in the distal, mid, and upper rectum respectively. Most of the cancers (81%) were staged as pT1; recurrence was 4%.

Some of the complications noted after TEM excision of both adenomas and cancers ($n = 186$) are listed below [6]:

1 Bleeding (4)
2 Rectovaginal fistula (2)
3 Rectal stenosis (7)
4 Peritoneal entry (1)
5 Bladder dysfunction (5)
6 Incontinence (1)

At the 1995 annual meeting of the American Society of Colon and Rectal Surgeons, the centers in the United States presented their pooled initial data [7]. Of 153 TEM procedures, eight were converted to laparotomy because the lesion was not accessible in its entirety and in one case an inadvertent entry into the peritoneum necessitated a laparotomy. Approximately half of the lesions were considered beyond reach of conventional instruments. Of the 82 adenomas, mean size was 4 cm. Recurrence rate following TEM was 11%, most were treated with cautery or snare excision, and repeat TEM was rarely required. Of the 54 cancers, mean size was 3 cm; there were 30 T1, 15 T2, and 6 T3 lesions. Recurrence rate following TEM increased in relation to tumor depth: 10% for T1, 40% for T2, and 66% for T3 cancers. Overall complications were experienced infrequently; only three patients reported mild incontinence which was temporary in two.

TEM has been utilized at Rush University Medical Center since 1991. From 1991 to June 2005, 260 cases have been performed; average patient age was 65.7 years and the average distance from the dentate line was 7.4 cm. The mean estimated blood loss was approximately 24 cc and in only 12% of cases did the estimated blood loss exceed 50 cc. The mean operative time was 75 min; 17% of cases lasted less than 30 min and only 9% of cases lasted longer than 2 h. During this time period, 112 adenomas and 135 cancers were removed; the remainder consisted of gastrointestinal stroma tumors and carcinoids. For the adenomas, 65% were above 6 cm from the anus (21% above 10 cm), 57% were 2–4 cm in size (22% were >4 cm), and 93% took less than 2 h to perform (39% took <1 h). For the cancers, 62% were above 6 cm from the anus (23% above 10 cm), 52% were 2–4 cm in size (24% were >4 cm), and 86% took less than 2 h (38% took <1 h). Of the cancers, 26% were carcinoma *in-situ*, 47% were pT1, 23% pT2, and 4% were pT3.

The number of new rectal cancers treated by all means at Rush over the last 10 years has remained fairly stable at 30–45 cases per year and the use of TEM for cancer has remained constant as well. This reflects our policy of strict patient selection when using TEM for cure. We have used TEM to treat 53 patients with pathologic T1 cancers. Forty-six percent were located 5–10 cm from the anus, and 25% were greater than 10 cm. Forty-four percent of the cancers were between 2 and 4 cm in maximum diameter. Thirteen percent were larger than 4 cm. With a mean follow-up of 2.84 years, the recurrence rate has been 7.5%, occurring at 9 months, 15 months, 16 months, and 11 years. Of the recurrences, three were salvaged with radical surgery, and one was treated with simple fulguration because of advanced age. During this period of follow-up, there have been no cancer-related deaths and we attribute this in part to our close follow-up program as outlined above.

Registry and prospective series have shown similar morbidity rates compared with traditional local excision, comparable short lengths of stay, and low local recurrence rates [7,13,14]. Sengupta *et al.* [15] performed a meta-analysis that demonstrated recurrence rates from 4.2 to 25% for lesions excised by TEM. For pT1 lesions, recurrence rates have been reported from 0 to 12.5% (Table 6.1).

Comparison of TEM with radical surgery

A retrospective comparison of TEM and radical surgery was performed by Lee *et al.* [14]. In this study, neither group received adjuvant chemoradiation and there were no significant differences in age, gender, tumor location,

Table 6.1 Oncologic results for pT1 lesions excised with TEM.

References	N	Local recurrence %	5-year disease-free %	5-year survival %
Lee, W [14]	52	4.1	95.9	100
Buess, G [4]	12	0		
Langer, C [16]	16	12.5		
Winde, G [17]	24	4.2		96.0
Demartines, N [18]	9	8.3		
Buess, G [6]	25	4.0		
Smith, L [7]	30	10		
Saclarides, TJ [13]	53	7.5	100	

or follow-up period between the two groups. Fifty-two patients had pT1 cancers removed by TEM, local recurrence was 4.1%, and 5-year disease-free survival was 95.9%. Neither was statistically different than the results noted in the group undergoing radical surgery. Twenty-two patients had pT2 cancers removed by TEM, local recurrence was 19.5%, and 5-year disease-free survival was 80.5%. This local recurrence rate was higher than that noted in the radical surgery group (9.4%, $p = 0.04$); however, 5-year disease-free survival was not statistically different.

Winde *et al.* [17] prospectively randomized 52 patients with ultrasound stage uT1N0 rectal cancers into TEM or anterior resection groups. Patient and tumor demographics were similar. Local recurrence rates (4.2%) and 5-year survival rates (96%) did not differ significantly. Early postoperative mortality was zero. Significant differences were noted comparing time of hospitalization (10 days longer for anterior resection, $p < 0.0001$), blood loss ($p < 0.001$), operative time (45 min longer for anterior resection, $p = 0.0021$), and need for narcotic analgesia (3 times higher after anterior resection, $p < 0.0001$). Various early complications were noted in 21% of the TEM group and in 35% of the anterior resection group [17].

Conclusions

TEM is safe and there are few complications. Most patients can be treated on an outpatient basis. Virtually any adenoma can be removed with this technique, even large circumferential lesions that necessitate sleeve resections. Regarding cancers, strict selection criteria must be used to avoid compromising recurrence rates and survival. Transrectal ultrasound may help identify those lesions which are appropriate for TEM. If TEM is selected, close follow-up is necessary to detect cancer recurrences; if they occur, radical surgery is indicated. TEM is not superior to conventional instrumentation for removing lesions in the distal rectum; however, it has distinct advantages for excising lesions in the mid and upper rectum.

Because of the high cost of the equipment, the relative infrequency with which it is used, and the difficulty in mastering the technique, TEM will probably become the domain of only a few surgeons. Over the last several years at our institution, we have performed 25–30 cases each year (benign and malignant), and since its arrival in 1991, referrals for rectal cancer have increased steadily. However, in comparison to the portion of cancers treated with low anterior resection or APER, the relative percentage of cancers treated with TEM has remained stable. This reflects our policy of adhering to strict selection criteria. Having the technology at hand is not a license to use it inappropriately.

Local (transanal) excision of rectal tumors has been part of the surgeon's armamentarium for over 100 years. All agree that benign disease can be safely addressed with this approach. However, debate has recently surfaced that cancers are best approached by more radical means. It is unlikely that randomized studies will ever be done comparing TEM with conventional transanal surgery. Comparison with radical surgery has been done in both a retrospective and prospective fashion, and the results suggest that TEM is a safe and effective means of treating pT1 cancers. Winde *et al.* [17] prospectively found operating time, blood loss, length of hospital stay, and analgesia requirements following TEM to be significantly less than for anterior resection. Local recurrence rates for pT1 tumors following APER are low (0 to 10%) with a 0% local recurrence rate reported in some series [19,20]. Overall 5-year survival rates for pT1 rectal cancers radically excised range from 78 to 100%. Local recurrence rates following conventional transanal excision without chemoradiation range from 0 to 33% for pT1 disease [15,21]. In our hands, local recurrence rate of pT1 lesions excised by TEM is 7.5%, and thus far we have not had any cancer-related deaths. In retrospect, the initial size and distance of pT1 lesions that did recur did not preclude safe removal by TEM, and it is unlikely that technical aspects played a role in these recurrences apart from one instance with a positive margin (patient refused further treatment).

In summary, therefore, TEM has emerged as another means of transanal excision of adenomas and selected cancers. These selection criteria have been embraced for decades, and if one assumes that they are appropriate for distal lesions, then logic demands that these same criteria are appropriate for cancers in the mid and upper rectum as well. TEM, or any form of local excision, is not recommended as the sole form of therapy for pT2 cancers unless one is participating in a clinical trial investigating the role of chemotherapy and radiation either before or after excision. For pT1 cancers, a close surveillance program is essential in order to detect many of those which can be salvaged with radical surgery.

References

1 Chorost MI, Petrelli NJ, McKenna M et al. Local excision of rectal cancer. Am Surgeon 2001; 67: 774–9.

2 Mellgren A, Sirivongs P, Rothenberger DA et al. Is local excision adequate therapy for early rectal cancer? Dis Colon Rectum 2000; 43: 1064–74.

3 Graham RA, Garnsey L, Jessup JM. Local excision of rectal carcinoma. Am J Surg 1990; 160: 306–12.

4 Buess G, Kipfmuller K, Ibald R et al. Clinical results of transanal endoscopic microsurgery. Surg Endosc 1988; 2: 245–50.

5 Mentges B, Buess G. Transanal endoscopic microsurgery in the treatment of rectal tumors. Perspect Colon Rectal Surg 1991; 4: 265–79.

6 Buess G, Mentges B, Manncke K et al. Technique and results of transanal endoscopic microsurgery in early rectal cancer. Am J Surg 1992; 163: 63–70.

7 Smith LE, Ko ST, Saclarides T et al. Transanal endoscopic microsurgery: initial registry results. Dis Colon Rectum 1996; 39: 579–84.

8 Taylor RH, Hay JH, Larsson SN. Transanal local excision of selected low rectal cancers. Am J Surg 1998; 175: 360–3.

9 Bleday R, Breen E, Jessup M et al. Prospective evaluation of local excision for small rectal cancers. Dis Colon Rectum 1997; 40: 338–92.

10 Saclarides TJ, Bhattacharyya AK, Britton-Kuzel C et al. Predicting lymph node metastases in rectal cancer. Dis Colon Rectum 1994; 37: 52–7.

11 Bianchi PP, Ceriani C, Rottoli M et al. Endoscopic ultrasonography and magnetic resonance in preoperative staging of rectal cancer: comparison with histologic findings. J Gastrointest Surg 2005; 9: 1222–8.

12 Kim NK, Kim MJ, Yun SH et al. Comparative study of transrectal ultrasonography, pelvic computerized tomography, and magnetic resonance imaging in preoperative staging of rectal cancer. Dis Colon Rectum 1999; 42: 770–5.

13 Saclarides, TJ. Transanal endoscopic microsurgery: a single surgeon's experience. Arch Surg 1998; 133: 595–9.

14 Lee W, Lee D, Choi S et al. Transanal endoscopic microsurgery and radical surgery for T1 and T2 rectal cancer. Surg Endosc 2003; 17: 1283–7.

15 Sengupta S, Tjandra JJ. Local excision of rectal cancer: what is the evidence? Dis Colon Rectum 2001; 44: 1345–61.

16 Langer C, Markus P, Liersch T et al. Ultracision or high frequency knife in transanal endoscopic microsurgery (TEM)? Advantages of a new procedure. Surg Endosc 2001; 15: 513–17.

17 Winde G, Nottberg H, Keller R et al. Surgical cure for early rectal carcinomas (T1): transanal endoscopic microsurgery vs anterior resection. Dis Colon Rectum 1996; 39: 969–76.

18 Demartines N, vonFlue MO, Harder FH. Transanal endoscopic microsurgical excision of rectal tumors: indications and results. World J Surg 2001; 25: 870–5.

19 Willet CG, Lewandrowski K, Donnelly S et al. Are there patients with stage I rectal

carcinoma at risk for failure after
abdominoperineal resection? *Cancer*
1992; 69: 1651–5.

20 Sticca RP, Rodriguez-Bigas M,
Penetrante RB *et al.* Curative resection
for stage I rectal cancer: natural history,
prognostic factors, and recurrence
patterns. *Cancer Invest* 1996; 14: 491–7.

21 Wagman RT, Minsky BD. Conservative
management of rectal cancer with local
excision and adjuvant therapy. *Oncology*
2001; 15: 513–19.

7: What is the best strategy for the management of hereditary colorectal cancer?

Seung-Yong Jeong, David Chessin, Susan Ritchie, John H. Scholefield, and José G. Guillem

Introduction

Five to ten percent of all cases of colorectal cancer (CRC) are believed to have a hereditary component [1]. Because hereditary CRCs are due to germline mutations, these patients have clinical features distinct from sporadic CRC. Generally, these features include (1) early age-of-onset of cancer, (2) frequent association with synchronous or metachronous tumors, and (3) characteristic extraintestinal manifestations. Due to these differences, the management strategy for patients with hereditary CRC is quite different from that for sporadic CRC. Additionally, there are important screening and surveillance implications for family members. Our aim is to review the most common hereditary CRC syndromes, namely familial adenomatous polyposis (FAP) syndrome, hereditary nonpolyposis colorectal cancer (HNPCC) syndrome, Peutz-Jeghers syndrome (PJS), juvenile polyposis syndrome (JPS), and MYH polyposis syndrome, with an emphasis on management strategies (Table 7.1).

Familial adenomatous polyposis

Familial adenomatous polyposis is an autosomal dominant hereditary CRC syndrome caused by a germline mutation of the *APC* gene [1]. FAP occurs in one of 10,000 live births and accounts for 1% of all CRC [2,3]. The majority of patients have a family history of FAP, but 20–30% of cases arise from a de novo *APC* mutation [4].

Clinical features

The FAP is characterized by at least 100 adenomatous polyps in the colon and rectum, but an attenuated form with fewer polyps has been

Table 7.1 Hereditary CRC syndromes.

	Inheritance	Causative gene	Frequency (% of total CRC)	Polyp Location	Prevalence	Number	CRC Risk	Mean age
FAP	AD	APC	1	Colorectum	100%	>1000	100%	39
HNPCC	AD	hMLH1, hMSH2, hPMS1, hPMS2, hMSH6	2–6	Colorectum	20–40%	1–10	80%	45
PJS	AD	STK11	0.1	Small intestine	>90%	10–100	20%	46
JPS	AD	SMAD4, BMPR1A	0.1	Colorectum	>90%	3–200	10–38%	34
MYH polyposis	AR	MYH	1–3 (?)	Colorectum	?	3–100	?	50

FAP, familial adenomatous polyposis; HNPCC, hereditary non-polyposis colorectal cancer; PJS, Peutz–Jeghers syndrome; JPS, juvenile polyposis syndrome; AD, autosomal dominant; AR, autosomal recessive; CRC, colorectal cancer; ? denotes that the values are still not clearly defined.

described [5,6]. Attenuated FAP (AFAP) is a variant characterized by fewer colorectal polyps (<5–100), later age of onset of polyps and cancer, infrequent rectal involvement, and a more proximal colonic distribution than classic FAP [5,6].

Colorectal cancer develops in nearly all FAP individuals with their colon and rectum in situ by age 40–50 [1]. In addition to colorectal polyps and CRC, patients with FAP also develop characteristic extracolonic manifestations. These include benign lesions of the stomach (adenoma and fundic gland retention polyps), small bowel (adenoma), skin (lipoma, fibroma, sebaceous, and epidermoid cysts), bone (osteoma), retina (congenital hypertrophy of the retinal pigment epithelium), teeth (supernumerary teeth), and soft tissue (desmoid) [7]. Extracolonic malignancies also develop at increased incidence in patients with FAP. These include cancers of the liver (hepatoblastoma), stomach, duodenum, pancreas, thyroid, biliary tract, and brain [8–11]. As increasing numbers of patients with FAP have been treated with prophylactic proctocolectomy, mortality from CRC has decreased. However, patients with FAP continue to have a reduced life expectancy after colectomy, largely due to mortality from desmoid tumors or upper gastrointestinal (GI) cancers [12].

Genetics and genetic testing

The FAP is caused by germline mutation of the *APC* gene on chromosome 5q21 [1]. *APC* is a tumor suppressor gene that inhibits the Wnt signaling pathway [13]. The key component in this pathway is β-catenin, which activates the transcription of growth-regulatory genes. The *APC* gene product targets β-catenin for degradation. However, when *APC* is mutated excess β-catenin is translocated to the nucleus, with resultant decreased regulation of cell growth [13].

Currently, several tests are available to test for an *APC* germline mutation, including sequencing of the entire gene, a combination of conformation strand gel electrophoresis (CSGE) and protein truncation test (PTT), PTT alone, and linkage analysis. Sequencing of the entire gene is the most sensitive test (95% mutation detection rate), but it is the most expensive. The mutation detection rate of the combination of CSGE and PTT, and PTT alone is 80–90%, and 70–80%, respectively. Linkage analysis can be performed when more than one affected family member is available and has a 95–99% accuracy [14]. As with all genetic testing, pre- and post-test counseling is strongly recommended [6].

Attenuated FAP is also due to a germline mutation in the *APC* gene that is inherited in an autosomal dominant fashion. However, it has been suggested that the mutated locus in AFAP is further toward the 5′ and 3′ ends of the *APC* gene than that reported for classic FAP [6].

Screening and surveillance

At-risk individuals should begin screening for FAP at age 10–12 [14]. The screening tests available for FAP include genetic testing for a mutation of the *APC* gene and endoscopy. Flexible sigmoidoscopy has been regarded as the procedure of choice for FAP screening [14]. However, it may be replaced by a genetic test when an *APC* mutation has been documented in an individual's family. In addition, colonoscopy may be used when screening is performed at an older age or when there is suspicion for AFAP [14].

If an individual has multiple polyps or a positive genetic test, referral of all first-degree relatives for genetic counseling is recommended. Patients with FAP should be followed by annual colonoscopic examinations until the time of colectomy. In addition, upper GI endoscopy should be performed beginning at age 21 and repeated at 6-month intervals or longer depending on the polyp burden [15]. Screening guidelines for the other extracolonic cancers associated with FAP are less well defined.

Management

Because 5% of untreated patients with FAP develop colorectal cancer by the age of 20 years [16], prophylactic surgery is advised shortly after FAP is diagnosed. However, the timing and type of prophylactic surgery in patients younger than age 20 are often influenced by educational, developmental, and self-image concerns. When polyps are small (<6 mm) and there is no evidence of dysplasia, cancer, or symptoms, prophylactic surgery may be delayed until after high school [16].

The optimal surgical management of FAP should include (1) removal of all at-risk colorectal mucosa, and (2) maintenance of anorectal function. Current surgical options for FAP include total proctocolectomy (TPC) with an ileal pouch-anal anastomosis (IPAA), total colectomy and ileorectal anastomosis (IRA), and TPC with ileostomy.

Total proctocolectomy with IPAA is the operation of choice for most patients with FAP, as it nearly eliminates the risk of CRC and maintains per-anal fecal evacuation. However, in a selected subset of individuals, a total colectomy with IRA and close endoscopic surveillance is an option, as IRA is associated with better functional results and lower perioperative morbidity [16]. Patients unable or unwilling to have aggressive postoperative surveillance are not suitable for IRA. TPC with permanent ileostomy results in a permanent stoma. However, it may be necessary when patients present with a distal rectal cancer, where a sphincter-preserving procedure may compromise oncologic results.

Patients with AFAP are also at increased risk for the development of CRC. However, given their lower polyp burden and potential for rectal sparing, management may be tailored to the individual. In very selected patients with very few adenomas, colonoscopic polypectomy and subsequent close endoscopic surveillance may be acceptable in patients not willing to undergo a prophylactic colectomy. When resection is required, a total colectomy with IRA may be appropriate in patients with AFAP who have rectal sparing [6].

Hereditary non-polyposis colorectal cancer

Hereditary non-polyposis colorectal cancer is an autosomal dominant hereditary CRC syndrome with an 80% penetrance, caused by mutations in one of several DNA mismatch-repair (MMR) genes [1]. It is the most common hereditary CRC syndrome and accounts for 2–6% of all CRC.

Clinical features

Hereditary non-polyposis colorectal cancer is characterized by early age-of-onset cancers in multiple family members. CRC is the most common tumor in HNPCC patients, but extracolonic cancers of the endometrium, small bowel, urinary tract, stomach, biliary tract, ovary, pancreas, and brain also can occur. CRC in HNPCC differs from sporadic CRC in that there is an increased incidence of synchronous and/or metachronous tumors and a predilection for the proximal colon [1]. CRC in HNPCC more frequently has mucinous or poorly differentiated histology and peritumoral lymphocytic infiltration [17]. In addition, patients with HNPCC have improved survival when compared to patients with sporadic CRC of similar stage [18]. Adenomas in HNPCC differ from sporadic adenomas in that there is an increased incidence of villous architecture, high-grade dysplasia, and morphologically flat lesions [19,20]. In addition, malignant transformation in adenomas in patients with HNPCC may be more rapid than sporadic adenomas [21]. In 1990, the International Collaborative Group on HNPCC

Table 7.2 Revised Amsterdam criteria for diagnosis of HNPCC.

There are at least three relatives diagnosed with an HNPCC-associated cancer (colorectal, endometrial, small bowel, ureter, or renal pelvis but not including stomach, ovary, brain, bladder, or skin)
One affected person is a first-degree relative of the other two
At least two successive generations are affected
At least one person was diagnosed before the age of 50 years
Familial adenomatous polyposis has been excluded
Tumors have been verified by pathologic examination

Source: Vasen HF, Watson P, Mecklin JP, Lynch HT. *Gastroenterology* 1999; 116: 1453–6.

developed the Amsterdam criteria (revised in 1999), which defines HNPCC by clinical findings and family history (Table 7.2) [22].

Genetics and genetic testing

Hereditary non-polyposis colorectal cancer is caused by a germline mutation in DNA MMR genes, which play a critical role in repairing mismatched nucleotides pairs during DNA replication [1]. The majority (more than 95%) of germline mutations have been found in the hMLH1 and hMSH2 genes, whereas mutations in hMSH6, hPMS1, and hPMS2 have been reported, but are rare [23,24].

Tumors due to MMR gene mutations exhibit a unique molecular phenotype termed microsatellite instability (MSI), which is characterized by accumulation of single nucleotide mutations and alterations in the length of simple repetitive sequences found throughout the genome. Over 90% of tumors in HNPCC exhibit MSI [25].

Initial screening for HNPCC may be performed with MSI testing or immunohistochemistry (IHC) for MMR proteins. MSI is identified using DNA extracted from tumor tissue. In 1997, the National Cancer Institute Workshop on HNPCC recommended a panel of five microsatellite markers for determination of MSI [26]. The tumor is defined as MSI-high when two or more markers display instability.

Selection of patients for testing for HNPCC is a major clinical issue. To date, the most well-accepted guidelines for MSI testing are the Bethesda Guidelines, which were developed in 1996 and revised in 2002 (Table 7.3) [27]. IHC for MMR proteins may also be used to screen for HNPCC. It has lower sensitivity than MSI testing, especially for inherited hMLH1 mutations [28]. However, it has distinct advantages over MSI testing in

Table 7.3 Revised Bethesda guidelines for testing of colorectal tumors for MSI.

Colorectal tumors should be tested for MSI in the following situations:
1 CRC diagnosed in a patient less than 50 years of age
2 Presence of synchronous, metachronous, or other HNPCC-associated tumors,* regardless of age
3 CRC with MSI-H histology in a patient less than 60 years of age
4 CRC diagnosed in one or more first-degree relatives with an HNPCC-related tumor, with one of the cancers diagnosed before 50 years of age
5 CRC diagnosed in two or more first- or second-degree relatives with HNPCC-related tumors,† regardless of age

* Includes tumors of the colorectum, endometrium, stomach, ovary, pancreas, ureter, renal pelvis, biliary tract, brain, sebaceous glands, and small bowel.
† Includes presence of tumor infiltrating lymphocytes, Crohns-like lymphocytic reaction, mucinous histology, signet ring cell differentiation, or medullary growth pattern.
Source: Umar A, Boland CR, Terdiman JP. *J Natl Cancer Inst* 2004; 96: 261–8.

terms of simplicity and availability. If it is used to complement MSI testing, IHC may reduce the cases to be tested by MSI and simplify the subsequent steps for mutation analysis. This approach may further decrease the cost for analysis and turnaround time. An algorithm for diagnosing HNPCC is provided in Fig. 7.1.

Management

HNPCC with verified germline mutation

Total colectomy with IRA may be offered to patients with a verified germline mutation in a MMR gene, due to the high risk of metachronous CRC [29]. Following total colectomy, close surveillance of the rectal remnant is required [30]. TPC with IPAA may be an option for patients who present with rectal cancer and sparing of the sphincter complex. In the highly unusual case of sphincter involvement with rectal cancer and synchronous colon polyps, a TPC and end ileostomy may be indicated.

Management of a known MMR gene mutation carrier with adenomas but no CRC is controversial. Prophylactic colectomy should be considered in an individual with multiple, high-grade adenomas or when colonoscopic follow-up is not possible. In mutation carriers without any clinical features of HNPCC, there is an 80% lifetime risk of CRC, as well as other extracolonic tumors. Cancer surveillance, including colonoscopy and extracolonic screening, should be conducted in these patients. Currently,

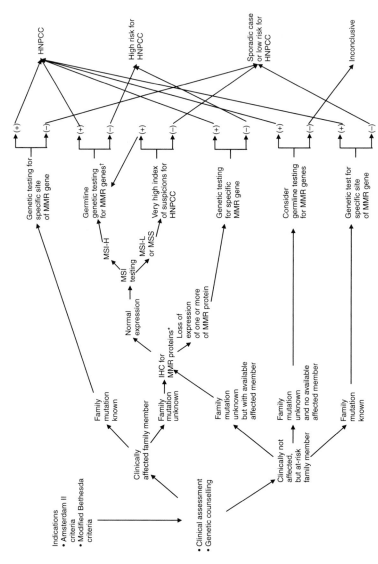

Fig. 7.1 Algorithm for identification of hereditary non-polyposis CRC.

* Initially for MLH1 and MSH2 protein. If these are negative, then MSH6 and PMS2 can be pursued.
† Initially for hMLH1 and hMSH2 genes. If these are negative, then hPMS1, hPMS2, and hMSH6 can be pursued. When clinically indicated, additional mutational analysis, including searching for a large deletion or changing the method of mutation detection, can be added.

some suggest prophylactic colectomy in patients with a MMR gene mutation, but no clinical features of HNPCC [30,31]. However this is controversial as the lifetime risk for developing CRC is 80% and not 100%.

Currently, there is insufficient evidence to definitively recommend prophylactic hysterectomy and oophorectomy in female patients with HNPCC. However, when women with HNPCC have surgery for CRC they may be offered these procedures, particularly if they are postmenopausal [30].

High risk for HNPCC

Patients at high risk for HNPCC include individuals with clinical suspicion of HNPCC who have (1) CRC with positive IHC or MSI testing but no verified germline mutation, and (2) CRC but negative IHC, MSI, and germline testing. Individuals with CRC and clinical suspicion for HNPCC should be managed as those with HNPCC, even when genetic testing is negative.

Non-informative genetic testings

Individuals in a HNPCC-kindred group who have negative genetic testing may be managed as the average risk population. Individuals in a HNPCC-kindred group with non-informative (no mutation identified) genetic testing should be managed according to the guidelines for HNPCC [32]. However, in these cases, the clinician should be aware of the potential for laboratory errors.

Surveillance

Germline mutation carriers and patients with the clinical diagnosis of HNPCC should undergo colonoscopic screening at intervals of 1–2 years beginning at age 20–25 years, or 10 years earlier than the youngest CRC diagnosis in the family [1,33]. Since HNPCC patients are also at risk for extracolonic tumors, screening may include abdominal sonography and urine cytology every 1–2 years. Female gene carriers should undergo screening for endometrial and ovarian cancer, which may include annual gynecological exams, transvaginal sonography, endometrial aspiration, and serum CA-125 levels beginning at age 25–35 years.

Peutz-Jeghers syndrome (PJS)

Peutz-Jeghers syndrome is an autosomal dominant harmartomatous polyposis syndrome caused by a germline mutation in the *STK11 (LKB1)* gene, which encodes for a multifunctional serine–threonine kinase [34,35]. It occurs in 1 in 120,000–200,000 live births [36,37].

Clinical features

Peutz-Jeghers syndrome is characterized by GI hamartomatous polyps and melanin hyperpigmentation of the lips, buccal mucosa, and digits [38]. The polyps are located mainly in the small intestine but may be found in the stomach and colorectum. PJS polyps may cause abdominal pain, intussusception, bleeding, or anemia [38]. A clinical diagnosis of PJS can be made if ≥2 Peutz-Jeghers polyps are found in the GI tract or if one Peutz-Jeghers polyp is found in association with classic pigmentation or a family history of the syndrome [39]. PJS is associated with an increased risk of colorectal (20%), gastric (5%), small bowel, pancreas, breast, ovary, lung, cervix, uterus, and testis cancer [40].

Genetics and genetic testing

Peutz-Jeghers syndrome is caused by a germline mutation in the *STK11 (LKB1)* gene that is located on chromosome 19p13.3 [34,35], which has been documented in 18–63% of cases [41–43]. Genetic testing for PJS is performed by DNA sequencing of the *STK11* gene. Individuals with PJS and their first-degree family members are candidates for genetic testing.

Management and surveillance

Currently, prophylactic colectomy is not recommended for patients with PJS. However, surveillance for CRC and extracolonic cancer is important. Most experts recommend colonoscopy at intervals of 2–3 years beginning during the late teenage years, with upper GI endoscopy and small-bowel radiography at intervals of 2–3 years and annual hemoglobin level beginning at age 10 [38]. Surveillance for pancreatic cancer with endoscopic or transabdominal ultrasonography, or CT scan may begin at 30 years of age and be repeated every 1–2 years. Mammography at intervals of 2–3 years, annual clinical breast and pelvic exam, annual PAP smear, and annual pelvic ultrasound may begin at age 20–25 years in females. Because male patients with PJS are at risk for testicular tumors, annual clinical testicular exam beginning at age 10 is recommended.

Although most clinicians recommend endoscopic polypectomy when technically feasible, surgery is indicated in certain circumstances. Indications include symptoms (obstruction, intussusception, and bleeding) and large (≥ 15 mm) or adenomatous polyps that cannot be removed endoscopically [16]. During surgery, as much of the small bowel and colon as is feasible should be cleared of polyps, either by enterotomy or intraoperative endoscopic resection [38].

Juvenile polyposis syndrome (JPS)

Juvenile polyposis syndrome is an autosomal dominant GI hamartomatous polyposis syndrome associated with an increased risk of CRC and upper GI cancer. The incidence is one per 100,000 live births [44]. Juvenile polyps are defined histologically as hamartomas with dilated mucus-filled cysts and hyperplastic stroma [45].

Clinical features

Juvenile polyposis syndrome is diagnosed clinically using the following criteria: (1) more than 3–10 juvenile polyps in the colorectum, (2) juvenile polyps throughout the GI tract, or (3) juvenile polyps (any number) with a family history of JPS [46]. Polyps in JPS are most common in the colorectum but may be found throughout the GI tract. The number of juvenile polyps ranges from 50 to 200 [45], with symptoms usually associated with increasing polyp size. The most common symptom is chronic anemia, followed by acute GI bleeding, rectal prolapse of the polyp, protein-losing enteropathy, and intussusception with or without obstruction [47]. JPS is associated with a 10–38% lifetime risk of CRC and a 15–21% lifetime risk of gastric and duodenal cancer [48,49]. Malignant tumors appear to arise from adenomatous components present in some juvenile polyps and usually occur after the fourth decade [49].

Genetics and genetic testing

Juvenile polyposis syndrome has been associated with germline mutations of two genes; *SMAD4* (*DPC4*) located on chromosome 18q21 and *BMPR1A* on chromosome 10q21–22 [50,51]. *SMAD4* encodes for a protein which is an intracellular regulator of transforming growth factor (TGF)-β, and mediates growth inhibitory signals from the cell surface to the nucleus. *BMPR1A* mediates intracellular signaling through *SMAD4* and is a member of the TGF-β superfamily. Genetic testing involves DNA sequencing for mutations in these two genes and detects the genetic etiology of approximately 35–50% of cases [52,53]. Candidates for genetic testing are individuals who meet the clinical criteria for JPS and first-degree relatives of individuals with a *SMAD4* or *BMPR1A* mutation.

Management

Patients with GI bleeding, anemia, diarrhea, protein-losing enteropathy, or with high polyp burden may be treated surgically. Operative options include TPC with IPAA or total colectomy with IRA. Regardless of the surgery performed, patients require endoscopic surveillance due to the high rate of polyp formation in the remaining rectum or pouch [54]. In asymptomatic patients, surveillance colonoscopy with removal of all detectable polyps is recommended every 1–2 years [14]. First-degree relatives of patients with JPS should be screened with colonoscopy at 3-year intervals beginning at age 12 [32].

MYH polyposis

The MYH polyposis, first described in 2002, is an autosomal recessive colonic polyposis syndrome which is associated with biallelic mutations in the *MYH* gene [55]. It may account for up to 40% of patients with an FAP or AFAP phenotype in whom a germline mutation in the *APC* gene has not been detected [55–58].

Clinical features

The mean age of diagnosis of polyposis and cancer are 46 and 50 years, respectively [57,59]. Clinical features of MYH polyposis are similar to AFAP. However, MYH polyposis may be differentiated by its recessive pattern of inheritance.

Genetics and genetic testing

The *MYH* gene is involved in the base excision DNA repair process by removing adenine nucleotides misincorporated into DNA opposite guanine or oxoguanine [55]. Genetic testing for MYH polyposis is by sequencing and should be considered in patients with clinically suspected FAP or AFAP without a demonstrable germline *APC* mutation who have a family history compatible with recessive inheritance.

Management and surveillance

There are no established guidelines for management and surveillance of MYH polyposis. However, total colectomy with IRA may be considered in patients where germline mutations in both MYH alleles have been documented and in whom multiple adenomatous polyps have been detected. Endoscopic surveillance of the remaining rectum should be performed following IRA [44].

Average- (low) and moderate-risk groups

Those individuals at "average or low risk" for CRC (the majority of the population) are those with no family history of CRC. These individuals have a 1 in 35 lifetime risk of developing bowel cancer. Those with a weak family history – one first-degree relative (FDR) under 45 years or two over 70 years have a 1 in 17 lifetime risk of developing. Individuals with two first-degree relatives (e.g. 2 FDRs average age 50–60 years; see Table 7.4) may meet the criteria for the moderate-risk group. They have a lifetime risk of 1 in 12 or greater but do not fulfill the high-risk criteria.

There are differences in recommendations for screening in these groups between the United Kingdom and the United States, which will be discussed further.

The management of those individuals in families with an identified Cancer Predisposition Syndrome leading to a significantly high risk of colorectal cancer has been discussed in detail above. It is important to identify those at highest risk in order to allocate limited endoscopic resources appropriately. However, it has been estimated that in 20% or more of individuals with colorectal cancer, there may be a genetic component. Less than 5% of these will be attributable to the syndromes described so far.

In the vast majority of colorectal cancers (>95%), the genetic predisposition is much less clearcut. The majority are likely to result from mutations in frequent alleles of low penetrance, acting either alone or in combination. Included in this may be functional polymorphisms in genes responsible for DNA repair, the metabolism of carcinogens, or the anti-tumor immune response. The complex interaction of these within individuals and with

Table 7.4 Inherited risk of CRC with screening recommendations based on risk assessment.

Risk group	Family history	Action
Low risk	1 FDR > 45 years	No screening
	2 FDR > 70 years	No screening
Low to moderate risk	2 FDR average 60–70 years	Single colonoscopy at 55 years
Moderate risk	1 FDR < 45 years	Colonoscopy every 5 years from 5 years prior to age of index case
	2 FDR average 50–60 years	As above + refer for genetic testing
High to moderate risk	2 FDR < 50 years	Colonoscopy every 3–5 years beginning at 35 years + refer for genetic testing
	3 FDR (Amsterdam negative)	As above + gyne screening
High risk	3 FDR (Amsterdam positive)	Colonoscopy every 2–3 years beginning at 30 years
	FAP	Annual sigmoidoscopy/genetic screening

FDR – first-degree relative.

the environment is likely to lead to a widely variable phenotype both within and between families.

Determining the influence of such alleles at a population level presents a major challenge and makes individual risk-determination extremely complex. With the continuing new identification of more susceptibility alleles for different cancers provided by the human genome project, it is possible that in the future, using DNA chip technology, there may come a time when simultaneous assay for multiple susceptibility alleles may allow more individual, accurate risk-estimation and targeted-screening protocols.

At the present time, practice in the United Kingdom varies but most centers use empiric risk-data and varying guidelines in order to offer these individuals some level of surveillance. Recommendations for regular endoscopic screening as advocated in the United States are not feasible in the United Kingdom due to a lack of endoscopic manpower and facilities. Whether regular surveillance is necessarily required in the low-risk group is also debatable on a cost/benefit analysis.

Moderate-risk group

The moderate-risk group (Table 7.4) is significantly larger than the high-risk group and consists of those who have more than one affected relative (or one under 45 years of age) but do not fulfill the Amsterdam criteria (Table 7.1). The risk assessment and subsequent recommendation for screening depends on the number of affected relatives, how closely related they are, and the age of onset (Table 7.2).

Application of these criteria depends on a detailed family history but this may often be uncertain or incomplete. It is good practice to obtain consent and request the records of living relatives or obtain confirmation from the relevant Cancer Registry about those who are deceased. Many centers see this as an essential part of the process because in up to 15% of cases the diagnosis reported by the relative turns out to be incorrect, thus compromising the risk assessment and recommendation for lifelong screening [60]. It is therefore essential that appropriately trained staff are available to triage all referrals of those with a family history of CRC in order that they are assigned to the appropriate risk category.

This service is best placed in the screening units where surveillance can be arranged if necessary and the procedures as well as the risks and benefits are fully explained. There should be strong links with the Regional Genetics Service so that families with identifiable cancer predisposition syndromes can be referred for consideration of genetic-mutation analysis. Ideally, a database should be established to ensure that patients obtain their screening examinations and that the results are recorded so that the efficacy of screening can be reviewed. For those in whom polyps are identified, there should be mechanisms to alter their follow-up and amend their risk category where appropriate.

Genetic testing?

At present, no informative molecular-genetic tests are available in this group but there is an argument for storing DNA from an affected individual in the family. This may allow identification of other possibly lower-penetrance susceptibility genes in the future or testing may become indicated if the family history should change and fulfill the Amsterdam criteria for HNPCC. Also, in some small families with young-age-onset CRC, where the likelihood of a genetic predisposition is suspected (but the number of individuals in the family is too small to fulfill the high-risk criteria for HNPCC), it may be worth looking at the tumor tissue for evidence of microsatellite instability or carrying out immunohistochemistry studies for measurement of gene expression. If these point to a high likelihood of an inherited cancer then the family would be reassigned to a higher-risk group and mutation analysis for HNPCC is justified. However, currently there is limited availability of such techniques due to lack of financial resources for genetic testing.

Management and surveillance

After the risk level has been established, most centers in the United Kingdom offer colonoscopy (or barium enema) every 5 years to these moderate risk-individuals once a normal colon has been demonstrated (Table 7.2). Ages for commencing endoscopic screening, 35–40 years or 5 years before age of onset in youngest family member, and ceasing (>75 years) are controversial and should be discussed with the individual after taking into account any comorbidities. The reasoning behind this approach is that the adenoma–carcinoma sequence is likely to take more than 10 years (unlike the high-risk group) and that early lesions can be removed simply and progression to cancer prevented. The downside of this approach is that there is a high volume of repeat endoscopies which in some centers cannot be achieved.

An alternative approach adopted by some centers is a baseline colonoscopy at 35–40 years or at first contact (whichever is the later) and a further one at 55 years [61]. If adenomatous polyps are confirmed at either of these screening episodes, then appropriate adenoma surveillance should be arranged. This approach has gained support because it requires less endoscopic follow-up.

The rationale for having the two assessments at 35 and 55 years is as follows:
1 Full colonic evaluation at 35–40 years aims to identify those (very few) people who might have HNPCC but no significant family history (a new mutation). It also reassures those concerned about waiting until 55 years. However, the likelihood of identifying a polyp in the 35–39 years age group is only 2% and the likelihood of detecting a cancer is only 1 : 1660.
2 The benefit of full colonic evaluation at 55 years in this moderate-risk group is perhaps easier to justify as the proportion of people in this age group with a polyp is 17–21% and 1 : 181 people will have a large-bowel cancer detected. The reduction in cancer incidence would be appreciable since those identified as having polyps would be entered into an ongoing surveillance program.

However, this approach can understandably sometimes cause concern in families because of the 20-year "gap" between screening episodes.

Patient pressure sometimes leads to a further examination between these intervals.

In the United States the moderate group is defined slightly differently in that having one relative affected with colorectal cancer under the age of 60 years (as opposed to 45 years in the UK) or 2 relatives at any age (as opposed to average age <70 years in the UK) puts you in this category. The recommendation would be a Total Colorectal Examination (colonoscopy or Double Contrast Barium Enema (DCBE) with Flexible Sigmoidoscopy (FS)) every 5 years in the first group and every 10 years in the second group starting at age 40 or 10 years before the youngest familial CRC.

Evaluation

Randomized controlled trials of screening strategies for family history are highly unlikely because of the numbers required and the accepted benefit of detecting polyps at an early stage; therefore it is important to continue to audit the outcomes of the screening protocols in place including total number of referrals, adenoma, and carcinoma prevalence in those recommended screening- and surveillance-related morbidity/mortality.

The financial costs and feasibility of providing the recommended screening should also be carefully considered, for example, appropriately trained staff, endoscopy costs, treatment of the complications of surveillance, and so on. Inevitably there will be variations from one center to another depending on resources. The production of national guidelines by National Institute for Clinical Excellence (NICE) over the next few years may set clearer standards.

Average- (low) risk group

This group includes those with no family history (who are at the population risk of 1 in 35) and those with one relative affected with CRC over 45 years or two close relatives affected over 70 years (1 in 17). None of these individuals would currently be considered at high enough risk to warrant screening by colonoscopy and no genetic investigations would be indicated or possible at present.

However, it should be remembered that even in those with a weak family history, their risk is slightly raised above the population and it is worth counseling them about diet and lifestyle measures to minimize this. Also they should be aware of any change in bowel habit or symptoms which may suggest a problem and report this at an early stage to their family doctor.

Additionally, it should be borne in mind that family histories are dynamic and that people should report any potentially relevant new diagnoses in the family as it may alter the risk assessment.

Management

Ideally this group should be managed in primary care but GPs and their support staff will require education and training in taking family histories and making a preliminary risk assessment. Any family where the situation is borderline or unclear should be referred to an assessment unit so that anxious family members can receive appropriate advice and reassurance.

Population screening

Colorectal cancer is a common condition with a known pre-malignant lesion (adenoma). The incidence of adenomatous polyps in the colon increases with age, and although these polyps can be identified in up to 20% of the population, most of these are small and unlikely to undergo malignant change.

The best available evidence suggests that only 10% of 1 cm adenomas undergo malignant change after 10 years [62]. The vast majority (90%) of adenomas can be removed at colonoscopy. Therefore, there is great potential for reducing the mortality from this disease by detecting adenomas and early cancers by screening asymptomatic individuals.

The single greatest risk factor for the development of CRC is advancing age as over 90% of CRCs occur in the over 60 age group. Due to the estimated 10 year timescale for the adenoma–carcinoma sequence, most experts agree that screening should target those over 50 years of age.

Population screening for bowel cancer will be introduced for the over 50s in the United Kingdom starting in 2006 (coordinated through Primary Care) and of course all individuals over 50 would be eligible for this. Fecal occult blood (FOB) testing will be used as a first-line screening tool and there is increasingly compelling evidence to show that such programs can save lives at a cost similar to that of the existing breast screening program [63–65].

A single FS is a potentially promising alternative to FOB testing, but conclusive data will not be available for a few years [66]. For this to be possible in the United Kingdom there would need to be a considerable investment in endoscopy facilities and expertise. Currently, this service is already stretched beyond capacity in many centers.

In the United States, the recommendation for those over 50 years who do not fit either the moderate-or high-risk criteria varies from:

Either FOB or Fecal Immunochemical Testing (FIT) – every year
Or Flexible Sigmoidoscopy (FS) – every 5 years
Or Double Contrast Barium Enema (DCBE) – every 5 years
Or Colonoscopy – every 10 years [67–69].

Summary

There are clearly a large number of people who have an increased lifetime risk of CRC which is difficult to quantify. Triaging procedures and risk assessment will vary from center to center and from one country to another. However, it is important to aim toward a consistent approach to avoid confusion and make sure that the allocation of resources is done according to risk and the results of screening are audited.

Population screening will soon be available for the over 50s in the United Kingdom and should address the concerns of those in the lower-risk groups. In the United States there are a number of options for these individuals and presumably this will depend to some extent on where they live and what health care services are available to them.

Genetic testing will not provide the answer for the majority of these low- and moderate-risk patients in the short term and indeed resources are extremely limited even for the higher-risk groups currently in the United Kingdom. In the future we may be able to tailor screening on a more individual basis as the relevance of an individual's lifestyle, genetic profile, and therefore susceptibility becomes more apparent.

References

1 Lynch HT, de la Chapelle A. Hereditary colorectal cancer. *N Engl J Med* 2003; 348: 919–32.
2 Campbell WJ, Spence RA, Parks TG. Familial adenomatous polyposis. *Br J Surg* 1994; 81: 1722–33.
3 Jarvinen HJ. Epidemiology of familial adenomatous polyposis in Finland: impact of family screening on the colorectal cancer rate and survival. *Gut* 1992; 33: 357–60.
4 Rustin RB, Jagelman DG, McGannon E *et al.* Spontaneous mutation in familial adenomatous polyposis. *Dis Colon Rectum* 1990; 33: 52–5.

5 Lynch HT, Smyrk T, McGinn T *et al.* Attenuated familial adenomatous polyposis (AFAP). A phenotypically and genotypically distinctive variant of FAP. *Cancer* 1995; 76: 2427–33.

6 Hernegger GS, Moore HG, Guillem JG. Attenuated familial adenomatous polyposis: an evolving and poorly understood entity. *Dis Colon Rectum* 2002; 45: 127–34; discussion 134–6.

7 Jagelman DG. Extra-colonic manifestations of familial adenomatous polyposis. *Oncology (Huntingt)* 1991; 5: 23–7; discussion 31–6.

8 Giardiello FM, Offerhaus GJ, Krush AJ *et al.* Risk of hepatoblastoma in familial adenomatous polyposis. *J Pediatr* 1991; 119: 766–8.

9 Giardiello FM, Offerhaus GJ, Lee DH *et al.* Increased risk of thyroid and pancreatic carcinoma in familial adenomatous polyposis. *Gut* 1993; 34: 1394–6.

10 Hamilton SR, Liu B, Parsons RE *et al.* The molecular basis of Turcot's syndrome. *N Engl J Med* 1995; 332: 839–47.

11 Debinski HS, Spigelman AD, Hatfield A *et al.* Upper intestinal surveillance in familial adenomatous polyposis. *Eur J Cancer* 1995; 31A: 1149–53.

12 Nugent KP, Spigelman AD, Phillips RK. Life expectancy after colectomy and ileorectal anastomosis for familial adenomatous polyposis. *Dis Colon Rectum* 1993; 36: 1059–62.

13 Chung DC. The genetic basis of colorectal cancer: insights into critical pathways of tumorigenesis. *Gastroenterology* 2000; 119: 854–65.

14 Grady WM. Genetic testing for high-risk colon cancer patients. *Gastroenterology* 2003; 124: 1574–94.

15 Giardiello FM, Brensinger JD, Petersen GM. AGA technical review on hereditary colorectal cancer and genetic testing. *Gastroenterology* 2001; 121: 198–213.

16 Guillem JG, Smith AJ, Calle JP, Ruo L. Gastrointestinal polyposis

syndromes. *Curr Probl Surg* 1999; 36: 217–323.

17 Gryfe R, Kim H, Hsieh ET *et al.* Tumor microsatellite instability and clinical outcome in young patients with colorectal cancer. *N Engl J Med* 2000; 342: 69–77.

18 Myrhoj T, Bisgaard ML, Bernstein I *et al.* Hereditary non-polyposis colorectal cancer: clinical features and survival. Results from the Danish HNPCC register. *Scand J Gastroenterol* 1997; 32: 572–6.

19 Jass JR. Colorectal adenomas in surgical specimens from subjects with hereditary non-polyposis colorectal cancer. *Histopathology* 1995; 27: 263–7.

20 Watanabe T, Muto T, Sawada T, Miyaki M. Flat adenoma as a precursor of colorectal carcinoma in hereditary nonpolyposis colorectal carcinoma. *Cancer* 1996; 77: 627–34.

21 De Jong AE, Morreau H, Van Puijenbroek M *et al.* The role of mismatch repair gene defects in the development of adenomas in patients with HNPCC. *Gastroenterology* 2004; 126: 42–8.

22 Vasen HF, Watson P, Mecklin JP, Lynch HT. New clinical criteria for hereditary nonpolyposis colorectal cancer (HNPCC, Lynch syndrome) proposed by the International Collaborative group on HNPCC. *Gastroenterology* 1999; 116: 1453–6.

23 Peltomaki P, Vasen HF. Mutations predisposing to hereditary nonpolyposis colorectal cancer: database and results of a collaborative study. The International Collaborative Group on Hereditary Nonpolyposis Colorectal Cancer. *Gastroenterology* 1997; 113: 1146–58.

24 Peterlongo P, Nafa K, Lerman GS *et al.* MSH6 germline mutations are rare in colorectal cancer families. *Int J Cancer* 2003; 107: 571–9.

25 Liu B, Parsons R, Papadopoulos N *et al.* Analysis of mismatch repair genes in hereditary non-polyposis colorectal

cancer patients. *Nat Med* 1996;
2: 169–74.

26 Boland CR, Thibodeau SN, Hamilton SR
et al. A National Cancer Institute
Workshop on Microsatellite Instability
for cancer detection and familial
predisposition: development of
international criteria for the
determination of microsatellite instability
in colorectal cancer. *Cancer Res* 1998;
58: 5248–57.

27 Umar A, Boland CR, Terdiman JP *et al.*
Revised Bethesda Guidelines for
hereditary nonpolyposis colorectal
cancer (Lynch syndrome) and
microsatellite instability. *J Natl
Cancer Inst* 2004; 96: 261–8.

28 Shia J, Ellis NA, Klimstra DS. The utility
of immunohistochemical detection of
DNA mismatch repair gene proteins.
Virchows Arch 2004; 445:
431–41.

29 Vasen HF, Nagengast FM, Khan PM.
Interval cancers in hereditary
non-polyposis colorectal cancer
(Lynch syndrome). *Lancet* 1995;
345: 1183–4.

30 Church J, Simmang C. Practice
parameters for the treatment of patients
with dominantly inherited colorectal
cancer (familial adenomatous polyposis
and hereditary nonpolyposis colorectal
cancer). *Dis Colon Rectum* 2003;
46: 1001–12.

31 Lynch HT. Is there a role for
prophylactic subtotal colectomy among
hereditary nonpolyposis colorectal
cancer germline mutation carriers? *Dis
Colon Rectum* 1996; 39: 109–10.

32 Half EE, Bresalier RS. Clinical
management of hereditary
colorectal cancer syndromes. *Curr Opin
Gastroenterol* 2004; 20: 32–42.

33 Burke W, Petersen G, Lynch P *et al.*
Recommendations for follow-up
care of individuals with an inherited
predisposition to cancer. I. Hereditary
nonpolyposis colon cancer. Cancer
Genetics Studies Consortium. *JAMA*
1997; 277: 915–9.

34 Jenne DE, Reimann H, Nezu J *et al.*
Peutz-Jeghers syndrome is caused by

mutations in a novel serine
threonine kinase. *Nat Genet* 1998;
18: 38–43.

35 Hemminki A, Markie D, Tomlinson I
et al. A serine/threonine kinase gene
defective in Peutz-Jeghers syndrome.
Nature 1998; 391: 184–7.

36 Boardman LA. Heritable colorectal
cancer syndromes: recognition
and preventive management.
Gastroenterol Clin North Am 2002;
31: 1107–31.

37 McGarrity TJ, Kulin HE, Zaino RJ.
Peutz-Jeghers syndrome.
Am J Gastroenterol 2000; 95:
596–604.

38 Chessin DB M, AJ, Guillem JG.
Peutz-Jeghers syndrome, 1st edn.
Sao Paulo: Lemar-Livraria Editoria
Marina; 2005.

39 Tomlinson IP, Houlston RS.
Peutz-Jeghers syndrome. *J Med Genet*
1997; 34: 1007–11.

40 Giardiello FM, Brensinger JD,
Tersmette AC *et al.* Very high risk of
cancer in familial Peutz-Jeghers
syndrome. *Gastroenterology* 2000;
119: 1447–53.

41 Jiang CY, Esufali S, Berk T *et al.*
STK11/LKB1 germline mutations are not
identified in most Peutz-Jeghers
syndrome patients. *Clin Genet* 1999;
56: 136–41.

42 Boardman LA, Couch FJ, Burgart LJ
et al. Genetic heterogeneity in
Peutz-Jeghers syndrome. *Hum Mutat*
2000; 16: 23–30.

43 Westerman AM, Entius MM, Boor PP
et al. Novel mutations in the
LKB1/STK11 gene in Dutch
Peutz-Jeghers families. *Hum Mutat*
1999; 13: 476–81.

44 Jarvinen HJ. Hereditary cancer:
guidelines in clinical practice. Colorectal
cancer genetics. *Ann Oncol* 2004;
15: iv127–31.

45 Jass JR, Williams CB, Bussey HJ, Morson
BC. Juvenile polyposis – a precancerous
condition. *Histopathology* 1988; 13:
619–30.

46 Giardiello FM, Hamilton SR, Kern SE
et al. Colorectal neoplasia in juvenile

polyposis or juvenile polyps. *Arch Dis Child* 1991; 66: 971–5.

47 Coburn MC, Pricolo VE, DeLuca FG, Bland KI. Malignant potential in intestinal juvenile polyposis syndromes. *Ann Surg Oncol* 1995; 2: 386–91.

48 Desai DC, Murday V, Phillips RK *et al.* A survey of phenotypic features in juvenile polyposis. *J Med Genet* 1998; 35: 476–81.

49 Howe JR, Mitros FA, Summers RW. The risk of gastrointestinal carcinoma in familial juvenile polyposis. *Ann Surg Oncol* 1998; 5: 751–6.

50 Howe JR, Roth S, Ringold JC *et al.* Mutations in the SMAD4/DPC4 gene in juvenile polyposis. *Science* 1998; 280: 1086–8.

51 Howe JR, Bair JL, Sayed MG *et al.* Germline mutations of the gene encoding bone morphogenetic protein receptor 1A in juvenile polyposis. *Nat Genet* 2001; 28: 184–7.

52 Sayed MG, Ahmed AF, Ringold JR *et al.* Germline SMAD4 or BMPR1A mutations and phenotype of juvenile polyposis. *Ann Surg Oncol* 2002; 9: 901–6.

53 Solomon CH, Pho LN, Burt RW. Current status of genetic testing for colorectal cancer susceptibility. *Oncology (Huntingt)* 2002; 16: 161–71; discussion 176, 179–80.

54 Oncel M, Church JM, Remzi FH, Fazio VW. Colonic surgery in patients with juvenile polyposis syndrome: a case series. *Dis Colon Rectum* 2005; 48: 49–55; discussion 55–6.

55 Al-Tassan N, Chmiel NH, Maynard J *et al.* Inherited variants of MYH associated with somatic G:C–>T:A mutations in colorectal tumors. *Nat Genet* 2002; 30: 227–32.

56 Isidro G, Laranjeira F, Pires A *et al.* Germline MUTYH (MYH) mutations in Portuguese individuals with multiple colorectal adenomas. *Hum Mutat* 2004; 24: 353–4.

57 Kairupan CF, Meldrum CJ, Crooks R *et al.* Mutation analysis of the MYH gene in an Australian series of colorectal polyposis patients with or without germline APC mutations. *Int J Cancer* 2005; 116: 73–7.

58 Sieber OM, Lipton L, Crabtree M *et al.* Multiple colorectal adenomas, classic adenomatous polyposis, and germ-line mutations in MYH. *N Engl J Med* 2003; 348: 791–9.

59 Sampson JR, Dolwani S, Jones S *et al.* Autosomal recessive colorectal adenomatous polyposis due to inherited mutations of MYH. *Lancet* 2003; 362: 39–41.

60 Fiona Douglas, Lindsay C O'Dair, Marion Robinson *et al.* The Accuracy of diagnoses as reported in families with cancer: a retrospective study. *J Med Genet* 1999; 36: 309–12.

61 Malcolm G Dunlop. Guidance on large bowel surveillance for people with two first degree relatives with colorectal cancer or one first degree relative diagnosed with colorectal cancer under 45 years. *Gut* 2002; 51: v17–v20.

62 Stryker SJ, Wolff BG, Culp CE *et al.* Natural history of untreated colonic polyps. *Gastroenterology* 1987; 93: 1009–13.

63 Hardcastle JD, Chamberlain JO, Robinson MH *et al.* Randomised controlled trial of faecal occult blood screening in colorectal cancer. *Lancet* 1996; 348: 1472–7.

64 Mandel JS, Bond JH, Church TR *et al.* Reducing mortality from colorectal cancer by screening for Faecal occult blood. *N Engl J Med* 1993; 328: 1365–71.

65 Winawer SJ, Schottenfield D, Felhinger BJ. Colorectal cancer screening. *J Natl Cancer Inst* 1991; 83: 243–53.

66 UK Flexible Sigmoidoscopy Screening Trial Investigation. Single flexible sigmoidoscopy screening to prevent colorectal cancer: baseline finding of a UK multicentre randomised trial. *Lancet* 2002; 359: 1291–300.

67 Winawer S, Fletcher R, Rex D *et al.* Colorectal cancer screening and surveillance: clinical guidelines and rationale – update based on new

evidence. *Gastroenterology* 2003;
124: 544–60.

68 Smith RA, von Eschenbach AC,
Wender R *et al.* American Cancer Society
guidelines for the early detection of
cancer: update of early detection
guidelines for prostate, colorectal, and
endometrial cancers. Also: update 2001 –

testing for early lung cancer detection.
CA Cancer J Clin 2001; 51: 38–75.

69 Simmang CL, Senatore P, Lowry A *et al.*
Practice parameters for detection of
colorectal neoplasms. The Standards
Committee, the American Society of
Colon and Rectal Surgeons. *Dis Colon
Rectum* 1999; 42: 1123–9.

8: Adjuvant radiotherapy and chemoradiotherapy in the treatment of rectal cancer

Rachel Cooper and David Sebag-Montefiore

Introduction

Although surgery is the predominant treatment for rectal cancer, over the last few decades, radiotherapy (RT) and more recently chemoradiotherapy (CRT) have been increasingly used as adjuvant treatments.

There are three basic indications for adding adjuvant radio(chemo)therapy to surgery. The first is to reduce local recurrence in resectable tumors, second, to shrink locally advanced tumors in order to allow surgical resection, and third, to improve the chance of sphincter preservation surgery in low-lying tumors. Reducing local recurrence is important because it is rarely salvaged, often painful, and greatly reduces the patient's quality of life. The purpose of this review is to address a number of important questions related to adjuvant treatment for rectal cancer which might assist when making decisions about patient management.

What is the evidence base for adjuvant radiotherapy?

Two meta-analyses have addressed the value of adjuvant RT for rectal cancer [1,2]. Both concluded that the addition of RT to surgery significantly reduced the risk of local recurrence with a more modest effect on survival which was statistically significant in one of the analyses [2]. Tables 8.1 and 8.2 summarize the results of studies of preoperative and postoperative RT and CRT [3–29].

The study from the Colorectal Cancer Collaborative Group (CCCG) included 8507 individual patient data from 22 randomized trials of preoperative and postoperative RT vs surgery alone [1]. The absolute risk of local recurrence at 5 years in patients who received preoperative RT compared to those who received surgery was 12.5 vs 22.2% ($p < 0.00001$) and postoperative RT compared to surgery was 15.3 vs 22.9% ($p = 0.0002$).

Overall survival at 5 years was not significantly increased (45 vs 42%). There was also clear evidence of a dose response with a greater reduction in local recurrence risk with the use of higher doses of preoperative RT (biologically effective doses >30). The study of Camma *et al.* [2] was a literature-based meta-analysis of 14 trials comparing preoperative RT (without chemotherapy) with surgery alone. This showed a significant reduction in local recurrence. However, they also found a significant survival advantage for patients who received preoperative RT (Odds Ratio 0.84; 95% confidence interval 0.72–0.98; $p < 0.001$).

The findings that RT significantly reduces the rate of local recurrence but has less impact on overall survival are consistent with most of the published randomized trials. One of the largest trials, the Swedish Rectal Cancer Trial [23], showed a significant survival advantage for preoperative RT as well as a reduction in local recurrence. Interestingly, a report of the long term follow-up of the Swedish Rectal Cancer Trial confirms that the reduction in local recurrence and survival improvement are maintained at 13 years [30]. This data and the 10-year data from the CCCG overview suggest that adjuvant RT prevents rather than delays local recurrence.

What is the benefit of adjuvant radiotherapy in addition to total mesorectal excision surgery?

With widespread adoption of total mesorectal excision (TME) for rectal cancer, the outcome after surgery alone has improved significantly. Using this technique local recurrence rates as low as 4–8% have been reported from single institutions [31,32] and have been reproduced, following training, in the multi-institutional setting [33,34]. The studies included in the two meta-analyses [1,2] did not use TME and reported recurrence rates with the addition of RT are similar or higher than those reported for TME alone. This has led some to argue that with optimal surgery adjuvant RT is no longer necessary. In order to address this issue the Dutch Colorectal Cancer Group performed a randomized trial of TME with selective postoperative RT (50 Gy in 25 fractions for patients with an involved CRM) vs preoperative RT followed by TME in patients with resectable rectal cancer [24]. The preoperative RT consisted of 5 Gy × 5 fractions over 1 week with surgery within 2 weeks of completion of RT. No adjuvant chemotherapy was given. A program of surgical training and quality control of surgical techniques was used for surgeons and centers participating in the trial. At 5 years, a significantly lower local recurrence was observed in the patients receiving preoperative

Table 8.1 Randomized trials of postoperative radiotherapy alone or postoperative combined treatment.

Trial (reference)	Patient numbers	Randomization	XRT fraction/ dose Gy	BED	Local recurrence	Significance	Survival	Significance
Surgery vs surgery plus postoperative radiotherapy included in CCCG meta-analysis								
Denmark [3]	250	Surgery			44/250	NS	126/250	NS
	244	XRT	25/50*	35.4	38/244		117/244	
Rotterdam [4]	84	Surgery			28/84	NS	29/84	NS
	88	XRT	25/50	43.8	21/84		37/84	
MRC (UK) [5]	235	Surgery			79/235	p = 0.001	145/235	NS
	234	XRT	20/40	36	48/234		139/234	
EORTC [6]	88	Surgery			26/88	NS	56/88	NS
	84	XRT	23/46	40.8	19/84		51/84	
GITSG-71 [7]	62	Surgery			14/62	NS‡		
	55	CT†			13/55			
	58	XRT	23–25/40–48	36.6/42.6	10/58			
	52	XRT plus CT†	23–25/40–44	36.6/35.5	5/52			p < 0.009
NSABP-R-01 [8]	184	Surgery			45/184		95/184	
	187	CT§			40/187	NS	78/187	p = 0.05
	184	XRT	26–29/46–53	36.9/42.7	30/184	p = 0.06	92/184	NS
Surgery vs surgery plus postoperative radiotherapy or combined radio-chemotherapy not included in CCCG meta-analysis								
NCCTG [9]	100	XRT	25–28/45–50.4	37.5–40.9	25%	p = 0.036	38/100	p = 0.043
	104	XRT + CT			13.5%		51/100	

Trial	n	Treatment						
NCCTG [10]	332	Bolus 5-FU +XRT	28/50.4	40.9	47%		60%	
	228	PVI 5-FU + XRT	28/50.4	40.9	37%	p = 0.01		p = 0.005
CLG-B/	421	5-FU||	28/50.4	40.9			70%	
NCCTG [11]	425	5-FU + Lv	28/50.4	40.9		NS	78%	NS
	426	5-FU + Lev	28/50.4	40.9			80%	
	424	5-FU + Lv + Lev	28/50.4	40.9			79%	
							79%	
Norway [12]	72	Surgery			21/72		50%	
	72	XRT + CT	23/46	40.8	8/72	p = 0.01	64%	p = 0.05
NSABP-R02 [13]	348	CT		40.9	47/348		146/348	NS
	346	CT + XRT	28/50.4	40.9	27/348	p = 0.02	142/346	
Postoperative vs preoperative radio(chemo)therapy								
Uppsala [14]	236	Preop XRT	5/25.5	37.8	26/209			NS
	235	Postop XRT	30/60	52.2	43/204	p = 0.02		
German [27]	421	Preop CRT¶	28/50.4	40.9	6%		76%	
	402	Postop CRT	28/50.4	40.9	13%	p = 0.006	74%	p = 0.80

XRT, postoperative radiotherapy; CT, chemotherapy (all was given postoperatively); 5-FU, 5-fluorouracil; Lv, Leucovorin; Lev, Levamisole; PVI, protracted venous infusion; NS, not significant.

*Radiotherapy was given as a split course with 2 weeks' break after 30 Gy.

†Chemotherapy consisted of 5-FU days 1–5 and 36–40 and semustine day 1 and every 10 weeks; concomitant chemotherapy consisted of 5-FU on first three and last three days of radiotherapy.

‡There was a significant difference in time to recurrence for patients receiving adjuvant treatment which was most favorable in the group receiving combined modality treatment.

§Combination 5-FU, semustine, and vincristine.

||All patients received postoperative XRT concomitant with chemotherapy.

¶All patients received 5-FU in the first and fifth week of radiotherapy.

Table 8.2 Randomized trials of preoperative radiotherapy and combined treatment in operable rectal cancer.

Trial	Patient numbers	Randomization	XRT fraction/dose Gy	BED	Local recurrence	Significance	Survival	Significance
Trials of preoperative radiotherapy included in the CCCG meta-analysis								
VASOG I [15]	353	Surgery	10/20–25	21–28			38.8%	NS
	347	XRT					48.5%	
MRC I [16]	275	Surgery	1/5	7.5	56.8%	NS	38%	NS
	277	XRT	10/20	20.4	55.4%		41.7%	
	272	XRT			52.9%		40%	
Stockholm I [17]	425	Surgery	5/25	37.5	120/425	$p = 0.01$	293/425	NS
	424	XRT			61/424		295/424	
VASOG II [18]	181	Surgery	18/31.5	26.8			82/181	NS
	180	XRT					91/180	
EORTC [19]	175	Surgery	15/34.5	34.6	49/175	$p = 0.003$	49%	NS
	166	XRT			24/166		51.6%	
MRC II [20]	140	Surgery	20/40	36	65/140	$p = 0.04$	114/140	NS
	139	XRT			50/139	NS	103/139	
Essen [81]	78	Surgery	13/25	24				NS
	64	XRT						
Norway [21]	150	Surgery	18/31.5	26.8	21.1%	NS	57.5%	NS
	159	XRT			13.7%		56.7%	
St Marks [22]	239	Surgery	3/5	22.5	24%	$p < 0.05$	56%	NS
	228	XRT			17%		52%	
SRCT* [23]	557	Surgery	5/25	37.5	150/557	$p < 0.001$	28%	$p = 0.002$
	553	XRT			63/553		58%	
NW England [82]	141	Surgery	4/20	30		$p < 0.001$		NS
	143	XRT						

Trials of preoperative radiotherapy not included in CCCG meta-analysis								
DRCT† [24]	937	Surgery		37.5	8.2%	p < 0.001	81.8%	NS
	924	XRT	5/25		2.4%		82%	
Trials of preoperative chemoradiotherapy vs radiotherapy not included in CCCG meta-analysis								
EORTC [25]	121	Preop XRT	15/34.5	36		NS	59%	p = 0.06
	126	XRT + CT	15/34.5				46%	
EORTC	Total 1011	Preop XRT	25/45	36.9	17.1%	p = 0.002	65.6%	p = 0.798
22921 [28]		Preop CRT	25/45‡	36.9	8.8%		64.8%§	
		Preop XRT	25/45	36.9	9.6%			
		Postop CT						
		Preop CRT	25/45	36.9	8%			
		Postop CT						
FFCD 9203 [29]	363	Preop XRT	25/45	36.9	Not available		66.6%	NS
	370	Preop CRT	25/45‖	36.9			67.8%	
Preop SCRT vs CRT								
Polish study [26]	155	SCPRT	5/25	37.5	Not available¶		Not available	
	157	Preop CRT‖	28/50.4	40.9				

* Swedish Rectal Cancer Trial.
† Dutch Rectal Cancer Trial.
‡ The chemotherapy was 5-FU and leucovorin in the first and fifth week of radiotherapy. Postoperative chemotherapy consisted of four courses of 5-FU and leucovorin.
§ This is the survival for preoperative XRT vs CRT with or without post-op chemotherapy. There was also no significant difference in overall survival for postoperative chemotherapy vs none.
‖ The chemotherapy was 5-FU and leucovorin in the first and fifth week of radiotherapy.
¶ No local control or survival results available. The rate of sphincter preservation was not significantly different between the two arms.

RT compared to those undergoing TME alone (5.8 vs 11.4%, $p < 0.001$). However, no significant difference in survival was observed (64.3% in the group randomized to RT vs 63.5% in the group assigned surgery alone, $p = 0.84$). The preoperative RT was well tolerated although, as in previous studies, perineal-wound complications were significantly increased in those undergoing abdominoperineal excision of the rectum (APER) [35].

Subset analysis of this trial has highlighted groups of patients who are less likely to benefit from short-course preoperative RT (SCPRT), in particular patients with a positive CRM (circumferential resection margin) [36] and those with a high tumor (<10 cm from the anal verge) [24]. These findings, although interesting, require confirmation. In the United Kingdom, the Medical Research Council (MRC) CR07 has a very similar trial design [37] to the Dutch study. One important difference is the use of CRT for patients with an involved CRM after initial surgery. This trial is due to reach its accrual target in July 2005.

Is preoperative radiotherapy superior to postoperative radiotherapy?

The disadvantages and advantages of preoperative and postoperative RT have been widely discussed [38]. Biologically, preoperative RT is attractive as the pelvic anatomy is undisturbed and therefore tissues are likely to be better oxygenated and may be more radiosensitive. This is why a lower total dose appears to be more or as effective for preoperative RT than that used with postoperative RT [39]. Generally there is less small bowel in the radiation field and less risk of adhesions, resulting in decreased acute- and late-toxicity with higher compliance [40]. The main disadvantage of preoperative RT, if it is used routinely in all patients, is the risk of overtreatment exposing some patients to the risks of late toxicity without benefit. The main advantage of postoperative RT is the ability to select patients considered at high risk of recurrence.

The first trial to compare the two approaches randomized 471 patients with resectable rectal cancer to receive either preoperative RT (25.5 Gy over 1 week) followed by immediate surgery or surgery followed by a split course of postoperative RT (60 Gy over 8 weeks) for patients with Astler-Coller stages B2, C1, and C2 [14]. There was a significantly lower local recurrence rate in the preoperative arm compared with the postoperative arm (12 vs 21%, respectively). The postoperative treatment was less well tolerated and there was a delay of 6 weeks or more in starting treatment for 50% of patients. Postoperative mortality and morbidity were equal between the two groups apart from perineal wound sepsis following abdominoperineal excision of rectum (APER) which was higher for the preoperative group. A second trial, National Surgical Adjuvant Breast and Bowel Project (NSABP) R-03, asking the same question using chemoradiation was closed early following accrual of only 116 of the planned 900 patients [41]. No firm conclusions can be reported apart from similar toxicity in the two groups.

Recently, the German Rectal Cancer Trial (CAO/ARO/AIO-94) has reported [27] the results of patients with transrectal ultrasound (TRUS) defined uT3/4 or uN+ disease have been randomized to either preoperative or postoperative CRT of 50.4 Gy in 28 fractions over 5.5 weeks with continuous 5-FU infusion during the first and last week of RT. Importantly, surgery was standardized to include TME. The 5-year cumulative local relapse was 6% in the preoperative arm and 13% in the postoperative arm ($p = 0.006$) with no difference in survival (76 vs 74%, $p = 0.8$). Compliance was reduced in the postoperative arm with only approximately 50% of patients receiving the planned dose of either RT or chemotherapy. Reduced acute and late toxicity was seen in the preoperative RT arm. This trial is likely to have a major impact on North American practice (see below).

In general, less acute complications are reported for SCPRT compared with long-course preoperative or postoperative RT or CRT [27,35,42]. For example, in the Dutch Rectal Cancer Trial only 7% of patients experienced grade 2 or 3 complications [35]. This compares with 27% of patients in the preoperative CRT arm and 40% in the postoperative arm of the German Rectal Cancer Study experiencing grade 3 or 4 acute toxicity [27].

However, there has been some concern over an increase in postoperative mortality in patients receiving SCPRT. The Stockholm I trial [17] and the Imperial Cancer Research Fund trial [22] reported significantly higher postoperative mortality in the irradiated group (8 vs 2% and 12 vs 7%) when parallel opposed fields were used. However a change to a 3- or 4-field planned volume in more recent trials eliminated this problem [23].

In the CCCG meta-analysis for patients receiving preoperative RT at high biological effective doses (≥ 30 Gy) there was a significant excess of non-rectal cancer deaths in the first year (8 vs 4%). This effect was particularly evident in patients over 75 years such that at ages younger than 55 years the difference was only 1% (6 vs 5%) whereas at ages 75 or more this increased to 8%. The excess of non-rectal cancer deaths, especially in the first year, was due mainly to vascular and infective causes. On a subset analysis, a similar significant increase in deaths due to cardiac causes was observed in the RT arm of the Dutch Rectal Cancer Trial (10 vs 3, $p = 0.04$) [35]. The exact cause of this still is not known.

In summary, both direct comparisons and data from randomized studies support the use of preoperative RT rather than postoperative RT, in terms of local control, reduced acute toxicity, and compliance. However, where preoperative RT is used Biologically Equivalent Dose (BED) in excess of 30 Gy should be employed.

What is the benefit of the addition of chemotherapy to long-course radiotherapy?

Until recently only one trial of 247 patients compared preoperative RT with preoperative RT plus 5-FU for patients with resectable disease [14]. There was no difference in local control (85% at 5 years for both groups) and the overall survival was higher in the RT only arm. This might be attributable to an excess of postoperative deaths in the combined modality arm possibly due to poor RT techniques.

Two trials have recently reported a significant reduction in local recurrence but no difference in disease-free survival when chemotherapy is added to long-course radiation compared with long-course RT alone. The EORTC-22921 (European Organisation of Research and Treatment of Cancer) trial using a 2 × 2 factorial design evaluated the addition of chemotherapy (two 5-day courses of bolus 5-FU given as a short infusion over 1 hour and leucovorin) to 45 Gy in 25 fractions and plus or minus the addition of postoperative chemotherapy (4 cycles 5 FU/LV) [28]. Surgery was not standardized. There was an increase in grade 2 diarrhea in the CRT group but this did not lead to a reduction in RT compliance [42]. However, only 75% of patients randomized to postoperative chemotherapy received treatment. With a median follow-up of 5.4 years there is no improvement in either overall survival or progression-free survival at 5 years for the addition of either preoperative or postoperative chemotherapy. The 5-year local control was similar (around 9%) for all groups who received some form of chemotherapy, either preoperative, postoperative, or both compared to 17.1% for those patients who received preoperative RT alone ($p = 0.002$) [28].

The FFCD 9203 (Federation Francophone de Cancerologie Digestive Group) study had a similar design to the EORTC 22921 randomizing 762 patients to either preoperative RT or preoperative CRT (with the same regimen), but all patients received four cycles of adjuvant chemotherapy [29]. However, unlike the EORTC study all tumors were palpable on digital rectal examination. The local recurrence rate was reduced in the preoperative CRT arm (8 vs 16.5%). At a median follow-up of 69.3 months there was no difference in overall survival (66.6% for RT vs 67.8% for CRT).

These trials demonstrate that the addition of concurrent 5-FU chemotherapy to long-course preoperative RT reduces locoregional failure but has no significant impact on disease-free survival.

What is the evidence for the role of pelvic MRI in preoperative staging?

In the preoperative setting, a number of individual center studies have demonstrated the advantages of diagnostic pelvic magnetic resonance (MR) in staging rectal cancer, demonstrating the gross tumor and influencing the selection of patients for pelvic irradiation [43–45]. Some of the earliest work was performed by Gina Brown *et al.* who should that thin-section MRI could accurately stage rectal cancers providing information to guide clinical decision making [45]. The study of Beets-Tan *et al.* [44] was a retrospective study of 76 patients who underwent preoperative magnetic resonance imaging (MRI). In 35 of these patients a regression curve was constructed. From this a histological distance of at least 1 mm was predicted when the radiological distance was at least 5 mm. The findings from these retrospective studies prompted a prospective study. The MERCURY (Magnetic Resonance Imaging and Rectal Cancer Equivalence Study) study is a multicenter prospective international trial of pelvic MR in rectal cancer [46]. This large trial demonstrates equivalence between the extramural spread of primary tumor seen on the preoperative pelvic MR and that seen in the excised histopathological specimen. This trial establishes pelvic MR as the preoperative staging investigation of choice for rectal cancer. Patients may be selected for preoperative RT if there is evidence of the mesorectal margin being threatened (defined as primary tumor extending beyond or within 1–2 mm of the mesorectal fascia).

Pelvic MRI can clearly define patients in whom the primary tumor threatens or involves the mesorectal fascia, which leads to selection of such patients for preoperative RT. There remains some difficulty in its role in guiding the selection for preoperative radiation in low rectal cancer below the level of the levator origin where there is little of no mesorectal fascia. Although MRI can clearly define enlarged lymph nodes threatening the mesorectal fascia and those outwith the mesorectal envelope, further research is required to confirm the accuracy of the prediction of lymph node involvement.

What are the late effects of adjuvant radiotherapy?

Long-term bowel function is dependent on the type of surgery as well as the timing of assessment. Patients experience increased bowel frequency, clustering of bowel movements, incontinence, especially for loose stool, and may require continual use of a pad. Some patients become "toilet dependent" and have a significantly impaired social life. In the Swedish Rectal Cancer Trial (SRCT) all surviving patients were sent a questionnaire to assess late toxicity [47]. SCPRT was associated with a significant increase in bowel frequency, incontinence, and urgency. This compares with the Dutch Rectal Cancer Trial where the only difference reported was at 24 months with a significant increase in fecal incontinence (51.3 vs 36.5%, $p = 0.002$) [48]. This difference might relate to the omission of the anal sphincter, where possible, from the RT field in the Dutch Rectal Cancer Trial.

In non-randomized studies postoperative CRT compared with surgery alone has been reported to be associated with increased frequency and incontinence [49]. Compared with postoperative therapy, preoperative short-course RT is associated with fewer symptoms. In the Uppsala trial of preoperative vs postoperative RT small-bowel complications were seen in 11% of patients receiving postoperative therapy compared to 5% receiving preoperative treatment [14]. In the German Rectal Cancer Trial late gastrointestinal toxicity (chronic diarrhea and small-bowel obstruction) was more common in patients receiving postoperative CRT (15 vs 9%, $p = 0.07$) [27].

The rate of small-bowel obstruction appears to relate to the treatment technique and the amount of small bowel within the field. In both the preoperative and postoperative setting large two-field techniques are associated with higher rates of obstruction compared to smaller three or four-field "box"-techniques [50,51]. This is illustrated by the findings of the two Stockholm studies of SCPRT. The overall incidence of small-bowel obstruction was 13.3% for patients receiving SCPRT compared with 8.5% for those who had surgery alone. The incidence was comparable for all groups during the first 2 years and in the Stockholm II study, where a smaller volume was irradiated the cumulative incidence which stayed the same over 5 years. However, in the Stockholm I study, while irradiating a larger volume and using large opposed fields including para-aortic nodes and the pelvis, the cumulative incidence increased in those patients receiving SCPRT [51]. Less detailed data are available for preoperative or postoperative RT and CRT. For postoperative CRT, rates of 1–6% have been reported [ref], although the follow-up in these studies is relatively short. The German Rectal Cancer Trial group have reported a 2% incidence of small-bowel obstruction in the post-operative treatment group with a median follow-up of 46 months [27].

Other late effects of RT have mainly been reported in relation to SCPRT. Significantly more patients experienced femoral neck or pelvic fractures following short-course RT compared to controls (5.3 vs 2.4%, $p = 0.03$) [51]. The increased risk was mainly during the first 3 years. SCPRT has also been shown to lead to more sexual dysfunction in both males and females [48,52]. Long term follow-up of the Dutch Rectal Cancer Trial suggests that male patients are more likely suffer from erectile dysfunction and ejaculation disorders following SCPRT [48]. It is important to recognize that there is very little published information on the late toxicity after preoperative CRT. This lack of information and the published poor functional outcome after SCPRT using relatively simple radiation techniques should not lead to the conclusion that CRT is less toxic for functional outcome. It should lead researchers to study this area in more detail.

Why do international differences in selection policy in patients with resectable rectal cancer persist?

There are considerable differences internationally in adjuvant RT policy. The North American standard of care was determined in 1990 [53] and recommends postoperative CRT and chemotherapy for all patients with stage II and III rectal cancer. This was based on limited trial evidence, particularly two phase III trials [9,10]. This approach only spares stage I patients from postoperative radiation. The NSABP R-02 trial attempted to answer the question of the benefit of adding postoperative chemoradiation to systemic chemotherapy [54]. Six hundred and ninety-four patients with stage II or III disease were randomized with no difference in disease-free or overall survival for those patients receiving RT in addition to chemotherapy but locoregional relapse was reduced from 13 to 8% at 5 years ($p = 0.02$).

In Scandinavia and the Netherlands, the results of the trials of SCPRT have led to a relatively unselective use of SCPRT whereas mainland Europe has tended to either adopt the North American standard of care or extrapolate from this data to use preoperative CRT.

For those patients in whom the mesorectal fascia is not threatened there are a number of options. The first is to give SCPRT to all patients. The Dutch TME study demonstrates an absolute reduction in local recurrence of 6%. Thus if 100 patients are irradiated, then six local recurrences will be prevented, so the number of patients treated to prevent one local recurrence is 16.7. This policy would expose a large proportion of patients to the risk of late morbidity (discussed below) without any benefit. Therefore, an alternative policy in patients with a predicted negative CRM would be to perform surgery followed by selective postoperative CRT for these patients in whom the CRM is unexpectedly positive.

The German rectal cancer trial is very likely to result in a significant shift towards the use of preoperative CRT for resectable T3 and T4 rectal cancer. There remains a significant concern that not all T3 rectal cancers require adjuvant RT at all.

In the United Kingdom there is an increasing use of a selective policy for preoperative radiation based on the preoperative pelvic MRI. An example of the approach used in the Leeds MDT is described. If the mesorectal fascia is not threatened and an anterior resection is planned, then patients proceed to mesorectal excision and are only considered for postoperative CRT in the unlikely event that the CRM is involved (<10–15% of patients). Where the mesorectal fascia is threatened, involved, or breached, there preoperative CRT is used.

This leaves a third group of patients who require an APER for a lower third tumor in whom preoperative radiation should be considered. There remains doubt as to whether all patients require CRT and whether SCPRT has a useful role in this patient group. For this group of patients SCPRT in addition to TME surgery did not appear to improve local control in the Dutch TME trial [24], although the opposite was found in the Swedish Rectal Cancer Trial where SCPRT reduced recurrences from 25 to 9% for patients undergoing non-TME curative resection [55]. At present, our policy is to use preoperative CRT for bulky T3/4 tumors and consider SCPRT for the mobile T2 tumor. A separate surgical option is to extend the current approach to APER and excise a wider cylinder of tissue to reduce the risk of margin involvement [56].

Preoperative chemoradiotherapy for locally advanced rectal cancer

The definition of "locally advanced disease" has been applied to a spectrum of disease that ranges from resectable T3N1 on TRUS to a fixed tumor invading the prostate and sacrum. Pelvic MRI has assisted in defining a group of patients where primary resection is likely to result in an involved CRM either macroscopically or microscopically. However despite the lack of a consistent definition there is general agreement that this group of patients should receive preoperative CRT.

There has been only one randomized trial comparing RT to combined treatment for this group of patients. Although radical resection rates were similar for the two groups, the local recurrence rate was 4% in the group receiving combined treatment compared to 35% in those receiving RT alone (the corresponding figures for the whole group was 17 vs 44%) [57]. There have been many non-randomized studies examining the use of CRT in locally advanced, initially unresectable rectal carcinoma [58–62]. There are several approaches to combining RT with chemotherapy for this group of patients. The commonly used CRT schedules combine 5-FU-based chemotherapy with 45–50.4 Gy of RT. 5-FU has been given either as a continuous infusion [61], bolus, or short infusion usually combined with leucovorin [29,42] or capecitabine [63,64]. One of the most commonly used regimens in the United Kingdom is the one evaluated in the EORTC-22921 study which combined 45 Gy in 25 fractions with a short infusion of 5-FU (350 mg/m^2) and leucovorin (20 mg/m^2) on days 1–5 and 29–33. This regimen is associated with low toxicity and high compliance. Recent data reports curative resection rates of over 70% and that involvement of the CRM predicts for local recurrence and survival after preoperative CRT [65–67].

Currently there is considerable interest in the integration of newer drugs to RT. Oral agents such as capecitabine have the potential to simplify CRT regimens. Two phase-I dose-finding studies have been performed with capecitabine with recommended doses of 900 mg/m^2 when given 5 days per week [64] throughout radiation or 825 mg/m^2 when given continuously [63]. Trials in metastatic colorectal cancer combining oxaliplatin and irinotecan with infused or oral 5-FU have reported improvements in survival or progression-free survival when compared to 5-FU alone [68–70]. The addition of biological agents such as bevacizumab [71] and cetuximab [72] have also shown benefits when added to conventional chemotherapy. All of these agents have the potential to interact with radiation with the hope of improved efficacy. So far the majority of studies of combination CRT have been dose finding and there remains considerable uncertainty as to the optimal balance between radiation and chemotherapy regime [73].

However, some conclusions can be drawn from the large number of phase II studies of combination CRT that have been performed by many groups. Higher rates of pCR and acceptable toxicity have been reported. Preliminary results with oxaliplatin and irinotecan combinations within the Colorectal Clinical Oncology Group (CCOG) portfolio suggest acceptable toxicity and histopathologically confirmed radical oncological (RO) resection rates of >80% when irinotecan or oxaliplatin are added to a fluoropyrimidine and 45 Gy pelvic radiation [74,75]. The next step is to evaluate the benefit of combination CRT compared with fluoropyrimidine CRT in phase III trials.

Can adjuvant treatment achieve sphincter preservation?

With improvements in surgical techniques it has become possible to perform more sphincter-preserving surgery (SPS) in patients with low-lying rectal tumors. However, many surgeons believe that low-lying tumors (3–6 cm from the anal verge) will require an APER particularly if the sphincter is invaded. In addition sphincter-sparing surgery may not be possible in bulky anterior tumors within a narrow pelvis.

There are two important factors to consider. Preoperative RT or CRT might shrink bulky tumors, allowing the surgeon to safely dissect around the mesorectal fascia onto the pelvic floor and therefore achieve a low-anterior resection. Second is the decision as to where the distal margin should be placed. For example, is it safe to place the distal resection margin 1 cm beyond visible tumor following major regression or is it safe to only use a margin based on the original tumor extent?

There have been a number of non-randomized studies which have tried to define the role of preoperative RT [76] or CRT [77–79] in SPS. Based on these studies sphincter preservation has been reported to be possible in 44–89% of patients who were clinically judged to require an APER. Three randomized trials have specifically examined the value of RT or CRT in SPS [26,76,80]. In the Lyon R90-01 patients received 39 Gy in 13 fractions followed by surgery within either 2 or 6–8 weeks of RT. SPS was achieved in 76% of patients following a long interval compared with 68% following a short interval ($p = 0.27$) [76]. A second study from the same group, Lyon 96-02, suggested that dose escalation of the RT might offer a higher rate of complete clinical response and therefore an increased chance of SPS (44 vs 76%) [80]. More recently Bujko et al. [26] published results of their randomized trial comparing 5×5 Gy followed by immediate surgery vs 50.4 Gy in 1.8 Gy per fraction combined with 5-FU chemotherapy in patients with resectable T3–4 tumors palpable on digital rectal examination. Surgeons declared what type of procedure was required before randomization, however the final decision on SPS was to be made at the time of surgery, following irradiation. Despite significant downsizing, an increased distance to the anorectal ring, and a better tumor response following CRT, the rate of SPS in this group was 58 vs 61% in the SCPRT group ($p = 0.57$). The local recurrence data are awaited. The authors of this study have suggested that the most likely explanation for these findings is the fact that surgeons violated the rule that the decision on sphincter preservation had to be made at the time of operation rather than at the pre-treatment assessment.

Although not the primary endpoint, four further trials have reported the impact of preoperative CRT on SPS. In the NSABP R-03, preoperative CRT appeared to improve the chance of SPS by 10% [41]. In the German Rectal Cancer Study the rate of SPS did not differ between preoperative CRT and postoperative CRT (69 vs 71%, respectively); however, in the patients where the surgeon declared that an APER was necessary the rate of SPS increased from 19 to 39% ($p = 0.004$) for those undergoing preoperative CRT [27]. However, the EORTC 22921 [28] and the FFCD 9203 [29] reported no difference in SPS with preoperative CRT with rates of approximately 50% in all groups.

Ultimately, the decision to perform SPS will depend on the skill and experience of the surgeon along with tumor and patient characteristics. However, whether preoperative RT or CRT can increase the chance of SPS is still an area of debate.

Conclusion

Current evidence suggests that some patients with rectal cancer will benefit from the addition of adjuvant therapy even when optimal surgery has been performed. However, the selection and timing of adjuvant therapy remains controversial and differs internationally.

Two recent trials have shown that the addition of preoperative chemotherapy to long-course RT has been shown to reduce local recurrence whereas a further trial demonstrates that preoperative CRT significantly reduces local recurrence with reduced acute and late toxicity when compared to postoperative CRT. These findings are likely to further increase the use of preoperative RT.

The use of pelvic MRI appears to help considerably in the selection of patients for RT in UK practice. This approach clearly identifies patients where radiological and clinical evaluation suggests that an R1 or R2 is likely and where preoperative CRT is indicated. It can also identify patients with mid- and upper-third rectal cancer where the tumor is free of the mesorectal margins in whom the role of RT is uncertain. The results of the MRC CR07 (Medical Research Council) trial are awaited with interest.

Combination chemoradiation regimens show promise in phase II trials. There is a need for phase III trials to compare fluoropyrimidine-based CRT with combination schedules.

References

1 Colorectal Cancer Collaborative Group. Adjuvant radiotherapy for rectal cancer: a systematic overview of 8,507 patients from 22 randomised trials. *Lancet* 2001; 358: 1291–304.

2 Camma C, Giunta M, Fiorica F *et al.* Preoperative radiotherapy for resectable rectal cancer. *JAMA* 2000; 284: 1008–15.

3 Balslev I, Pederson M, teglbjaerg PS *et al.* Postoperative radiotherapy in Dukes' B and C carcinoma of the rectum and rectosigmoid. A randomized multicenter study. *Cancer* 1986; 58: 22–8.

4 Treurniet-Donker AD, van Putten WLJ, Wereldsma JCJ *et al.* Postoperative radiation therapy for rectal cancer. An interim analysis of a prospective, randomized multicenter trial in The Netherlands. *Cancer* 1991; 67: 2042–8.

5 Medical Research Council Rectal Cancer Working Party. Randomised trial of surgery alone versus surgery followed by radiotherapy for mobile cancer of the rectum. *Lancet* 1996; 348: 1610–14.

6 Arnaud JP, Nordlinger B, Bosset JF *et al.* Radical surgery and postoperative radiotherapy as combined treatment in rectal cancer. Final results of a phase III study of the European Organization for Research and Treatment of Cancer. *Br J Surg* 1997; 84: 352–7.

7 Gastrointestinal Tumour Study Group. Prolongation of the disease-free interval in surgically treated rectal carcinoma. *N Engl J Med* 1985; 312: 1465–72.

8 Fisher B, Wolmark N, Rockette H *et al.* Postoperative adjuvant chemotherapy or radiation therapy for rectal cancer: results from NSABP protocol R-01. *J Natl Cancer Inst* 1988; 80: 21–9.

9 Krook JE, Moertel CG, Gunderson LL *et al.* Effective surgical adjuvant therapy for high-risk rectal carcinoma. *N Engl J Med* 1991; 324: 709–15.

10 O'Connell MJ, Martenson JA, Wieand HS *et al.* Improving adjuvant therapy for rectal cancer by combining protracted-infusion fluorouracil with radiation therapy after curative surgery. *N Engl J Med* 1994; 331: 502–7.

11 Tepper JE, O2Connell JM, Petroni GR *et al.* Adjuvant postoperative fluorouracil-modulated chemotherapy combined with pelvic radiation therapy for rectal cancer: initial results of intergroup 0114. *J Clin Oncol* 1997; 15: 2030–9.

12 Tveit KM, Guldvog I, Hagen S *et al.* Randomized controlled trial of postoperative radiotherapy and short-term time-scheduled 5-fluorouracil against surgery alone in the treatment of Dukes B and C rectal cancer. *Br J Surg* 1997; 84: 1130–5.

13 Wolmark N, Wieand HS, Hyams DM *et al.* Randomized trial of postoperative adjuvant chemotherapy with or without radiotherapy for carcinoma of the rectum: National Surgical Adjuvant Breast and Bowel Project Protocol R-02. *J Natl Cancer Inst* 2000; 92: 388–96.

14 Pahlman L Glimelius B. Pre- or postoperative radiotherapy in rectal and rectosigmoid carcinoma. *Ann Surg* 1989; 211: 187–95.

15 Higgens GA, Conn JH, Jordan PH *et al.* Preoperative radiotherapy for colorectal cancer. *Ann Surg* 1975; 181: 624–31.

16 Medical Research Council. The evaluation of low dose pre-operative therapy in the management of operable rectal cancer; results of a randomly controlled trial. *Br J Surg* 1984; 71: 21–5.

17 Cedermark B, Johansson BA, Rutqvist LE, Wilking N. The Stockholm I trial of preoperative short term radiotherapy in operable rectal carcinoma. A prospective randomized trial. *Cancer* 1995; 75: 2269–75.

18 Higgens GA, Humphrey EW, Dwight RW *et al.* Preoperative radiation and surgery for cancer of the rectum. Veterans Administration Surgical Oncology Group Trial II. *Cancer* 1986; 58: 352–9.

19 Gerard A, Butse M, Nordlinger B et al. Preoperative radiotherapy as adjuvant treatment in rectal cancer. Final results of a randomized study of the European Organization for Research and Treatment of Cancer (EORTC). Ann Surg 1988; 208: 606–14.

20 MRC Randomised trial of surgery alone versus radiotherapy followed by surgery for potentially operable locally advanced rectal cancer. Lancet 1996; 348: 1605–10.

21 Dahl O, Horn A, Morild I et al. Low-dose preoperative radiation postpones recurrences in operable rectal cancer. Results of a randomized multicenter trial in western Norway. Cancer 1990; 66: 2286–94.

22 Goldberg PA, Nicholls RJ, Porter NH et al. Long-term results of a randomised trial of short-course low-dose adjuvant pre-operative radiotherapy for rectal cancer: reduction in local treatment failure. Eur J Cancer 1994; 30A: 1602–6.

23 Anon. Improved survival with preoperative radiotherapy in resectable rectal cancer. Swedish Rectal Cancer Trial. N Engl J Med 1997; 336: 980–7.

24 Kapiteijn E, Marijnen CAM, Nagtegaal ID et al. Preoperative radiotherapy combined with total mesorectal excision for resectable rectal cancer. N Engl J Med 2001; 345: 638–46.

25 Boulis-Wassif S, Gerard A, Loygue J, Camelot D et al. Final results of a randomized trial on the treatment of rectal cancer with preoperative radiotherapy alone or in combination with 5-fluorouracil, followed by radical surgery. Trial of the European Organization on Research and Treatment of Cancer Gastrointestinal Tract Cancer Cooperative Group. Cancer 1984; 53: 1811–18.

26 Bujko K, Nowacki MP, Nasierowska-Guttmejer A et al. Sphincter preservation following preoperative radiotherapy for rectal cancer: report of a randomised trial comparing short-term radiotherapy vs conventionally fractionated radiochemotherapy. Radiother Oncol 2004; 72: 15–24.

27 Sauer, R, Becker H, Hohenberger W et al. Preoperative versus postoperative chemoradiotherapy for rectal cancer. N Engl J Med 2004; 351: 1731–40.

28 Bosset JF, Calais G, Mineur L et al. Pre-operative radiation in rectal cancer: effect and timing of additional chemotherapy 5 year results of the EORTC 22921 trial. J Clin Oncol 2005; 23(Proceedings of the ASCO 2005): p. 247s. Abstract 3505.

29 Gerard JP, Bonnetain F, Conroy T et al. Preoperative radiotherapy + 5FU/folinic acid in T3–4 rectal cancers: results of the FFCD 9203 trial. J Clin Oncol 2005; (Poceedings of the ASCO 2005): p. 247s. Abstract 3504.

30 Folkesson J, Birgisson H, Pahlman L et al. Swedish Rectal Cancer Trial: long lasting benefits from radiotherapy on survival and local recurrence rate. J Clin Oncol. 2005 20; 23: 5644–50.

31 Heald RJ, Moran BJ, Ryall RD et al. Rectal cancer: the Basingstoke experience of total mesorectal excision, 1978–1997. Arch Surg 1998; 133: 894–9.

32 MacFarlane JK, Ryall RDH, Heald RJ. Mesorectal excision for rectal cancer. Lancet 1993; 342: 457–60.

33 Carlsen E, Schlichting E, Guldvog I et al. Effect of the introduction of total mesorectal excision for the treatment of rectal cancer. Br J Surg 1998; 85: 526–9.

34 Wibe A, Moller B, Norstein J et al. A national strategic change in treatment policy for rectal cancer – implementation of total mesorectal excision as routine treatment in Norway. A national audit. Dis Colon Rectum 2002; 45: 857–66.

35 Marijnen CAM, Kapiteijn E, van de Velde CJH et al. Acute side effects and complications after short-term preoperative radiotherapy combined with total mesorectal excision in primary rectal cancer: report of a multicenter randomised trial. J Clin Oncol 2002; 20: 817–25.

36 Marijnen CAM, Nagtegaal ID, Kapiteijn E et al. Radiotherapy does not compensate for positive resection

margins in rectal cancer patients: report of a multicenter randomised trial. *Int J Radiat Oncol Biol Phys* 2003; 55: 1311–20.

37 Steele RJ, Sebag-Montefiore D. Adjuvant radiotherapy for rectal cancer. *Br J Surg* 1999; 38: 1233–52.

38 Marijnen CA, Glimelius B. The role of radiotherapy in rectal cancer. *Eur J Cancer* 2002; 38: 943–52.

39 Glimelius B, Isacsson U, Jung B, Pahlman L. Radiotherapy in addition to radical surgery in rectal cancer: evidence for a dose-response effect favoring preoperative treatment. *Int J Radiat Oncol Biol Phys* 1997; 37: 281–7.

40 Minsky BD, Conti JA, Huang Y, Knopf K. Relationship of acute gastrointestinal toxicity and the volume of irradiated small bowel in patients receiving combined modality therapy for rectal cancer. *J Clin Oncol* 1995; 13: 1409–16.

41 Hyams DM, Eleftherios PM, petrelli N *et al*. A clinical trial to evaluate the worth of preoperative multimodality therapy in patients with operable carcinoma of the rectum. A progress report of NSABP R-03. *Dis Colon Rectum* 1997; 40: 131–9.

42 Bosset JF, Calais G, Daben A *et al*. Preoperative chemoradiotherapy vs preoperative radiotherapy in rectal cancer patients: assessment of acute toxicity and treatment compliance. Report of the 22921 randomised trial conducted by the EORTC Radiotherapy Group. *Eur J Cancer* 2004; 40: 219–24.

43 Botterill ID, Blunt DM, Quirke P *et al*. Evaluation of the role of pre-operative magnetic resonance imaging in the management of rectal cancer. *Colorectal Dis* 2001; 3: 295–303.

44 Beets-Tan RGH, Beets GL, Vliegen RFA *et al*. Accuracy of magnetic resonance imaging in prediction of tumour-free resection margin in rectal cancer surgery. *Lancet* 2001; 357: 497–504.

45 Brown G, Richard CJ, Newcombe RG *et al*. Rectal Carcinoma: Thin-section MR imaging for staging in 28 patients. *Radiology* 1999; 211: 215–22.

46 Daniels I. MRI accurately predicts the CRM status of rectal cancer in a multicentre multidisciplinary European study. *Colorectal Dis* 2005; 7: 1 Abstract 001.

47 Dahlberg M, Glimelius B, Graf W, Pahlman L. Preoperative irradiation affects functional results after surgery for rectal cancer: results from a randomized study. *Dis Colon Rectum* 1998; 41: 543–9; discussion 549–51.

48 Marijnen CA, van de Velde CJ, Putter H *et al*. Impact of short-term preoperative radiotherapy on health-related quality of life and sexual functioning in primary rectal cancer: report of a multicenter randomized trial. *J Clin Oncol* 2005; 23: 1847–58.

49 Kollmorgen CF, Meagher AP, Wolff BG *et al*. Ilstrup DM. The long-term effect of adjuvant postoperative chemoradiotherapy for rectal carcinoma on bowel function. *Ann Surg* 1994; 220: 676–82.

50 Mak AC, Rich TA, Schultheiss TE *et al*. Late complications of postoperative radiation therapy for cancer of the rectum and rectosigmoid. *Int J Radiat Oncol Biol Phys* 1994; 28: 597–603.

51 Holm T, Sinnomklao T, Rutqvist LE, Cedermark B. Adjuvant preoperative radiotherapy in patients with rectal carcinoma. Adverse effects during long term follow-up of two randomized trials. *Cancer* 1996; 78: 968–76.

52 Allal AS, Gervaz P, Gertsch P *et al*. Assessment of quality of life in patients with rectal cancer treated by preoperative radiotherapy: a longitudinal prospective study. *Int J Radiat Oncol Biol Phys* 2005; 61: 1129–35.

53 NIH consensus conference. Adjuvant therapy for patients with colon and rectal cancer. *JAMA* 1990; 264: 1444–50.

54 Wolmark N, Wieand HS, Hyams DM *et al*. Randomized trial of postoperative adjuvant chemotherapy with or without radiotherapy for carcinoma of the rectum: National Surgical Adjuvant Breast and Bowel Project Protocol R-02. *J Natl Cancer Inst* 2000; 92: 388–96.

55 Dahlberg M, Glimelius B, Pahlman L. Improved survival and reduction in local failure rates after preoperative radiotherapy: evidence for the generalisability of the results of Swedish Rectal Cancer Trial. *Ann Surg* 1999; 229: 493–7.

56 Marr R, Birbeck K, Garvican J *et al.* The modern abdominoperineal excision: the next challenge after total mesorectal excision. *Ann Surg* 2005; 242: 74–82.

57 Frykholm GJ, Pahlman L, Glimelius B. Combined chemo- and radiotherapy vs radiotherapy alone in the treatment of primary, nonresectable adenocarcinoma of the rectum. *Int J Radiat Oncol Biol Phys* 2001; 50: 427–34.

58 Landry JC, Koretz MJ, Wood WC *et al.* Preoperative irradiation and fluorouracil chemotherapy for locally advanced rectosigmoid carcinoma: phase I–II study. *Radiology* 1993; 188: 423–6.

59 Minsky BD, Cohen AM, Enker WE *et al.* Preoperative 5-FU, low-dose leucovorin, and radiation therapy for locally advanced and unresectable rectal cancer. *Int J Radiat Oncol Biol Phys* 1997; 37: 289–95.

60 Mohiuddin M, Regine WF, John WJ *et al.* Preoperative chemoradiation in fixed distal rectal cancer: dose time factors for pathological complete response. *Int J Radiat Oncol Biol Phys* 2000; 46: 883–8.

61 Rich TA, Skibber JM, Ajani JA *et al.* Preoperative infusional chemoradiation therapy for stage T3 rectal cancer. *Int J Radiat Oncol Biol Phys* 1995; 32: 1025–9.

62 Videtic GM, Fisher BJ, Perera FE *et al.* Preoperative radiation with concurrent 5-fluorouracil continuous infusion for locally advanced unresectable rectal cancer. *Int J Radiat Oncol Biol Phys* 1998; 42: 319–24.

63 Dunst J, Reese T, Sutter T *et al.* Phase I trial evaluating the concurrent combination of radiotherapy and capecitabine in rectal cancer. *J Clin Oncol* 2002; 20: 3983–91.

64 Ngan SY, Michael M, Mackay J *et al.* A phase I trial of preoperative radiotherapy and capecitabine for locally advanced, potentially resectable rectal cancer. *Br J Cancer* 2004; 91: 1019–24.

65 Sebag-Montefiore D, Hingorani M, Cooper R, Chesser P. Circumferential resection margin status predicts outcome after pre-operative chemoradiation for locally advanced rectal cancer. *J Clin Oncol* 2005 (Proceedings of GI ASCO symposium): p. 180. Abstract 193.

66 Mawdsley S, Glynne-Jones R. The importance of pathological downstaging and a negative circumferential margin in rectal carcinomas treated with neoadjuvant chemoradiation. *J Clin Oncol* 2005; Proceedings of GI ASCo symposium: p.189. Abstract 211.

67 Sebag-Montefiore D, Glynne-Jones R, Mortensen N *et al.* Pooled analysis of outcome measures including the histopathological R0 resection rater after pre-operative chemoradiation for locally advanced rectal cancer. *Colorectal Dis* 2005; 7: abstract 020.

68 Douillard JY, Cunningham D, Roth AD *et al.* Irinotecan combined with fluorouracil compared with fluorouracil alone as first-line treatment for metastatic colorectal cancer: a multicentre randomised trial. *Lancet* 2000; 355: 1041–7.

69 de Gramont A, Figer A, Seymour M *et al.* L Leucovorin and fluorouracil with or without oxaliplatin as first-line treatment in advanced colorectal cancer. *J Clin Oncol* 2000; 18: 2938–47.

70 Saltz LB, Cox JV, Blanke C *et al.* Irinotecan plus fluorouracil and leucovorin for metastatic colorectal cancer. Irinotecan Study Group [see comment]. *N Engl J Med* 2000; 343: 905–14.

71 Hurwitz H, Fehrenbacher L, Novotny W, Cartwright T, Hainsworth J, Heim W, Berlin J, Baron A, Griffing S, Holmgren E, Ferrara N, Fyfe G, Rogers B, Ross R, Kabbinavar F. Bevacizumab plus Irinotecan, Fluorouracil, and Leucovorin for Metastatic Colorectal Cancer. *N Engl J Med* 2004; 350: 2335–42.

72 Cunningham D, Humblet Y, Siena S *et al.* Cetuximab Monotherapy and Cetuximab plus Irinotecan in Irinotecan-Refractory Metastatic Colorectal Cancer. *N Engl J Med* 2004; 351: 337–345.

73 Glynne-Jones R, Sebag-Montefiore D. Chemoradiation schedules – what radiotherapy? *Eur J Cancer* 2002; 38: 258–69.

74 Sebag-Montefiore D, Falk S, Glynne-Jones R *et al.* Preoperative radiation and irinotecan in combination with 5fluorouracil and low dose leucovorin in locally advanced rectal cancer. *J Clin Oncol* 2005; 23(Proceedings of ASCO 2005): p.265s. Abstract 2576.

75 Glynne-Jones R, Sebag-Montefiore D, Samuel L *et al.* Socrates phase II study results: capecitabine combined with oxalilatin and pre-operative radiation in patients with locally advanced rectal cancer. *J Clin Oncol* 2005; 23(Proceedings of ASCO 2005): p.252s. Abstract 3527.

76 Francois Y, Nemaz CJ, Baulieux J *et al.* Influence of the interval between preoperative radiation therapy and surgery on downstaging and on the rate of sphincter-sparing surgery for rectal cancer: the Lyon R90–01 randomized trial. *J Clin Oncol* 1999; 17: 2396–2402.

77 Grann A, Feng C, Wong D *et al.* Preoperative combined modality therapy for clinically resectable uT3 rectal adenocarcinoma. *Int J Radiat Oncol Biol Phys* 2001; 49: 987–95.

78 Janjan NA, Khoo VS, Abbruzzese J *et al.* Tumor downstaging and sphincter preservation with preoperative chemoradiation in locally advanced rectal cancer: the M. D. Anderson Cancer Center experience. *Int J Radiat Oncol Biol Phys* 1999; 44: 1027–38.

79 Mohiuddin M, Regine WF, Marks GJ, Marks JW. High-dose preoperative radiation and the challenge of sphincter-preservation surgery for cancer of the distal 2 cm of the rectum. *Int J Radiat Oncol Biol Phys* 1998; 40: 569–74.

80 Gerard JP, Chapet O, Nemoz C *et al.* Improved sphincter preservation in low rectal cancer with high-dose preoperative radiotherapy: the lyon R96–02 randomized trial. *J Clin Oncol* 2004; 22: 2404–9.

81 Niebel W, Schulz U, Ried M *et al.* Five year results of a prospective randomized study: experience with combined radiotherapy and surgery for primary rectal carcinoma. *Recent Results Cancer Res* 1988; 110: 111–13.

82 Marsh PJ, James RD, Schofield PF. Adjuvant pre-operative radiotherapy for locally advanced rectal carcinoma: results of a prospective randomized trial. *Dis Colon Rectum* 1994; 37: 1205–14.

9: Current challenges in the adjuvant therapy of colon cancer

George P. Kim and Axel Grothey

Introduction

Over the past several years, significant advances have been made in the treatment of colorectal cancer (CRC) patients with metastatic disease. The introduction of oxaliplatin and irinotecan and their preferential use with infusional 5-fluorouracil (5-FU) has nearly doubled the survival in this patient population. The incorporation of biologic agents such as bevacizumab and cetuximab into treatment regimens provides additional improvements in response and survival. The benefits seen in patients with stage IV disease consequently led to exploration of these novel agents in earlier stage disease such as with stage II and III patients. These ongoing trials will likely translate into greater numbers of patients being cured and further reductions in overall mortality. The present challenge is to thoroughly assess these agents and predict which patients benefit most from which treatment.

The most pertinent issues to consider in the adjuvant treatment of CRC are:

- How is 5-FU best administered in the adjuvant setting?
- What survival outcome should be the primary endpoint for adjuvant colorectal trials?
- What is the role of oxaliplatin in the adjuvant setting?
- Should irinotecan be used in adjuvant treatment?
- What is the role of capecitabine in stage III colon cancer adjuvant treatment?
- Should stage II colon cancer patients receive treatment?
- Does microsatellite instability predict which patients will benefit from adjuvant treatment?
- Should the biologic agents cetuximab or bevacizumab be added to treatment regimens?

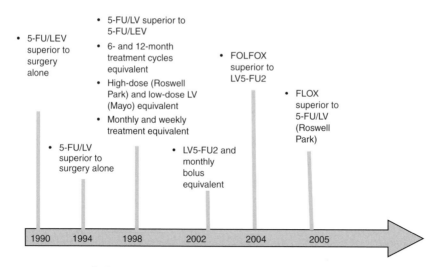

Fig. 9.1 History of adjuvant therapy of colon cancer.

How is 5-FU best administered in the adjuvant setting?

The importance of systemic chemotherapy in improving patient survival was demonstrated in a series of studies combining 5-FU with leucovorin (LV) or levamisole (LEV) (Fig. 9.1). The United States Intergroup 035 study is of historic importance as it reported a 41% reduction in the relapse rate ($p < 0.0001$) and a decrease in overall cancer mortality by 33% ($p = 0.0007$) [1,2]. This study led a National Institutes of Health consensus panel to recommend that 5-FU-based adjuvant therapy be administered to all resected stage III colon cancer patients. In this trial, 929 patients with stage III colon cancer were randomly assigned to receive either surgery alone or surgery followed by 12 months of 5-FU (bolus 450 mg/m^2 intravenously daily for 5 days and then, beginning at 28 days, weekly for 48 weeks) and the antihelminthic LEV (50 mg orally three times/day for 3 days, repeated every 2 weeks for 1 year). A third arm included treatment with LEV alone but demonstrated no activity. After a median follow-up of 6.5 years, the 5-year survival in the 5-FU/LEV patients was 60.2 vs 46.7% in the surgery alone arm. The trial also included 318 stage II patients with the 5-FU/LEV patients experiencing a 31% reduction in recurrence rate (79 vs 71%, $p = 0.01$) and a similar 72% 5-year survival as their surgery alone counterparts [3].

The Intergroup 0089 trial is a landmark study that established the equivalence of the Mayo Clinic and Roswell Park regimens and also determined the duration of postoperative treatment [4]. Three thousand, seven hundred and fifty-nine stage II or III patients were randomized to one of four arms – 5-FU LEV, Mayo Clinic regimen (5-FU 425 mg/m^2 and LV 20 mg/m^2 for five consecutive days, repeated every 28 days for six cycles), Roswell Park regimen (5-FU 500 mg/m^2 and LV 500 mg/m^2 weekly for 6 weeks, repeated every 8 weeks for four cycles), and the Mayo regimen with LEV. The results demonstrated similar disease-free and overall 5-year survival among all four arms. In the stage III patients, the two 5-FU/LV containing schedules (Mayo Clinic and Roswell Park) were equivalent while the three-drug regimen, 5-FU/LV and levamisole, had more associated toxicity. The 5-FU/LEV arm was effective but, because of its 12-month schedule, was considered less favorable than the 6-month 5-FU/LV regimens. This trial established the standard practice for the adjuvant treatment of stage III colon cancer in the United States for many years.

The QUASAR trial from the United Kingdom confirmed the equivalence of various 5-FU-based schedules in the adjuvant setting [5]. In this large, multi-arm trial with 4927 patients, no difference in efficacy was found between weekly bolus 5-FU/LV and the bolus 5-FU/LV Mayo Clinic schedule. Likewise, higher-dose LV did not produce extra benefit compared with lower dose, and finally, the use of LEV was not associated with better outcome.

Another 5-FU and LV combination evaluated in the adjuvant setting involves the administration of 5-FU as a continuous infusion [6]. This LV5-FU2 regimen developed in France consists of a 2-h LV injection followed by a 5-FU bolus and then a 22-h 5-FU continuous infusion. Treatment is given on days 1 and 2 and repeated every 14 days. A study comparing the LV5-FU2 with a modified Mayo Clinic regimen (bolus 5-FU/LV) in 905 stage II (43%) and III (57%) patients has been reported. The survival endpoints were similar in both arms and toxicity trended in favor of the LV5-FU2 regimen. After 6 years of follow-up, the 5-year overall survival rates were an identical 80% for both LV5-FU2 and 5-FU/LV. Similarly, no difference in disease-free survival (DFS) was seen (67.2% LV5-FU2 and 67.7% 5-FU/LV). Survival outcomes were the same with the two regimens in stage II as well as stage III patients. Importantly, overall grade 3/4 toxicities were significantly lower in the LV-FU2 patients than in the 5FU/LV group (11 vs 26%, $p = 0.001$). In particular, neutropenia (7 vs 16%), diarrhea (4 vs 9%), and mucositis (2 vs 7%) were less frequent in the LV5-FU2 arm (all $p < 0.001$) with nausea and emesis also trending in favor of the continuous infusion approach ($p = 0.093$). Accounting for an underpowered statistical analysis, the conclusion from the study is that the LV5-FU2 regimen is a comparable alternative to bolus 5-FU/LV approaches in the adjuvant treatment of colon cancer.

These trials clearly establish a role for LV-modulated 5-FU in the adjuvant treatment of colorectal cancer. All evaluated 5-FU/LV regimens produce an improvement in survival over surgical resection alone in stage III patients. The schedules are likely similar in terms of survival outcomes although different but manageable side effects are seen. Future trials and advances in the adjuvant setting focused on improving the outcomes over 5-FU/LV alone.

What survival outcome should be the primary endpoint for adjuvant colorectal trials?

The measurement of success for a given chemotherapy regimen in the adjuvant treatment of CRC is the percentage of patients alive at 5 years – the 5-year overall survival rate (OS). The limitation of this endpoint is the length of time required for follow-up and the potential delays in drug approval and availability that this creates. In an effort to identify alternative endpoints to OS, Sargent and colleagues explored the role of disease free survival (DFS) [7]. Available data from eighteen randomized phase III clinical trials (total of 20,898 patients) from 1977 to 1999, that included at least one arm with a 5-FU-based regimen, was compiled. In the by-study-arm analysis, the relationship between the DFS rate after 3 years of median follow-up and the 5-year OS rate was shown to have a R^2 value of 0.85 from a weighted linear regression (Fig. 9.2). The Spearman rank correlation coefficient between DFS and OS was 0.88. Similar findings for the relationship between within-study hazard ratios comparing experimental vs control arms for DFS and OS were found (R^2 value – 0.90; the Spearman rank correlation coefficient – 0.94). These data demonstrate a consistent association between DFS and OS. This permits DFS to be used as a primary endpoint in future colorectal trials, as statistically significant observed differences in DFS, assessed after 3 years, correlate with 5-year OS. Based on these findings and the notion that a longer time to recurrence is of inherent value to the patient, the FDA recognized 3-year DFS as appropriate endpoint for full approval of a regimen in adjuvant colon cancer.

What is the role of oxaliplatin in the adjuvant setting?

The superior efficacy of oxaliplatin and 5-FU regimens in the treatment of advanced CRC provided the rationale for trials assessing oxaliplatin-based

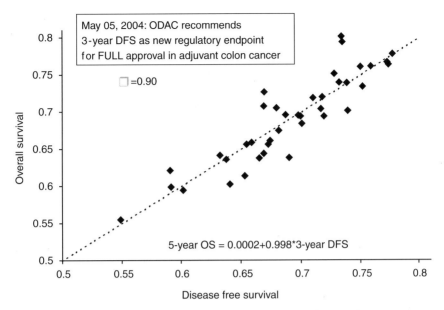

Fig. 9.2 Three-year DFS vs 5-year OS. (Reprinted from Sargent *et al.* [7], with permission from the American Society of Clinical Oncology.)

combination regimens in the adjuvant setting. A large trial conducted in Europe used an oxaliplatin/5-FU/LV regimen as adjuvant therapy for stage II and III colon cancer [8] (Table 9.1). The MOSAIC trial randomized 2246 patients with stage II and III colon cancer to receive either 6 months of LV5-FU2 (bolus plus infusional 5-FU/LV) or FOLFOX4 (oxaliplatin 85 mg/m^2 on day 1 only with bolus 5-FU 400 mg/m^2 and LV 200 mg/m^2 followed by 5-FU 600 mg/m^2 as a 22-h continuous infusion on days 1 and 2. Cycles repeated every 2 weeks). FOLFOX4 was found to be superior to LV5-FU2 in terms of 3-year DFS, a parameter which is highly predictive of 5-year OS. A combined analysis for stage II and III patients demonstrated a 23% risk reduction for 3-year recurrence (hazard ratio [HR] 0.77, 95% confidence interval [CI] 0.65–0.91, $p = 0.002$). DFS after 3 years was 78.2% in the FOLFOX4 arm and 72.9% in the LV5-FU2 arm. An updated DFS analysis at 4 years has recently been reported at the American Society of Clinical Oncology (ASCO) meeting in 2005, and FOLFOX4 continues to demonstrate about a 24% reduction in relapse ($p = 0.0008$) [9]. However, a stage-based subgroup analysis showed that the difference in DFS was significant only for stage III patients (3-year DFS 72.2 vs 65.3%; HR 0.76, CI 0.62–0.92) and not for stage II (87.0 vs 84.3%; HR 0.80, CI 0.56–1.15). As with previously reported studies with stage II patients, this result can be attributed to the study being statistically underpowered.

Table 9.1 Efficacy results of recent adjuvant trials.

Study	Stage	N pts	Arms	3-year DFS	DFS Δ%	P-value/HR (95% CI)
Oxaliplatin-based						
MOSAIC* [8,9] (N = 2246)	II/III	1123 1123	LV5FU2 FOLFOX4		6.6	p < 0.001 HR 0.77 (0.65–0.90)
	II	448 451	LV5FU2 FOLFOX4		3.5	HR 0.82 (0.60–1.13)
	High Risk II	290 286	LV5FU2 FOLFOX4		5.4	HR 0.76
	III	675 672	LV5FU2 FOLFOX4		8.6	HR 0.75 (0.62–0.89)
NSABP C-07 [10] (N = 2407)	II/III	1207 1200	Roswell Park FLOX	71.6 76.5	4.9	p < 0.004 HR 0.79 (0.67–0.93)
Irinotecan-based						
CALGB 89803 [14] (N = 1264)	III	629 635	Roswell Park IFL			p = 0.89
PETACC3 [15] (N = 3005)	II/III	1509 1496	LV5FU2 FOLFIRI	66.8 69.6	2.8	HR 0.88 (0.77–1.00)
	II	451 443	LV5FU2 FOLFIRI	82.0 84.8	2.8	HR 0.80 (0.58–1.11)
	III	1058 1053	LV5FU2 FOLFIRI	60.3 63.3	3.0	p = 0.091 HR 0.89 (0.77–1.11)
ACCORD [16] (N = 400)	High Risk III	200 200	LV5FU2 FOLFIRI	60 51	−9.0	p = 0.22 HR 1.19 (0.90–1.59)
Capecitabine-based						
X-ACT [19] (N = 1987)	III	983 1004	Mayo Clinic Capecitabine	61.0 64.6	3.6	p = 0.0525 HR 0.87 (0.75–1.00)

*MOSAIC data after median follow-up of 56 months.
HR – hazard ratio.

The main side effect of FOLFOX4 was anticipated sensory neuropathy with grade 3 toxicity affecting 12.4% of patients overall and 18% of patients that received the entire planned 1020 mg/m^2 dose of oxaliplatin. However, the neurotoxicity proved reversible in the vast majority of patients so that 12 and 18 months after discontinuation of therapy only 1.1 and 0.5%

of patients, respectively, had residual grade 3 neurotoxicity. Based on the results of the MOSIAC trial, FOLFOX4 has emerged as the new standard of care in the adjuvant treatment of stage III and high-risk stage II patients.

Another study conducted by the National Surgical Adjuvant Breast and Bowel Project (NSABP C-07), and reported at the ASCO meeting in 2005, supports the importance of oxaliplatin in the adjuvant setting [10]. In this study, 2407 stage II and III patients were randomized to either 5-FU/LV (500 mg/m^2 of both given weekly for 6 weeks followed by 2 weeks rest for 3 cycles) versus the same 5-FU/LV regimen and oxaliplatin (FLOX). The oxaliplatin was administered at 85 mg/m^2 every 2 weeks but only on weeks 1, 3, and 5 of the 8-week cycle (cumulative dose 765 mg/m^2). Seventy-three percent of patients received the planned oxaliplatin treatment. The primary endpoint, 3-year DFS, favored the FLOX arm (76.5 vs 71.6%) with a HR of 0.79 ($p = 0.004$). Importantly, the regimen was tolerable, as grade 3 and 4 toxicities were similar in the two arms (Gr 3/4 – 50%/10% FLOX vs 41%/9% 5-FU/LV). Only 8% of patients experienced grade 3 neurotoxicity, and after 12 months, this decreased to 0.5% of patients. Enteritis leading to diarrhea and dehydration was higher in the experimental arm (4.5 vs 2.7%). Additional efficacy and toxicity data are awaited to fully define whether FLOX is as effective but more tolerable than FOLFOX.

The results from these phase III adjuvant trials clearly demonstrate the superiority of oxaliplatin-containing arms over conventional 5-FU/LV controls (Table 9.2). The decision to use the FOLFOX4 or the FLOX schedule remains unclear. An additional factor to consider is whether a modified regimen, FOLFOX6, which omits the day 2 bolus 5-FU/LV and increases the continuous infusion dose, is equivalent to conventional FOLFOX4. The Tournigand study in advanced disease which showed equivalence in the use of infusional 5-FU regimens with either oxaliplatin or irinotecan supports the use of FOLFOX6 (oxaliplatin at 100 mg/m^2 every 2 weeks) [11]. Modified FOLFOX6 (mFOLFOX6: oxaliplatin at 85 mg/m^2 every 2 weeks) is currently being used as standard arm in all ongoing cooperative group studies in the United States (Intergroup/NCCTG N0147 and NSABP C-08) so that eventually cautious historical comparisons between mFOLFOX6 and FOLFOX4 can be made.

Should irinotecan be used in adjuvant treatment?

In the 1990s, the topoisomerase I inhibitor, irinotecan, was found to have significant activity in advanced colorectal cancer [12]. Irinotecan combined

Table 9.2 Standard adjuvant therapy in colon cancer

- FOLFOX remains standard adjuvant therapy in stage III and high
- FLOX is an alternative, but more toxicity data needed
- 5-FU/LV (Mayo or Roswell Park), LV5-FU2, or capecitabine or those patients who are not considered candidates for oxaliplatin
- Irinotecan-based combinations are NOT options in the adjuvant setting
- XELOX-A, bevacizumab and cetuximab are under investigation

with weekly bolus 5-FU/LV (IFL – irinotecan 125 mg/m^2 and bolus 5-FU 500 mg/m^2 with LV 20 mg/m^2 weekly for four consecutive weeks of an every 6-week cycle) significantly improved outcomes compared with Roswell Park 5-FU/LV. Positive outcomes (39% response rate [RR], 7-month time to progression, and median survival of 14.8 months) led to the FDA approval of irinotecan as first-line therapy for CRC in 2000. It is of note that at the same time IFL was found superior to bolus 5-FU/LV, a European phase III trial likewise showed that irinotecan in combination with infusional 5-FU/LV was significantly more effective than LV5-FU2 in terms of RR, PFS, and OS [13]. The consistent improvements seen in advanced disease logically led to the evaluation of irinotecan in the adjuvant setting.

The Cancer and Leukemia Group B (CALGB) 89803 trial was the first to test whether irinotecan-based chemotherapy was a valid option in adjuvant treatment [14]. This study compared the IFL regimen with a weekly 5-FU/LV (Roswell Park) control arm. Twelve hundred and sixty-four stage III patients were enrolled. Toxicity encountered in the IFL arm was significant with neutropenia (43 vs 5%), and febrile neutropenia (4 vs 1%) being significantly higher than with 5-FU/LV. In addition, early safety analysis of the trial identified an alarming increase in early treatment-related mortality for the experimental arm. Within the first 4 months of treatment, 18 deaths were seen with the IFL arm vs 6 deaths on the control arm ($p = 0.008$). Overall, 2.8% with IFL vs 1% deaths on treatment ($p = 0.008$) were reported. At a median follow-up of 3 years in each arm, no differences in either disease-free survival ($p = 0.80$) or overall survival ($p = 0.81$) were seen. Statistical analysis indicated that the futility boundaries for both of these efficacy parameters had been crossed meaning awaiting more mature data would not yield a positive outcome for either DFS or OS. The conclusion from this study was that irinotecan should not be used with bolus 5-FU in the adjuvant setting.

With the CALGB trial, the question remained whether the irinotecan or the treatment schedule contributed to the negative results. The IFL regimen uses an inferior and more toxic bolus 5-FU backbone whereas another irinotecan-based regimen, FOLFIRI, employs infusional 5-FU. FOLFIRI had demonstrated equal efficacy compared with FOLFOX in a small phase III trial in the palliative setting. Consequently, FOLFIRI was evaluated as adjuvant therapy for colon cancer and was predicted to have a positive impact. The Pan-European Trial Adjuvant Colon Cancer 3 (PETACC3) randomized 3005 stage II and III patients to FOLFIRI (irinotecan 180 mg/m^2 on day 1 only with bolus 5-FU 400 mg/m^2 and LV 200 mg/m^2 followed by 5-FU 600 mg/m^2 as a 22-h continuous infusion on days 1 and 2 [15]. Cycles repeated every 2 weeks) vs a standard 5FU/LV (LV5FU2 regimen). The primary endpoint was a 27% improvement in 3-year DFS with 2014 stage III patients required to achieve 90% power. Of note, an imbalance of T4 patients between the arms (17% FOLFIRI vs 13% LV5FU2, chi-squared, $p = 0.006$) was observed. The treatment was fairly well-tolerated with no increase in the 60-day all cause mortality although grade 3/4 neutropenia, neutropenic infection, and diarrhea were greater in the FOLFIRI arm. Unfortunately, in contrast to expectations, FOLFIRI failed to demonstrate superiority over the control arm in 3-year DFS in stage III patients (63.3 vs 60.3%, $p = 0.091$, HR 0.89 [0.77–1.11]). Only with adjustments for the T-stage imbalances was a borderline significant 3-year DFS result achieved (65.2 vs 60.4%, $p = 0.021$, HR 0.85). The PETACC3 study supported the conclusion that irinotecan had no role in the adjuvant treatment of colon cancer.

The final trial to consider in deciding to incorporate irinotecan in the adjuvant setting is the French ACCORD02/FFCD9802 trial which used the same treatment arms, LV5FU2, and FOLFIRI, as the PETACC3 study [16]. This trial focused on the impact of irinotecan on high-risk stage III colon cancer (N2 disease or N1 with tumors causing obstruction or perforation). The primary endpoint was 3-year DFS (improvement from 45 to 60% or HR > 0.64, 85% power) and 400 patients were enrolled. Oddly, an imbalance in T4 patients was again observed (31.2 FOLFIRI vs 22.7%, $p = 0.015$). After 46 months of follow-up, an inferior DFS with FOLFIRI was seen (51 vs 60%, $p = 0.22$, HR 1.19 [0.90–1.59]). This study in combination with the disappointing experiences with the CALGB and PETACC3 trials leads to the conclusion that irinotecan-based chemotherapy regimens are not a valid option in the adjuvant treatment of CRC.

What is the role of capecitabine in stage III colon cancer adjuvant treatment?

It is well-established that the anti-neoplastic activity of 5-FU is enhanced with protracted intravenous infusion. Unfortunately, this approach requires the placement of a central venous catheter device to enable treatment in the out-patient setting. Oral formulations of fluoropyrimidines mimic prolonged infusion of 5-FU and are more convenient without compromising clinical efficacy. Capecitabine is an oral fluoropyrimidine that undergoes a three-step enzymatic conversion to 5-FU with the final conversion catalyzed by the enzyme, thymidine phosphorylase [17]. This enzyme is preferentially expressed in tumor cells and has angiogenic properties.

A combined analysis of two randomized phase III trials including 1207 patients with metastatic disease demonstrated that capecitabine at a dose of 1250 mg/m^2 twice daily for 2 out of 3 weeks is as effective and less toxic than bolus 5-FU/LV, Mayo Clinic schedule [18]. Capecitabine was superior in terms of RR (25.7 vs 16.7%, $p < 0.0002$), although no differences were observed in TTP (capecitabine 4.6 vs 5-FU/LV 4.7 months; $p = 0.9535$) and OS (12.9 vs 12.8 months; $p = 0.48$). This combined analysis clearly establishes capecitabine as an equipotent and less toxic, oral alternative to LV-modulated, bolus 5-FU.

The role of capecitabine in the adjuvant setting has been defined by the most informative postoperative trial to date, the X-ACT study [19]. In this trial of stage III patients, a similar equivalence in efficacy and safety with capecitabine (1250 mg/m^2 days 1–14, every 3 weeks for 24 weeks) compared to the Mayo Clinic bolus regimen was demonstrated. This multinational trial of 1987 patients showed that capecitabine was at least equally effective compared with bolus 5-FU/LV. In fact, a trend towards superiority in terms of 3-year DFS (HR 0.87, 95% CI 0.75–1.00, $p = 0.0528$; 64.2 vs 60.6%) and OS (HR 0.84, 95% CI 0.69–1.01, $p = 0.0706$; 81.3 vs 77.6%) was observed. More mature data at 51 months of follow-up reveals persistence of the better DFS for capecitabine with an absolute difference at 3 years of 3.6%. Significantly less grade 3/4 neutropenia, stomatitis, and neutropenic fever/sepsis were seen with capecitabine vs 5-FU/LV.

A critical issue that remains unsettled is whether capecitabine can serve as a substitute for the infusional 5-FU/LV schedule that is an integral component of contemporary regimens using oxaliplatin (FOLFOX). Several phase II trials have reported a reasonable safety profile and significant activity of capecitabine/oxaliplatin combinations in the treatment of advanced CRC [20]. The results of ongoing phase III trials with metastatic patients comparing capecitabine-based combination protocols with infusional 5-FU/LV plus oxaliplatin are awaited. Similarly, adjuvant trials with capecitabine and oxaliplatin are ongoing. The XELOXA study compares the XELOX regimen (oxaliplatin 130 mg/m^2 and 1000 mg/m^2 capecitabine every 21 days for 8 cycles) to bolus 5-FU/LV regimens (either the Mayo Clinic or Roswell Park schedules) [21]. Early safety findings from the trial reveal acceptable side effects overall with grade 3/4 adverse events being reported in 39.3%/5.9%, respectively, within the XELOX cohort and 33.2%/8.9%, respectively, with the 5-FU/LV patients. There is less neutropenia (8 vs 15%) and stomatitis (8 vs <1%) with XELOX but, as expected, greater incidence of hand–foot syndrome (5 vs <1%) and neurotoxicity (11 vs 0%). This study is likely to demonstrate a benefit with the XELOX arm but whether the oxaliplatin or the capecitabine exert greater influence on this outcome will not be resolved. The true test will be a comparison of this capecitabine/oxaliplatin regimen with its infusional 5-FU/LV-based counterparts. If equivalence or superiority is seen in the metastatic trials and if the XELOXA trial is indeed positive without identifying any ominous side effects, then capecitabine will be declared the new 5-FU backbone for these regimens and become the new standard-of-care. The XELOX regimen is further explored in the ongoing AVANT trial in combination with bevacizumab.

Should stage II colon cancer patients receive treatment?

Despite an approximate 75% 5-year survival with surgery alone, some stage II patients have a higher risk of relapse, with outcomes similar to those of node-positive patients. Adjuvant chemotherapy in stage III patients provides at least a 33% overall survival advantage, resulting in an absolute treatment benefit of roughly 8%. Several analyses have reported varying outcomes in stage II patients who received adjuvant treatment.

• The NSABP summary of protocols (C-01 to C-04) with 1565 patients with stage II disease reported a 32% reduction in mortality (cumulative odds, 0.68; 95% CI, 0.50–0.92; $p = 0.01$) [22]. This reduction in mortality translated into an absolute survival advantage of 5%.
• A meta-analysis by Erlichman and colleagues detected a non-significant 2% benefit (82 vs 80%, $p = 0.217$) in 1020 patients with high risk T3 and T4 patients treated with 5-FU/LV for five consecutive days [23].

• Schrag reviewed Medicare claims for chemotherapy within the SEER Database and identified 3151 resected stage II patients in which 27% received adjuvant treatment [24]. No survival benefit with 5-FU vs surgery alone (78 vs 75%; HR 0.91; 95% CI, 0.77 to 1.09). Patients with T4 lesions, obstruction, or perforation were excluded from this analysis but 33% with these characteristics received treatment.

• In the MOSAIC study [8], a benefit from FOLFOX4 chemotherapy was seen in stage II patients albeit this was not statistically significant (86.6 vs 83.9% 5FU/LV; HR 0.82 [0.57–1.17], risk reduction, 18%).

• The Quasar Collaborative Group study reported an overall survival benefit of 1–5% in 3239 patients (92% Dukes' B) randomized to chemotherapy vs surgery alone [25]. With a median follow-up of 4.6 years, risk of death (5-year survival 80.3 vs 77.4%, $p = 0.02$, HR 0.83, 95%CI 0.71–0.91) and recurrence rate (recurrence-free survival 77.8 vs 73.8%, $p = 0.001$, HR 0.78, 95%CI 0.67–0.91) favored 5-FU/LV chemotherapy.

• The American Society of Clinical Oncology Panel recently concluded that the routine use of adjuvant chemotherapy for stage II patients could not be recommended [26]. A review of 37 randomized controlled trials and 11 meta-analyses found no evidence of a statistically significant survival benefit with postoperative treatment. For specific subsets of patients (T4 lesions, perforation, poorly differentiated histology, or inadequately sampled nodes), treatment needed to be considered and patient input was critical.

Does microsatellite instability predict which patients will benefit from adjuvant treatment?

Microsatellite instability is one of two forms of genetic instability contributing to colon carcinogenesis [27]. High-degree microsatellite instability (MSI-H) is observed in approximately 15% of non-hereditary patients and is the consequence of a defective DNA mismatch repair (MMR) system. Typically, the proteins MLH1 and MSH2 are lost and their absence leads to decreased DNA repair, anti-apoptosis and drug resistance [28–30]. Preclinical studies revealed specific resistance to 5-FU creating the dilemma of whether administration of 5-FU-based adjuvant treatment is potentially detrimental to MSI-H patients [31,32]. Several groups of investigators have evaluated the predictive role of MSI-H in the context of 5-FU treatment and reported contrasting results. One group of researchers reported a clear

Table 9.3 High-degree microsatellite instability (MSI-H) as predictor of outcome from adjuvant therapy.

Study	% MSI-H pts	5-year OS	Outcome P-value HR or RR (95% CI)
Watanabe *et al.* [37]	21	74 vs 46% MSI-H/TGF-β mutated 5-FU treatment	$p = 0.03$ RR 2.90* (1.14–7.35)
		74 vs 50% MSS/18q loss 5-FU treatment	$p = 0.006$ RR 2.75 (1.34–5.65)
Elsaleh *et al.* [34]	20	90 vs 35% MSI-H- 5-FU treatment	$p = 0.0007$ HR 0.07 (0.01–0.53)
Elsaleh *et al.* [33]	20	NR MSI-H/mutant p53 5-FU treatment	$p = 0.023$ RR 0.65 (SE 0.122)
Ribic *et al.* [35]	16.7	88.0 vs 68.4% MSI-H-surgery alone	$p = 0.004$ HR 0.31 (0.14–0.72)
		70.7 vs 88.0% MSI-H-5-FU treatment	$p = 0.10$ HR 2.17 (0.84–5.55)
Kim *et al.* [30]	18	NR MSI-H-5FU treatment	$p = 0.51$ HR 0.82 (0.44-1.50)
		RFS MSI-H/mutant p53 5-FU treatment	$p = 0.24$ HR 0.41

* Relative risk for control arm.
TGF-β – transforming growth factor beta; NR – not reported;
SE – standard error; RFS – relapse free survival.

survival benefit in MSI-H patients treated with 5-FU and LEV for 6 months [33,34] (Table 9.3). A second study using an international cohort of patients demonstrated a lack of survival benefit in MSI-H patients treated with post-operative 5-FU while those with microsatellite stability (MSS) derived the anticipated benefit from the use of adjuvant chemotherapy [35]. A National Cancer Institute-NSABP collaborative analysis of patients enrolled in the

NSABP C-01 through C-04 trials failed to identify any interaction between 5-FU/LV therapy and MSI status [36]. This analysis is noteworthy as a direct comparison was made between patients treated with surgery alone vs receiving 5-FU-based adjuvant treatment. In addition, MSI-H correlation with thymidylate synthase was studied although no interaction was detected. Similar to laboratory reports and retrospective clinical series [37], an inverse relationship with mutated p53 was seen and, in conjunction with MSS status, portended a poor outcome.

Based on these studies with varying conclusions, the routine use of MSI-H in treatment decision-making cannot be recommended. In addition, the importance of MSI-H status is further brought into question in the era of oxaliplatin-based regimens. One should recall that oxaliplatin circumvents the DNA MMR system [38], which governs platinum resistance in colorectal cell lines, and the resultant anti-tumor activity in this historically platinum-resistant cancer was the main reason for its clinical development. This means that oxaliplatin-DNA adducts do not elicit the same anti-apoptosis and drug resistance pathways, and thus sensitivity to oxaliplatin and MSI-H status are independent of one another. Another hesitation in the routine use of MSI-H status is that no data is available to suggest how MSI-H patients will do with targeted agents such as cetuximab and bevacizumab. In reviewing preclinical studies, no relationship between the EGFR or VEGFR pathways and MSI has been reported.

In an effort to prospectively validate the role of MSI-H in the prediction of adjuvant treatment benefit, the Eastern Cooperative Oncology Group (ECOG 5202) will decide to treat stage II patients based on their molecular marker status (Fig. 9.3). Patients will be categorized as having microsatellite or chromosomal instability (as measured by loss of 18q), the other form of genetic instability that uniformly predicts poor outcome. If patients have loss of 18q, they will receive FOLFOX treatment without or with bevacizumab

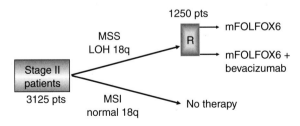

Fig. 9.3 Eastern Cooperative Oncology Group 5202 stage II high-risk.

while MSI-H patients will undergo only observation and no postoperative chemotherapy. This visionary study will answer several issues: will patients with a worse outcome due to their chromosomal instability status (18q loss) do better with the addition of bevacizumab? Will MSI-H patients do as well as non-MSI patients treated with an oxaliplatin- and bevacizumab-containing regimen? For the latter comparison, an 88% power to detect a 37% difference in median DFS (absolute difference of 5%, from 80 to 85%, at three years) is projected. Although this worthy endeavor falls short in not clarifying the straightforward question of what is the true role of MSI-H (randomization of all MSI-H patients to observation, surgery alone vs chemotherapy only), further guidance in the use of MSI-H as a predictor of postoperative chemotherapy benefit will be available.

Should the biologic agents cetuximab or bevacizumab be added to treatment regimens?

The superiority of oxaliplatin-containing arms over conventional 5-FU/LV controls is demonstrated by the MOSAIC and NSABP CO-7 phase III trials. The likelihood of an incremental survival benefit with the addition of cetuximab to these regimens is supported by intriguing phase II results showing high RRs when FOLFOX or FUFOX are combined with cetuximab [39,40] (Fig. 9.4). These studies provide an excellent rationale for using this combination in the adjuvant setting. The documented single-agent activity of cetuximab against CRC cells provides additional rationale for the use of this drug in the adjuvant setting. It is assumed that these high RRs translate

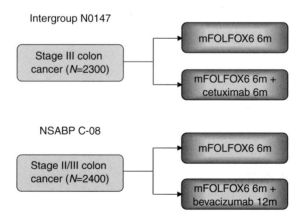

Fig. 9.4 Ongoing US cooperative group trials adjuvant therapy of colon cancer.

into greater efficacy in eradicating micrometastasis – a prerequisite for cure. The NCCTG/Intergroup is currently conducting a study (N0147) in stage III patients with modified FOLFOX6 without and with cetuximab for 6 months [41]. Modified FOLFOX6 uses an 85 mg/m^2 dose of oxaliplatin, omits the second day of bolus 5-FU/LV, and increases the dose of continuous infusion of 5-FU to 2400 mg/m^2 over 46 h. The goal is to compare the 3-year DFS between the two arms with overall survival being a secondary endpoint. A hazard ratio of 1.3 in terms of benefit is proposed in the N0147 trial.

Similar to the impressive RR seen with cetuximab, bevacizumab has clearly demonstrated its ability to impact survival – a remarkable 4.7 month overall survival benefit when combined with IFL [42]. Substantial biologic data supports the use of bevacizumab in preventing cancers from recurring through the blockade of angiogenesis essential to small tumor growth and to the promotion of metastasis. The NSABP is presently conducting a phase III trial (C-08) of a projected 2600 stage II and III patients with randomization to mFOLFOX6 or mFOLFOX6 and bevacizumab. This study also continues the bevacizumab for an additional 6 months (12 months total) as maintenance therapy. A similar trial, the AVANT trial, is being conducted in stage III colon cancer with international participation. A projected 3450 patients are being randomized to receive either FOLFOX4, FOLFOX4 plus bevacizumab, or XELOX plus bevacizumab. Similar to the NSABP design, bevacizumab will be administered for a total of 12 months. These trials are critical in defining the role of bevacizumab in the postoperative treatment setting. It is probable that the bevacizumab-containing arms will be positive which creates the future dilemma of whether to treat all patients with the additional 6-months of bevacizumab. Similarly, subsequent studies will be required to address the optimal duration of maintenance treatment; why not continue for 5 years analogous to tamoxifen in breast cancer?

Conclusions

In the past several years, the treatment of CRC has seen unprecedented advances. Median overall survivals in metastatic disease as reported in phase III trials have almost doubled and exceed the 2-year barrier. These advances are presently being applied to earlier-stage patients with the potential to increase the cure rate of these patients and force the mortality rate of this disease further downward. Oxaliplatin-based regimens (FOLFOX, FLOX) clearly have a role in this endeavor as does capecitabine. Studies

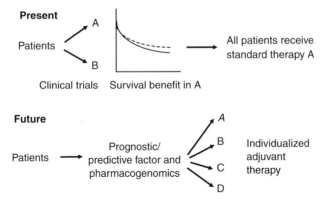

Fig. 9.5 What is the future adjuvant therapy in colon cancer? (Courtesy of Daniel Haller.)

evaluating the impact of biologic agents such as cetuximab and bevacizumab when combined with oxaliplatin will be reported in the near future and are likely to demonstrate incremental improvements in survival. In addition, exhaustive efforts by statisticians committed to reducing the suffering from CRC have led to the validation of surrogate clinical endpoints. This translates into patients having earlier access to promising newer agents. Finally, further progress in patient care will be possible with the individualization of cancer treatment through the understanding of molecular characteristics of a patient's cancer and the application of this information to predict toxicity and outcome (Fig. 9.5).

References

1 Moertel CG, Fleming TR, Macdonald JS et al. Levamisole and fluorouracil for adjuvant therapy of resected colon carcinoma. N Engl J Med 1990; 322: 352–8.

2 Moertel CG, Fleming TR, Macdonald JS et al. Fluorouracil plus levamisole as effective adjuvant therapy after resection of stage III colon carcinoma: a final report. Ann Intern Med 1995; 122: 321–6.

3 Moertel CG, Fleming TR, Macdonald JS et al. Intergroup study of fluorouracil plus levamisole as adjuvant therapy for stage II/Dukes' B2 colon cancer. J Clin Oncol 1995; 13: 2936–43.

4 Haller DG, Catalano PJ, Macdonald JS, Mayer RJ. Fluorouracil (FU), leucovorin (LV) and levamisole (LEV) adjuvant therapy for colon cancer: five-year final report of INT-0089. Proc Am Soc Clin Oncol 1998; 17: 256a: abstr. 982.

5 QUASAR Collaborative Group. Comparison of flourouracil with additional levamisole, higher-dose folinic acid, or both, as adjuvant chemotherapy for colorectal cancer: a randomised trial. Lancet 2000; 355: 1588–96.

6 Andre T, Colin P, Louvet C et al. Semimonthly versus monthly regimen of fluorouracil and leucovorin administered for 24 or 36 weeks as adjuvant therapy

in stage II and III colon cancer: results of a randomized trial. *J Clin Oncol* 2003; 21: 2896–903.

7 Sargent DJ, Wieand HS, Haller DG *et al.* Disease-free survival versus overall survival as a primary end point for adjuvant colon cancer studies: individual patient data from 20,898 patients on 18 randomized trials. *J Clin Oncol* 2005; 23: 8664–70.

8 Andre T, Boni C, Mounedji-Boudiaf L *et al.* Oxaliplatin, fluorouracil, and leucovorin as adjuvant treatment for colon cancer. *N Engl J Med* 2004; 350: 2343–51.

9 de Gramont A, Boni C, Navarro M *et al.* Oxaliplatin/5FU/LV in the adjuvant treatment of stage II and stage III colon cancer: efficacy results with a median follow-up of 4 years. *J Clin Oncol* 2005; 23: abstr. 3501.

10 Wolmark N, Wieand HS, Kuebler J *et al* A phase III trial comparing FULV to FULV + oxaliplatin in stage II or III carcinoma of the colon: results of NSABP Protocol C-07. *J Clin Oncol* 2005; 23: abstr. LBA3500.

11 Tournigand C, Andre T, Achille E *et al.* FOLFIRI Followed by FOLFOX6 or the Reverse Sequence in Advanced Colorectal Cancer: a Randomized GERCOR study. *J Clin Oncol* 2004; 22: 229–37.

12 Saltz LB, Cox JV, Blanke C *et al.* Irinotecan plus fluorouracil and leucovorin for metastatic colorectal cancer. Irinotecan Study Group. *N Engl J Med* 2000; 343: 905–14.

13 Douillard JY, Cunningham D, Roth AD *et al.* Irinotecan combined with fluorouracil compared with fluorouracil alone as first-line treatment for metastatic colorectal cancer: a multicentre randomised trial. *Lancet* 2000; 355: 1041–7.

14 Saltz LB, Niedzwiecki D, Hollis D *et al.* Irinotecan plus fluorouracil/leucovorin (IFL) versus fluorouracil/leucovorin alone (FL) in stage III colon cancer (intergroup trial CALGB C89803). *J Clin Oncol* 2004; 22: 3500.

15 Van Cutsem E, Labianca R, Hossfeld DK *et al.* Randomized phase III trial comparing infused irinotecan/5-fluorouracil (5-FU)/folinic acid (IF) versus 5-FU/FA (F) in stage III colon cancer patients (pts). (PETACC 3). *J Clin Oncol* 2005; 23: abstr. LBA8.

16 Ychou M, Raoul J, Douillard JY *et al.* A phase III randomized trial of LV5-FU2+CPT-11 vs LV5-FU2 alone in adjuvant high risk colon cancer (FNCLCC Accord02/FFCD9802). *J Clin Oncol* 2005; 23: abstr. 3502.

17 Schuller J, Cassidy J, Dumont E *et al.* Preferential activation of capecitabine in tumor following oral administration to colorectal cancer patients. *Cancer Chemother Pharmacol* 2000; 45: 291–7.

18 Van Cutsem E, Hoff PM, Harper P *et al.* Oral capecitabine vs intravenous 5-fluorouracil and leucovorin: integrated efficacy data and novel analyses from two large, randomised, phase III trials. *Br J Cancer* 2004; 90: 1190–7.

19 Twelves C, Wong A, Nowacki M *et al.* Updated efficacy findings from the X-ACT phase III trial of capecitabine (X) vs bolus 5-FU/LV as adjuvant therapy for patients (pts) with Dukes' C colon cancer. *J Clin Oncol* 2005; 23: abstr. 3521.

20 Grothey A, Jordan K, Kellner O *et al.* Capecitabine/irinotecan (CapIri) and capecitabine/oxaliplatin (CapOx) are active second-line protocols in patients with advanced colorectal cancer (ACRC) after failure of first-line combination therapy: results of a randomized phase II study. *J Clin Oncol* 2004; 22: 3534.

21 Schmoll HJ, Tabernero J, Nowacki M *et al.* Safety findings from a randomized phase III trial of capecitabine + oxaliplatin (XELOX) versus bolus 5-FU/LV as adjuvant therapy for patients (pts) with stage III colon cancer. 2006 Gastrointestinal Cancers Symposium, abs. 278.

22 Mamounas E, Wieand S, Wolmark N *et al.* Comparative efficacy of adjuvant chemotherapy in patients with Dukes' B versus Dukes' C colon cancer: results from four National Surgical Adjuvant

Breast and Bowel Project adjuvant
studies (C01, C02, C03, and C04)
[see comments]. *J Clin Oncol* 1999;
17: 1349–55.

23 IMPACT. Efficacy of adjuvant
fluorouracil and folinic acid in colon
cancer: International Multicentre Pooled
Analysis of Colon Cancer Trials
(IMPACT) investigators. *Lancet* 1995;
345: 939–44.

24 Schrag D, Rifas-Shiman S, Saltz L *et al.*
Adjuvant chemotherapy use for Medicare
beneficiaries with stage II colon cancer.
J Clin Oncol 2002; 20: 3999–4005.

25 Gray RG, Barnwell J, Hills R *et al.*
QUASAR: a randomized study of
adjuvant chemotherapy (CT) vs
observation including 3238 colorectal
cancer patients. *J Clin Oncol* 2004; 22:
abs 3501.

26 Benson AB 3rd, Schrag D, Somerfield
MR *et al.* American Society of Clinical
Oncology recommendations on adjuvant
chemotherapy for stage II colon cancer.
J Clin Oncol 2004; 22: 3408–19.

27 Lengauer C, Kinzler K, Vogelstein B.
Genetic instability in colorectal cancers.
Nature 1997; 386: 623–7.

28 Fishel R, Ewel A, Lee S, Lescoe MK,
Griffith J. Binding of mismatched
microsatellite DNA sequences by the
human MSH2 protein. *Science* 1994;
266: 1403–5.

29 Palombo F, Iaccarino I, Nakajima E *et al.*
hMutSbeta, a heterodimer of hMSH2
and hMSH3, binds to insertion/deletion
loops in DNA. *Curr Biol* 1996;
6: 1181–4.

30 Anthoney DA, McIlwrath AJ, Gallagher
WM *et al.* Microsatellite instability,
apoptosis, and loss of p53 function in
drug-resistant tumor cells. *Cancer Res*
1996; 56: 1374–81.

31 Meyers M, Wagner MW, Hwang HS
et al. Role of the hMLH1 DNA
mismatch repair protein in
fluoropyrimidine-mediated cell death and
cell cycle responses. *Cancer Res* 2001;
61: 5193–201.

32 Carethers JM, Chauhan DP, Fink D,
Nebel S *et al.* Mismatch repair
proficiency and in vitro response to

5-fluorouracil. *Gastroenterology* 1999;
117: 123–31.

33 Elsaleh H, Powell B, McCaul K, Grieu F
et al. P53 alteration and microsatellite
instability have predictive value for
survival benefit from chemotherapy in
stage III colorectal carcinoma. *Clin
Cancer Res* 2001; 7: 1343–9.

34 Elsaleh H, Joseph D, Grieu F *et al.*
Association of tumour site and sex with
survival benefit from adjuvant
chemotherapy in colorectal cancer.
Lancet 2000; 355: 1745–50.

35 Ribic CM, Sargent DJ, Moore MJ *et al.*
Tumor microsatellite-instability status as
a predictor of benefit from
fluorouracil-based adjuvant
chemotherapy for colon cancer. *N Engl J
Med* 2003; 349: 247–57.

36 Kim GP, Colangelo L, Wieand H *et al.*
Prognostic and predictive roles of
high-degree microsatellite instability
(MSI-H) in colon cancer: National
Cancer Institute (NCI)-National Surgical
Adjuvant Bowel Project (NSABP)
collaborative study. 2005
Gastrointestinal Cancers Symposium,
abstr. 227.

37 Watanabe T, Wu TT, Catalano PJ *et al.*
Molecular predictors of survival
after adjuvant chemotherapy for colon
cancer. *N Engl J Med* 2001;
344: 1196–206.

38 Fink D, Zheng H, Nebel S *et al.* In vitro
and in vivo resistance to cisplatin in cells
that have lost DNA mismatch repair.
Cancer Res 1997; 57: 1841–5.

39 Diaz Rubio E, Tabernero J, van Cutsem E
et al. Cetuximab in combination with
oxaliplatin/5-fluorouracil (5-FU)/folinic
acid (FA) (FOLFOX-4) in the first-line
treatment of patients with epidermal
growth factor receptor
(EGFR)-expressing metastatic colorectal
cancer: an international phase II study.
J Clin Oncol 2005; 23: 3535.

40 Seufferlein T, Dittrich C, Riemann J
et al. A phase I/II study of cetuximab in
combination with 5-fluorouracil
(5-FU)/folinic acid (FA) plus weekly
oxaliplatin (L-OHP) (FUFOX) in the
first-line treatment of patients with

metastatic colorectal cancer (mCRC) expressing epidermal growth factor receptor (EGFR). Preliminary results. *J Clin Oncol* 2005; 23: 3644.

41 Alberts SR, Sinicrope FA, Grothey A. N0147: a randomized phase III trial of oxaliplatin plus 5-fluorouracil/leucovorin with or without cetuximab after curative resection of stage III colon cancer. *Clin Colorectal Cancer* 2005; 5: 211–3.

42 Hurwitz H, Fehrenbacher L, Novotny W, *et al*. Bevacizumab plus irinotecan, fluorouracil, and leucovorin for metastatic colorectal cancer. *N Engl J Med* 2004; 350: 2335–42.

10: The role of the colorectal nurse specialist in the management of colorectal cancer

Jill Dean

Introduction

The role of the colorectal nurse specialist is continually evolving and each multidisciplinary Team (MDT), Unit, Hospital, or Trust has developed roles in line with local needs, priorities, and funding. Throughout this chapter you will find the words *sometimes, usually, may*, and so on in association with the responsibilities of the nurse specialist role. This is because while the core components of specialist nurse roles remain fairly standard, the way roles are implemented and the actual responsibilities for individual nurses varies enormously from unit to unit.

In my role as Lead Nurse for the Pelican National MDT Development Programme I have been in a position to discuss roles and responsibilities with colorectal nurses from all areas of the country, which has provided a unique insight. In some units nurses have developed roles with advanced responsibilities in diagnosing, breaking bad news, presenting the patient's case at MDT meetings, even chairing meetings in one area, and in coordinating the pathway, but this is not standardized in every MDT.

The aim of this chapter is to demonstrate the core clinical roles and responsibilities of a colorectal nurse specialist within the MDT and to highlight some of the advancing nursing roles in the management of colorectal cancer.

Colorectal cancer nursing

The role of the colorectal nurse specialist in the management of colorectal cancer is a relatively recent development that has evolved, mainly over the last decade, following implementation of the Calman-Hine Report [1]. This report highlighted for the first time the role specialist nurses play in the pathway of care and the need for information and support throughout the patient's journey from diagnosis onward [1]. Prior to this, the only colorectal patient groups to benefit from specialist nurses were those with either inflammatory bowel disease or stoma formation [2]. The stoma nurse remit at that time (rather sadly) only included patients with a stoma. In reality this meant a situation, for example, where a patient having an abdominoperineal excision of rectum for rectal cancer would be given preoperative and postoperative information, support, and counselling. However, a patient having surgery for a right-sided cancer would often not be referred to the nursing service, despite the fact that they might have been desperately in need of support. Clearly there was inequality of services.

However, since the government provided direction on the development of cancer services through key documents such as the Calman-Hine Report [1] and the Cancer Plan [3], the role of specialist nursing has developed specifically to support patients with colorectal cancer within the framework of the MDT. McIllmurray [4] highlights the important role specialist cancer nurses play in service provision, providing patients with regular support and advice, and in coordinating the multidisciplinary team. This is supported by the findings of a study by Bousfield [5] investigating the role of the clinical nurse specialist and suggesting that, as experienced practitioners, nurses work hard to be in a position to influence patient care by using their knowledge, expertise, and leadership skills in a multidisciplinary setting. However, an investigation by the Commission for Health Improvement suggested that as many as a quarter of Trusts did not have a nurse specialist for colorectal cancer and that 40% of the nurse specialists who were in post felt they were unable to give sufficient time to patients with colorectal cancer [6].

Development of the multidisciplinary team

It is in the development of MDT that changes in cancer service delivery are most clearly seen, where colorectal nurse specialists, surgeons, medical colleagues from cancer related disciplines, and other healthcare professionals work together as a team to deliver effective patient treatment and care. Rapid growth and sub-specialization in nursing has seen an increase in the number of roles and where, pre Calman-Hine, a single specialist nurse managed the patient caseload, most colorectal MDTs now have a team of nurses with complementary roles. However, sub-specialization has made the business of defining the role of a colorectal nurse specialist a complex affair. Two current health policy documents – Guidance on Cancer Services: Improving

Outcomes in Colorectal Cancer [7] and Manual for Cancer Services 2004: Colorectal Measures [8] – help to provide definition by outlining the core roles and responsibilities of the nurse specialist in the management of patients with colorectal cancer.

Core elements of specialist colorectal nursing roles

The core elements of colorectal nursing are included in the roles of the colorectal cancer nurse and the stoma care nurse. In some Trusts the two specialist roles are amalgamated in a dual colorectal/stoma role although other units have post holders with separate responsibilities for each aspect of the role.

Colorectal cancer nurse

The main colorectal cancer nursing role is centered on the aspect of being a "key-worker" for patients, providing information, psychological support, practical help, and clinical expertise in colorectal and stoma care nursing. Campbell and Borwell [9] sum the role up nicely by saying:

> The specialist nurse often represents a constant factor for the patient, providing ongoing support and encouragement, backed up by clinical knowledge and understanding of the individual's situation [9, p. 197]

The philosophy of a key-worker is to provide support and continuity of care for patients as they move through the different stages of a complex patient journey from home, clinic appointments, in-patient episodes (possibly in different hospitals or wards), and back home into the community. The need for a "constant factor" is reinforced in the measures for peer review where it is recommended that patients should see the same nurse both before and after surgery [7]. Colorectal nurses have a clear role in providing support, encouragement and information for patients, family, or carers, and, according to Elcoat [10], it is this level of communication that is fundamental to nursing care. Nurses are challenged to communicate and provide information to patients at times when it would be most beneficial, in a form that is acceptable and understandable, and tailored to individual patient's specific wants and needs [7].

Colorectal nurses have taken the lead in most MDTs in developing specific information booklets and leaflets to help patients and their relatives understand the disease process, pathway, surgery, and treatment options. Written information should be evidence based and tailored to the needs of the individual patient, using terminology and forms that can be easily understood [11]. Written material and forms of communication also need to take into account disability (poor vision, comprehension, etc.), language, and ethnic diversity. Individual written information including diagrams and pictures, test results, and so on to build a personal record for patients is desirable [7] and helps to reduce the volume and complexity of literature. Taking a strategic view to produce patient literature for use across cancer networks helps to standardize the information given.

A vital component of the colorectal nursing role is not only to pass on information but also to listen to, and provide psychological support and practical help for patients and relatives, and to refer appropriately to other agencies. Support and information is vital for patients, as highlighted by Wright and Myint [12] who acknowledge that following the fear and anxiety associated with a cancer diagnosis, patients have numerous adjustments to make at each stage of the journey. In response, nurses provide support for patients through a variety of means – telephone help-line, home visits, or clinic appointments – to maintain patient contact at times when it is most needed.

Colorectal nurses in some units take on the main role of "breaking bad news," discussing the diagnosis and treatment plan with patients and their relatives after decisions have been made at MDT meetings. In other units the specialist nurse is present as the doctor gives the information and then provides further support for patients and relatives.

Stoma care

Once a diagnosis is made, a treatment pathway determined, and if a stoma is a possibility, the stoma care role becomes important. According to figures from the Office for National Statistics [13] there are approximately 34,000 newly diagnosed cases of colorectal cancer annually in the United Kingdom. This figure includes 11,000 rectal cancers where there is greatest risk of stoma formation. In fact, according to Medicare Audits, in 2001 there were approximately 11,800 new colostomies with 45% temporary ones and 55% permanent ones [14]. However, advances in the management of colorectal cancer continue to reduce the number of patients requiring a permanent stoma. Surgery for rectal cancer with total mesorectal excision and the use of stapling devices now facilitate restorative resections even in cases of low rectal tumors. Due to the negative effect of a stoma on quality of life, surgeons have been urged to conserve the anal sphincter wherever possible [7]. However, in response there has been a rise in the number of temporary stomas, commonly a loop ileostomy, although alternatively a transverse loop colostomy may be formed. The benefits of one type of defunctioning stoma over another remains contentious with some studies concluding that a loop ileostomy is the stoma of choice [15–18] while other studies report in favor of a transverse loop colostomy [19,20]. Despite the configuration, and whether a stoma is temporary or permanent, all require expert stoma care nursing to minimize the effect of complications and maximize patient adaptation and recovery.

The value of expert stoma care nurses has long been acknowledged and a landmark study by Wade in 1989 [21] compared the progress of patients who had access to a stoma nurse against those who did not. The study reported that where patients had access to a stoma nurse they were

- better informed;
- a greater proportion of patients knew what to expect;
- were more satisfied with the information they were given;
- had more family involvement;
- were more expert in stoma management prior to discharge;
- were discharged earlier from hospital;
- had greater satisfaction with their stoma appliance; and
- had less appliance leakages in the early follow-up period.

Wade concludes: "All these findings were statistically significant and they are clearly nursing outcomes" [21, p. 171].

To facilitate positive outcomes stoma nurses have contact with patients in the preoperative setting either in clinic or the patient's home to discuss key topics, such as the configuration, position and output of the stoma, and the type of appliance needed. Some centers are encouraging practical stoma care instruction prior to admission to aid stoma education postoperatively and to reduce length of stay in hospital. To help with the changes to life that having a stoma brings, stoma nurses also discuss the implications of a stoma on lifestyle, employment, diet, sexuality, and body image. Some of the key issues surround preconceived myths and beliefs and the challenge of trying to change negative attitudes. Introducing the patient to someone who already has a stoma and is a positive role model can help alleviate anxieties and perceptions [7,10].

Stoma nurses have a specific responsibility in marking a suitable site for the stoma following criteria designed to improve management postoperatively and reduce postoperative complications [22]. This includes observing abdominal contours, scars from previous surgery, the proposed incision site, waistline, umbilicus, bony prominences, and skin creases, allowing the site to be marked in an appropriate place visible to the patient [10,23,24]. It is common practice to place the stoma site within the rectus abdominus muscle sheath as it is thought to offer more support to the site and possibly reduce the incidence of parastomal hernia. Parastomal hernia is one of the most problematical long-term postoperative complications, occurring in up to 50% of colostomists [25]. Prevention of parastomal hernia has long been the goal and two recent studies have had some success. The first, a study by Thompson and Trainor [26], successfully reduced the incidence of parastomal hernia through a program of postoperative interventions including instructing patients to avoid lifting for the first 3 months and from then on instigating daily abdominal exercises and an abdominal support garment. The second is a study by Janes *et al.* [24] who have shown promising results in reducing the incidence of parastomal hernia through insertion of a mesh at the time of surgery.

In the early postoperative period following stoma formation complications can occur such as necrosis, mucocutaneous dehiscence, high output, and skin problems. Stoma complications frequently need individualized complex wound and appliance systems to provide a good healing environment and a leak-free appliance. This has prompted the introduction of computerized digital photography as an education and communication tool, to ensure that high quality care can be continued despite shift patterns, and in community care, when the nurse specialist is not available [28]. Education in managing the stoma is designed to ensure a secure appliance system and speed the confidence and recovery of patients. Following discharge the stoma nurse provides continuity of care and maintains support and practical help through phone calls, home visits, and outpatient contact. The unique role of stoma specialists as they work across boundaries between hospital and community is becoming more important as the pressure to improve waiting times for treatment gathers strength and the challenge to enhance recovery and reduce length of hospital stay increases.

Colorectal nursing in the MDT meeting

Colorectal and stoma nurses have a major role to play in MDT meetings but the specifics of the role are evolving as MDT working becomes more established and support for organization and administration is increasingly provided by MDT coordinators. The shift in focus allows nurses to concentrate more on the important treatment-planning aspect of the meeting by

- presenting/contributing to discussions on patient cases,
- being an advocate for patients, and
- providing information from a nursing assessment to help inform decision making.

Increasingly colorectal nurses have a deep and expert knowledge base, both in the management of colorectal cancer and in the specialty and art of nursing, to contribute to MDT discussion and decisions.

During the process of talking to a patient about the cancer diagnosis, and the possible pathway of preoperative and postoperative chemotherapy/radiotherapy, surgery, and stoma formation, the patient will often disclose their wishes and fears. The information disclosed gives the colorectal nurse a special role as advocate in the MDT discussion, protecting and promoting the patient's interests [20], because at an MDT meeting the colorectal nurse and surgeon may be the only two people who have actually met and talked to the patient and know their wishes [29]. Nurses also assess patients continuously, and at each contact gather knowledge about physical, psychological, and social problems, helping them to anticipate how well a patient will cope and what their needs will be.

Following MDT discussions the colorectal nurse may also be the person who communicates the discussion and decisions of the meeting to the patient – preoperatively to discuss diagnosis, neoadjuvant treatment, surgery, and stoma formation and postoperatively to communicate decisions about histological staging, adjuvant therapy and the follow-up process. The role of nurse specialists within the MDT is recognized as becoming increasingly significant and according to Campbell and Borwell [9]: "The provision of a uniformly high standard of specialist nursing care and psychological support is now a requirement for all providers of cancer services" [9, p. 197].

Specialist colorectal nursing roles

The core aspects of colorectal nurse specialist roles are now enhanced by new and developing roles. Nurses have diversified in response to changes in healthcare provision and advances in the treatment of colorectal cancer.

A wide variety of innovative nursing sub-specialties now work collectively together with key role titles including

- colorectal nurse specialist,
- stoma care nurse,
- nurse endoscopist/practitioner,
- colorectal cancer nurse,
- oncology/chemotherapy nurse,
- colorectal research nurse,
- genetics nurse or family history counselor, and
- colorectal surgical assistant.

The list is almost endless with an array of different titles varying from unit to unit. While larger centers may contain a number of nurses with distinct responsibilities, local needs and funding often drive the development and emergence of more generic colorectal nursing roles encompassing aspects of several role titles. Indeed there seems to be no distinct job description for colorectal nurse specialists and no national guidelines, with the result that even when nurses have the same job title the components of the role often vary widely from unit to unit [9].

New and expanding roles

Specialist nursing roles continue to expand into new areas of practice and frequently overlap with responsibilities that traditionally have been in the remit of medical staff. However, ideally none of the roles work in isolation but function as a result of MDT working where the MDT members together develop protocols for care based on current evidence and safe practice. The process is more about deciding which member of the MDT is most appropriate to be involved with patients at each part of the pathway based on skills, training, staff availability, and cost effectiveness.

While most people see the benefits in continuity and efficiency of a multi-skilled nursing workforce there is an argument that as a result junior doctors are being de-skilled and not receiving the training and practice they require in diagnostic and practical skills [30]. However, nurses play an important role in education for health professionals of all disciplines, including medicine. As part of a cohesive team the MDT can utilize skilled nurses as educators to share expertise by teaching practical skills in the working environment or in more formal teaching sessions [31].

Nurse endoscopist/practitioners

Several new nursing roles fit the criteria of advanced/expanded role and a prime example is that of the nurse endoscopist where there is a growing workforce of nurses who have undergone extensive training. In many units nurses perform flexible sigmoidoscopy and have advanced to become skilled colonoscopists, taking on therapeutic as well as diagnostic work. A wealth of evidence shows that the expertise of nurses as colorectal endoscopists equals that of their medical colleagues [32–38].

Nurse-led "one stop" clinics

To meet demand and improve services, 50% of networks have introduced rapid access and fast-track clinics [39]. The majority of clinics are hospital based but similar services offering flexible sigmoidoscopy can also be successfully established in a primary care setting [40]. Colorectal nurse endoscopists/practitioners run nurse-led clinics and increasingly see new patients, take a history, examine, and diagnose. Depending on findings the nurse may instigate a series of outcomes to
- discharge the patient if no further action is required,
- treat minor anorectal conditions such as hemorrhoids or fissure, and
- instigate investigations or staging if more serious pathology is encountered or suspected.

Nurse-led "one stop" clinics are well established in many areas and evidence supports the expertise of nurses in this role [41,42].

Oncology colorectal nurse

As knowledge about colorectal cancer expands, management options become more complex and the role of radiotherapy and chemotherapy becomes more prominent. This has led to specialist nurses in the oncology setting where they have an increasingly important role in management, education and coordination for patients, especially those receiving chemotherapy [12]. Chemotherapy nurse specialists may be responsible for ensuring the safe administration of chemotherapeutic drugs and monitoring progress for complications [9]. Nurses play an important role in the management of specific problems such as anorexia, diarrhea, nausea/vomiting, mucositis, and fatigue. Specialist nurses support patients using interventions centered around prevention and management of problems, with practical information and advice on nutrition, hygiene, coping mechanisms, and expectations [12].

Nurse-led follow-up

Nurse-led colorectal cancer follow-up is also well established in many units. Patients attend nurse-led clinics postoperatively through the follow-up period, often for 5 years, and may not see a doctor during this time. Specialist nurses request radiology, endoscopy, and tumor-marker surveillance investigations at the appropriate time and review results. If recurrent or metastatic disease is suspected or diagnosed the nurse will ensure the case is discussed at the MDTM and that decisions are communicated and explained to the patient and their family, informing them of the diagnosis and treatment plan.

Support for advancing nursing roles

Nursing roles such as those described above are increasingly advocated. One recent document produced by the Cancer Service Collaborative Improvement Partnership [43] outlines how "High Impact Changes" in service delivery can be achieved to help meet government targets. The targets currently center on redesign of cancer services through three key areas:
• meeting targets for government waiting times (31 days from decision to treat to first treatment and 62 days from urgent GP referral to first treatment);
• peer review to achieve Cancer Center/Unit status; and
• implementing the Improving Outcomes Guidance.
The use of expanded nursing roles is advocated in three key stages of the patient pathway: at diagnosis with the use of nurse-led one stop clinics and nurse endoscopists; at treatment planning through involvement in discussion at MDT meetings and participation in decision making; and in nurse-led follow-up. It is anticipated that the use of nurse specialists in these three key stages of the patient pathway will help to provide continuity of care and release consultant capacity for other essential tasks [43].

Education and training

In nursing there is a move toward more academic training, especially for nurses in advanced and specialist roles, to provide the necessary skills and knowledge to function at a higher level of practice. Sparacino [44] highlights the need for advanced knowledge in addition to expert skill as pivotal in the role of a clinical nurse specialist and Koetlers [45] puts this into context:

> As patients' needs in hospitals and homes become more complex and as the care patients receive increases in sophistication, the education and knowledge of the person they turn to for help and information also needs to be specialised and timely [45, p. 109]

As a result we have seen an increase in the number of nurses who have gone through rigorous courses providing specialist post-registration training at degree, masters, or doctorate level.

However, we have also seen a rapid increase in the United Kingdom in the last decade of the number and variety of specialist colorectal nurse posts being developed to meet the needs of the service [46]. According to Bousfield [5] many clinical nurse specialist roles have developed with no set career structure and with varied levels of preparation. The government health policy document Colorectal MDT Measures [47] concurs with this, highlighting that there are no official role definitions or training requirements for nurse MDT members and that this is in contrast to the clear national training requirements provided for the medical profession. To redress the balance, further training requirements for specialist nurses have been incorporated in the Manual for Cancer Services 2004; Colorectal Measures [8] and mandatory review of Cancer centers and units requires Trusts to adopt the policy. To comply with the directive, nurses must provide evidence to show they hold (or are enrolled to undertake) a qualification in their specialist area of nursing practice of at least 20 level-3 (degree level) CAT points. A second national requirement is to have completed (or be enrolled on) an accredited course/module (level unspecified) in communication skills to include aspects of counselling and in breaking bad news. If the unit/center has more than one nurse then they must all undergo training in the areas described above to be compliant with the measures.

Discussion

Colorectal nurses working in traditional or innovative new roles are charged with bringing to the role something that is unique to nursing, about connecting with the patient and building an individualized, patient-centered service. If nurses undertake a role originally in the medical domain then there is an onus to improve and optimize the service provided and to ensure that the new service is an improvement in quality care. Consider the role of cancer follow-up where these aspects are clearly demonstrated. Nurses now frequently undertake the role instead of surgeons and arrange surveillance to protocol. However, as well as making sure clinical review and surveillance investigations are completed in a timely and appropriate manner, nurses also address the psychological and practical aspects, assessing how the patient is coping and whether further support is required. Referral to psychological, complementary cancer care, day services, and to services providing practical advice, support, and benefits is an integral part of nurse-led follow-up but considered only rarely in a medical follow-up service.

The technical side of the new and expanding roles described, while highly skilled, is only part of the overall specialist nursing involvement with colorectal cancer patients. In a joint RCN/DoH document [48] specialist nurses have been described as maxi nurses not mini doctors, a description sure to delight many advanced nurses. The key elements that make our roles "special" are in providing continuity of care, support, and information along the care pathway from diagnosis onward, with practical assistance and clinical expertise before and after surgery and into follow-up. The vital ingredient to make it work is in ensuring a cohesive approach to patient management across the MDT.

Summary

The role of colorectal nurses is evolving with greater emphasis on high quality patient-centered care but with no single model for the nursing role or mode of delivery. Nurses continue to push the boundaries of nursing, taking on more advanced roles in the management of patients with colorectal cancer. Emphasis is placed on the importance of MDT working and developing protocols for patient-care management.

References

1 Department of Health. The Calman-Hine Report: A Policy Framework for Commissioning Cancer Services: *A Report by the Expert Advisory Group on Cancer to the Chief Medical Officers of England and Wales.* Department of Health, London, 1995.

2 McCallum J. The role of the nurse endoscopist. *Hosp Med* 2003; 64: 337–9.

3 DOH 2000.

4 McIllmurray MB. Cancer support nurses; a co-ordinating role in cancer care. *Eur J Cancer Care* 1998; 7: 125–8.

5 Bousfield C. A phemonenological investigation into the role of the clinical nurse specialist. *J Adv Nurs* 1997; 25: 245–56.

6 Commission for Health Improvement, Audit Commission. *NHS Cancer Care in England and Wales*. The Stationery Office, London, 2001.

7 National Institute for Clinical Evidence (NICE) (2004). *Guidance on Cancer Services: Improving Outcomes in Colorectal Cancer: Manual Update*. NICE, London.

8 Department of Health *Manual for Cancer Services 2004: Colorectal Measures*. Department of Health, London, 2004.

9 Campbell T, Borwell B. Colorectal cancer part 4: specialist nursing roles. *Prof Nurse* 1999; 15: 197–200.

10 Elcoat C. *Stoma Care Nursing*, Bailliere Tindall. Surrey, GB, 1986.

11 National Institute for Health and Clinical Excellence (NICE) (2005). *Referral Guidelines for Suspected Cancer*. Clinical Guideline 27, Developed by the National Collaborating Centre for primary Care. NICE.

12 Wright K, Myint Sun A. The colorectal cancer clinical nurse specialist in chemotherapy. *Hosp Med* 2003; 64: 333–6.

13 Office for National Statistics. Rectal cancer. In: Philips RKS, ed. *Colorectal Surgery*, 2nd edn. London: W.B. Saunders, 2001: 89–109.

14 IMS Health Incorporated Group. *New Stoma Patient Audit*. IMS Health Incorporated Group, London, 2003.

15 Fasth S, Hulten L, Palselius I. Loop ileostomy – an attractive alternative to a temporary transverse colostomy. *Acta Chir Scand* 1980; 146: 203–7.

16 Williams NS, Nasmyth DG, Jones D, Smith AH. De-functioning stomas: a prospective controlled trial comparing loop ileostomy with transverse loop colostomy. *Br J Surg* 1986; 73: 566–70.

17 Khoury GA, Lewis MC, Meleagros L, Lewis AAM. Colostomy or ileostomy after colorectal anastomosis?: a randomised trial. *Ann R Coll Surg Engl* 1986; 68: 5–7.

18 Edwards DP, Leppington-Clarke A, Sexton R *et al*. Stoma related complications are more frequent after transverse colostomy than loop ileostomy: a prospective randomised clinical trial. *Br J Surg* 2001; 88: 360–3.

19 Law WL, Chu KW, Choi HK. Randomized clinical trial comparing loop ileostomy and loop transverse colostomy for faecal diversion following total nesorectal excision. *Br J Surg* 2002; 89: 704–8.

20 Gooszen AW, Geelkerken RH, Hermans J *et al*. Temporary decompression after colorectal surgery: randomised comparison of loop ileostomy and loop colostomy. *Br J Surg* 1998; 85: 76–9.

21 Wade B. A Stoma is for LIFE. Harrow, England: Scutari Press, RCN, 1989.

22 Bass EM, Del Pino A, Tan A et al. Does pre-operative stoma marking and education by the enterostomal therapist affect outcome? *Dis Colon Rectum* 1997; 40: 440–2.

23 Black PK. *Holistic Stoma Care*. Bailliere Tindall, Royal College of Nursing. London, 2000.

24 McCahon S. Faecal stomas. In: Porrett T, Daniel N, eds. *Essential Coloproctology for Nurses*. London: Whurr Publishers Ltd., 1999.

25 Londono-Schimmer E, Leong AP, Phillips RK. Life table analysis of stomal complications following colostomy. *Dis Colon Rectum* 1994; 37: 916–20.

26 Thompson MJ, Trainor B. Incidence of parastomal hernia before and after a prevention programme *Gastrointest Nurs* 2005; 3: 23–7.

27 Janes A, Cengiz Y, Israelsson L. A randomised clinical trial of the use of a prosthetic mesh to prevent parastomal hernia. *Br J Surg* 2004; 91: 280–2.

28 Fretwell I, Mallender E, Smith K. Computerised digital photography for stoma and wound management *Gastrointest Nurs* 2004; 2: 19–24.

29 Dean JM, Sharpe A. *Pelican Nursing Atlas* C21. Advertising and Marketing Ltd., Altrincham, 2004.

30 Newland B. Debate: is the clinical nurse specialist deskilling the junior doctor? Yes. *Nurs Times* 2001; 97: 17.

31 Burns N. Debate: is the clinical nurse specialist de-skilling the junior doctor? No. *Nurs Times* 2001; 97: 17.

32 Pathmakanthan S, Smith K, Thompson G *et al.* A comparison of nurse and doctor performed colonoscopy. *Gut* 2002; 50: A102.

33 Vance ME, Shah SG, Suzuki N *et al.* Nurse colonoscopy: a review of 160 cases. *Gut* 2002; 50: A98.

34 Hughes MAP, Keng V, Hartley JE *et al.* A randomised trial comparing nurses and doctors performing flexible sigmoidoscopy. *Colorectal Dis* 2000; 2: 21.

35 Duthie GS, Drew PJ, Hughes MAP *et al.* A UK training programme for nurse practitioner flexible sigmoidoscopy and a prospective evaluation of the practice of the first UK trained flexible sigmoidoscopist. *Gut* 1998; 43: 711–14.

36 Schoenfeld P, Lipscomb S, Crook J *et al.* Accuracy of polyp detection by gastroenterologists and nurse endoscopists during flexible sigmoidoscopy: a randomised trial. *Gastroenterology* 1999a; 117: 312–18.

37 Jain A, Falzarano J, Decker R *et al.* Outcome of 5,000 flexible sigmoidoscopies done by nurse endoscopists for colorectal screening in asymptomatic patients. *Hawaii Med J* 2002; 61: 118–20.

38 Shapero TF, Alexander PE, Hoover J *et al.* Colorectal cancer screening: video reviewed flexible sigmoidoscopy by nurse endoscopists: a Canadian community based perspective. *Can J Gastroenterol* 2001; 15: 441–5.

39 CancerBACUP *Living with Cancer: Waiting for Treatment*, A report by CancerBACUP, May 2004.

40 Maruthachalam K, Stoker E, Nicholson G, Horan AF. Flexible sigmoidoscopy in the community – a pilot project. *Br J Surg* 2005; 19: 107.

41 Basnyat PS, Gomez KF, West J *et al.* Nurse-led direct access endoscopy clinics: the future? *Surg Endosc Ultrason Interv Tech* 2002; 16: 166–9.

42 Taylor P. Clinical effectiveness of the colorectal service at St Mary's NHS trust. *Clin Govern Bull* 2000; 1: 10–12.

43 National Health Service (NHS) (2005). *Applying High Impact Changes to Cancer Care.* Produced by the Cancer Services Collaborative Improvement Partnership.

44 Sparacino P. Advanced practice: the clinical nurse specialist. *Nurs Practice* 1992; 5: 2–4.

45 Koetlers T. Clinical practice and direct patient care. In: Hamric A, Spross J eds. The *Clinical Nurse Specialist in Theory and Practice*, 2nd edn. London: W.B. Saunders, 1989.

46 Humphris D. *The Clinical Nurse Specialist Issues in Practice.* London: MacMillan Press, 1994.

47 MDT Standards for Accreditation of Cancer Centres and Units (2004).

48 Royal College of Nursing and Department of Health. *Maxi Nurses: Nurses Working in Advanced and Extended Roles Promoting and Developing Patient-Centred Health Care.* Royal College of Nursing, London, 2005.

49 Department of Health. *The NHS Cancer Plan.* Department of Health, London, 2001.

11: The role of the multidisciplinary team in the management of colorectal cancer

Julia Jessop and Ian Daniels

Multi ... *Prefix – more than or many*
Disciplinary ... *of promoting discipline, order, or a system of rules for conduct*
Team ... *set of persons working together*

Introduction

The organization and configuration of services within the National Health Service (NHS) has changed radically over the last decade, particularly within cancer services. The provision of clinical care within formalized multidisciplinary teams (MDTs), replacing the provision of care within "firms of individual disciplines," has been central in the drive to improve the quality of care that cancer patients receive. This is based upon the rationale that clinical decision-making is improved by the sharing of expertise across different disciplines and specialties.

In this chapter we will discuss the effect of this change on the management of colorectal cancer, the benefits to this approach, the limitations, and some thoughts on how this approach may adapt to changes in the future.

Background: the development of multidisciplinary teams in cancer services

Traditionally, rectal cancer was diagnosed and "staged" by a surgeon performing digital rectal examination and sigmoidoscopy. Following surgical excision of the tumor, the use of any further adjuvant (postoperative) treatment was based upon the pathologist's assessment and staging of the excised specimen. One of the most important prognostic factors in rectal cancer is the relationship of the tumor to the surgical or circumferential resection margin (CRM) [1,2]. If the pathologist discovers tumor at this margin, the patient is at high risk of developing local recurrence of the cancer. Tumor detected at the CRM is usually given adjuvant chemotherapy and radiotherapy but many of these patients still develop local recurrence, with rates up to 40% having been reported [3].

The International Agency for Research on Cancer (IARC) data from 1995 showing survival rates for colorectal cancer in England and Scotland are amongst the worst in Europe [4]. Denmark, the Netherlands, Finland, France, Germany, Italy, Spain, and Switzerland, all report significantly better outcomes for colon cancer, rectal cancer, or both. Selection bias may exaggerate the size of these differences. However, having identified the poor outcome in the United Kingdom, this study highlighted the need to standardize and optimize the management of the rectal cancer.

The Calman-Hine Policy Framework for Commissioning Cancer Services first highlighted the need to deliver improved and coordinated cancer services through a cancer network infrastructure [5].

Reviews of published medical literature in the late 1980s and early 1990s, supplemented by registry studies, revealed that there could be significant improvements in survival as a result of specialist care for a number of cancers including colorectal cancer [5,6]. With these developments in mind, the NHS Cancer Plan was introduced to improve the diagnosis and treatment for patients of the five most common cancers – breast, lung, bowel, ovarian, and prostate [7]. Following the Cancer Plan, Improving Outcomes Guidance (IOG) have been published for these five cancers, which all specify MDT working and meetings as a key recommendation.

The establishment of MDT working and regular meetings to discuss patients and coordinate care is seen as a central element for cancer care. The MDT is defined as

> a group of different health care disciplines, which meets together at a given time (whether physically in one place or by video or tele-conferencing) to discuss a given patient and who are able to contribute independently to the diagnosis and treatment decisions about the patients.

Individual MDTs are now subject to a peer review process whereby each zone (a collective of cancer networks) appoints a coordinating team of multidisciplinary health professionals, managerial and service-user peer reviewers who work with the cancer networks to assess the MDTs according to nationally standardized processes and criteria.

Multidisciplinary teams in colorectal cancer

Colorectal cancer is the second most common cancer in the United Kingdom with over 30,000 newly diagnosed cancers per annum. The incidence of colorectal cancer is gradually increasing. A major reason for this is our increasingly elderly and longer-living population. Survival rates (relative to age-matched groups without colorectal cancer) are now around 45% at 5 years after diagnosis, and beyond 5 years relative survival rates decline only slightly.

Colorectal was one of the leading sites to establish specific guidance emphasizing the importance of MDTs [8]. This guidance was updated in 2004 [3] reinforcing the role of cancer networks in ensuring specific arrangements are in place for rapid access of all patients to a member of a specialist colorectal cancer MDT. The minimum numbers for a viable MDT are suggested as a population of 200,000 with 120 new patients per year. The core members of the colorectal cancer MDT are:

- at least two specialist surgeons
- clinical oncologists
- diagnostic radiologist
- histopathology
- skilled colonoscopist
- clinical nurse specialists
- palliative care specialist
- clinical trials coordinator/research nurse
- meeting coordinator
- team secretary (clerical support).

The last four core members of the colorectal MDT which are listed above are disciplines added to the core MDT membership from the original 1997 IOG guidance [3]. (Gastroenterologist was also moved from a core member to an extended team member.)

The guidance also places more emphasis on networks to ensure:

1 guidelines are established and audited regarding referral to MDTs,
2 attendance at the meetings, and
3 provision of adequate resources and support.

Organization of the meeting is explicitly defined, including the requirement for a weekly meeting scheduled in sessional time and arranged by the MDT coordinator.

The following is a list of patients for consideration at an MDT meeting:
• Every new patient with a diagnosis of colorectal cancer.
• All patients having undergone resection with curative intent and pathology available.
• All patients with newly identified recurrent or metastatic disease.
• Patients referred back for management by the local colorectal MDT after referral to a specialist MDT.
• Any other patient thought by a member of the MDT to require discussion. All the information required for effective team functioning should be available at the meeting. Emphasis is put on hospital trusts to ensure that preparation for and attendance at MDT is recognized as "an important clinical commitment and time should be allocated accordingly."

The most important benefits of team working are improved coordination of care and the opportunity to consider each case from a variety of perspectives. Patients managed by a team are more likely to be offered a range of types of treatment at appropriate times and to receive seamless care through all stages of the disease [3].

When MDTs function well, they offer a supportive environment where individual members can share their concerns. MDT meetings also provide opportunities for surgeons to receive feedback from histopathologists and other team members on the results of their work.

Treatment by MDTs, which treat relatively large numbers of patients, rather than by individual surgeons who may only deal with a few, can be expected to produce substantial benefits for patients. There is accumulating evidence that hospitals that treat more than 20 new patients with rectal cancer per annum – the minimum number that would be treated by MDTs working in accordance with the recommendations – achieve better outcomes. Their patients are less likely to receive permanent colostomies, suffer fewer postoperative complications, have lower local recurrence rates, and are more likely to become long-term survivors [3]. Concentration of surgery in the hands of fewer, more specialized surgeons, working in the context of MDTs, can be expected to produce similar benefits though the evidence for this is generally weak.

It was also seen that patients who underwent emergency surgery by anyone other than a designated specialist working in an MDT were unlikely to be referred on to a specialist for subsequent management [3].

Potential disadvantages of MDTs include discussion of patients without any of those involved having seen the patient. This can result in inappropriate decisions which later need to be corrected, resulting in wasted appointments for the patient and unnecessary anxiety.

Coordination of the MDT, the availability of clinical notes, and appropriate radiological and histopathological input requires a dedicated member of staff. Chairing a large MDT also places considerable responsibility on that individual, particularly in communicating with colleagues and other team members.

The function of the MDT

The importance of input from each discipline into the management of colorectal cancer, particularly imaging, surgery, pathology, oncology, and nursing, has been highlighted in other chapters within this book. The MDT meeting is increasingly important as it is the process for presenting all the accumulated evidence in order that a multidisciplinary management decision can be made on how to proceed with a patient's treatment. The single most important principle in the management of colorectal cancer is the need to consider every patient as an individual.

It is essential that there is representation from all the core disciplines at the MDT meetings, that all the clinical information is available and presented to the rest of the team, and that this information is captured on an appropriate database in order to allow audit of the MDT to occur. All too often data collection is limited to managerial outcomes measures rather than clinical outcomes due to lack of personnel and facilities.

The multidisciplinary team has a number of managerial and clinical roles to fulfill. Beyond the assessment and planning of individual care, the MDT has responsibility for:

Protocols and guidelines. At the core of the management strategy are the guidelines themselves. Guidelines must be formulated based on the consensus of the team and should integrate the complementary areas of their expertise [9].

Planning local service delivery. Identification of gaps in current service provision in line with national guidelines should be identified and endorsed through the MDT to ensure equity of service across cancer networks. Each member has a responsibility to progress developments within their area.

Communication/co-ordination of care. Identification of a key worker for the patient throughout the patient pathway is a responsibility of the MDT to ensure effective communication between the MDT, the patient, and their primary healthcare services.

Service redesign and improvement. Process mapping, capacity and demand planning, and identification of areas for improvements in service should be undertaken by all MDTs.

Data collection and audit. Audit is a vital part of healthcare provision since only in this way can we monitor performance against the accepted standard. Audit should focus on case management and clinical outcomes as well as provide the required managerial information [9].

Research. Participation in trials benefits the patient. It has been shown that participation in clinical trials improves clinical outcome [9]. The principal reason for this is that meticulous pre-defined management algorithms and rigorous follow-up are routinely part of the trial procedure. All patients should therefore be considered for enrolment in current clinical trials. Currently, approximately 12% of patients are enrolled into colorectal clinical trials.

Evidence for improved outcome/benefits

Evidence for specialization

Studies of colorectal cancer in the United Kingdom show considerable variation in surgical outcome [6] and Scandinavian studies suggest that university hospitals have better survival rates than general hospitals [10]. Similar results were found in Germany and in France [11,12]. However, declared specialists working in district general hospitals in the North West of England were able to produce similar results to declared specialists in colorectal cancer work in teaching hospitals [13]. This last study suggests that high-quality specialist services can be successfully established in district hospitals when specific commitments to them are made. A recent survey showed that differences in outcome following apparently curative resection for colorectal cancer among surgeons appear to reflect the degree of specialization rather than case volume [14].

Evidence for multidisciplinary teamwork

Teamwork has been related to improved patient care by reducing hospital readmission rates [15–18]. A recent study of teamwork in UK breast cancer teams explored the relationship between components of teamwork and patient outcomes, reporting that the team size (larger) was associated with the provision of accurate and timely diagnoses and that higher breast cancer workloads and a greater proportion of breast care nurses within teams were associated with better clinical performance. Shared leadership within teams was also associated with better self-reported effectiveness [19].

The benefits of teamworking for colorectal cancer are generally recognized. Documented ways of working in multidisciplinary teams are needed to look after the quality control of all the disciplines involved and to be a platform to discuss the treatment plan for the individual patient [20].

The need for a multidisciplinary approach to the treatment of advanced colorectal cancer has also been recognized in maximizing the benefits of current treatment options. A multidisciplinary approach allows healthcare professionals to develop a clear understanding of each other's roles and an appreciation of the complementary treatment approaches [21].

Evidence for colorectal multidisciplinary teams

Most of the evidence for teamworking to date has been based upon breast-cancer MDTs. However, evidence that colorectal MDT working impacts on patient survival is currently being collated and the first papers are presently being published.

An audit undertaken by the Royal Marsden Hospital Colorectal MDT demonstrated that the MDT discussion of magnetic resonance imaging (MRI) and implementation of a preoperative treatment strategy resulted in significantly reduced positive CRM in rectal cancer patients. Overall, CRM positive rate for all potentially curative patients was reduced from 12.5 to 7% after mandating preoperative MRI-based MDT discussion of all rectal cancer patients. They conclude that CRM positive rate is reducible, but only in the presence of robust MRI staging, preoperative MDT discussion of all the staging investigations, optimal surgery, the availability of effective preoperative therapies, and standardized histopathology reporting with comprehensive data collection [22].

Limitations of the multidisciplinary team's process

A recent report by the Commission for Health Improvement and the Audit Commission in 2000/2001 showed that MDTs working is less well developed in colorectal cancer care than in breast cancer care [23]. Of 12 Trusts, which reported that they had colorectal cancer MDTs, half held weekly patient-planning meetings and a third held meetings fortnightly; the other two met monthly or less. It seems that the other six Trusts did not hold regular colorectal MDT meetings at which patient management was planned. This led to delays in the patients' treatment or treatment being given without a consensus MDT management plan.

In Trusts that did have colorectal cancer MDTs, surgeons who were not members nevertheless carried out operations. One-third of the lead consultants reported problems dissuading colleagues from occasional practice. In one Trust, for example, four out of eight surgeons who carried out operations for colorectal cancer attended MDT meetings; in a second, only one of the two main colorectal cancer surgeons attended MDT meetings and the patients treated by the second surgeon (about a quarter of the total) were not discussed by the MDT. Overall, 40% of lead consultants, working in 21 Trusts, reported that there were surgeons in their Trust who regularly carried out operations for colorectal cancer, but who did not attend MDT meetings [3].

Although MDTs have been given a high priority nationally in terms of being essential for the management of patients, this has not always been supported at a local level with provision of adequate basic requirements in terms of dedicated rooms with adequate facilities to enable effective meetings. The lack of real-time patient management systems exacerbates the time required to prepare for and conduct the meetings. Many teams are unaware of their own results as there is limited support for collection and analysis of clinical information.

In order for MDTs to function effectively they not only need appropriate support in terms of facilities and personnel, but also in access to resources. Many teams still struggle to gain access to MRI for routine rectal cancer staging even though it is a recommendation in current national guidelines [3]. Long waiting times for radiotherapy can also inhibit teams in achieving waiting time targets for non-surgical initial treatment.

There are a wide variety of roles being undertaken by clinical nurse specialists across the country with each developing according to the needs of the local team. The further development of nursing roles, for example nurse-led clinics, are often indicated following evaluation of services to improve efficiency.

Future developments in MDT management of colorectal cancer

The challenges to the MDT continue to appear with the introduction of minimum datasets, initially in histopathology, but now being developed for radiology and surgery. As we collect increasing amounts of data, these have to be put into the context of physiological correction of outcome results. Improved data collection can be attained through the use of standardized proformas.

The expansion of the different technologies – through different surgical techniques – newer oncological compounds, and different staging modalities has led to a large variation in reporting of results.

The development of internet-based datasets and proformas has been a revolution in data collection, although many local projects cannot be integrated into a national system. Other areas of interest include the following:

1 The future use of telemedicine to produce virtual MDTs enables all MDT members to participate fully in case reviews and agree treatment plans for patients. It also enables regular meetings increasing access to expert opinion and reducing delay in implementing treatment [24].

2 Improved prediction of tumor behavior through gene assessment of the biopsied tissues and the correlation to preoperative staging.

Conclusions

We began by defining "multi," "disciplinary," and "teams" as many individuals working together for a group that acts through clear guidelines with uniformity and reproducibility. The advent of MDT working has been a revolution in the provision of healthcare, not only in patients with malignant disease, but in all areas of medicine where disciplines interact to provide seamless care. Within the world of colorectal cancer we have seen the introduction of the MDT process, often with little or no evidence base. However, through research and audit the approach is benefiting patients. It has also led to an improvement in standards across the disciplines, together with record of the discussions that are involved in patient care. But with these changes have come challenges, both through the immediate provision of resources to allow the MDT to function efficiently and the highlighting of gaps in the knowledge of the management of colorectal cancer. As technology evolves, new drugs and surgical techniques become available, together with improvements in patient selection for therapy through staging; these areas must be assessed in a standardized way with accurate data collection. The MDT offers this forum, and although currently recognized as a static forum between meetings, the MDT process is dynamic through all aspects of patient care. The process is not without its problems and some clinicians feel that it reduces clinical freedom and does not involve the patient.

Since clinical governance is now a key target in healthcare the MDT process is probably here to stay and must be viewed as a method to improve standards and outcomes.

References

1 Nagtegaal ID, Marijnen CA, Kranenbarg EK *et al.* Circumferential margin involvement is still an important predictor of local recurrence in rectal carcinoma: not 1 mm but 2 mm is the limit. *Am J Surg Pathol* 2002; 26: 350–7.
2 Birbeck KF, Macklin CP, Tiffin NJ *et al.* Rates of circumferential resection margin involvement vary between surgeons and predict outcomes in rectal cancer surgery. *Ann Surg* 2002; 235: 449–57.
3 DoH. Guidance on Commissioning Cancer Services: Improving Outcomes in Colorectal Cancer. The Manual. London: Department of Health; 2004(b).
4 World Health Organization International Agency for research on Cancer – European Commission. Survival of cancer patients in Europe: the Eurocare Study. Lyon: IARC Scientific Publications 1995; No 132.
5 Calman K, Hine D. A Policy Framework for Commissioning Cancer Services. London: Department of Heath; 1995.
6 McArdle C, Hole D. Impact of variability among surgeons on post-operative morbidity and mortality and ultimate survival. *Br Med J* 1991; 302: 1501–5.
7 Health. Do. The NHS Cancer Plan. London: Department of Health; 2000.
8 DoH. Clinical Outcomes Group, Cancer Guidance Sub-group. Guidance on Commissioning Cancer Services: Improving Outcomes in Colorectal Cancer. The Manual. London: Department of Health; 1997.
9 The International Working Group in Colorectal Cancer. An International Multidisciplinary Approach to the Management of Advanced Colorectal Cancer. *Eur J Surg Oncol* 1997; 23 (Suppl A): 1–66.
10 Hakama M, Karjalainen S, Hakulinen T. Outcome-based equity in the treatment of colon cancer patients in Finland. *Int J Technol Assess Health Care* 1989; 5: 619–30.
11 Launoy G, Coutour X, Gignoux M, Pottier Dugleux G. Influence of rural environment on diagnosis, treatment, and prognosis of colorectal cancer. *J Epidemiol Community Health* 1992; 46: 365–7.
12 Mohner M, Slisow W. Effect of regional centralization treatment on chances of survival in rectal cancer in East Germany. *Zentralbl Chir* 1990; 115: 801–12.
13 Kingston RD, Walsh S, Jones AJ. Colorectal surgeons in district general hospitals produce similar survival outcomes to their teaching hospital colleagues: review of 5-year survivals in Manchester. *J R Coll Surg Edinb* 1992; 37: 235–7.
14 McArdle C, Hole D. Influence of volume and specialization on survival following surgery for colorectal cancer. *Br J Surg* 2004; 91: 610–17.
15 Sommers L, Marton K, Barbaccia J, Randolph J. Physician, nurse and social worker collaboration in primary care for

chronically ill seniors. *Arch Intern Med* 2000; 160: 1825–33.

16 Rafferty AM, Ball J, Aiken LH. Are teamwork and professional autonomy compatible, and do they result in improved hospital care? *Qual Health Care* 2001; 10 (Suppl II): ii32–ii37.

17 West MA, Borrill C, Dawson J et al. The link between the management of employees and patient mortality in acute hospitals. *Int J Hum Resour Manage* 2002; 13: 1299–310.

18 Knaus WA, Draper EA, Wagner DP, Zimmerman JE. An evaluation of outcome from intensive care in major medical centres. *Ann Intern Med* 1986; 104: 410–18.

19 Haward R, Amir Z, Borrill C et al. Breast cancer teams: the impact of constitution, new cancer workload, and methods of operation on their effectiveness. *Br J Cancer* 2003; 89: 15–22.

20 Wiggers T, van de Velde CJ. The circumferential margin in rectal cancer. Recommendations based on the Dutch total mesorectal excision study. *Eur J Cancer* 2002; 38: 973–6.

21 Rougier P, Neoptolemos JP. The need for a multidisciplinary approach in the treatment of advanced colorectal cancer: a critical review from a medical oncologist and surgeon. *Eur J Surg Oncol* 1997; 23: 385–96.

22 Burton S, Daniels IR, Norman AR et al. MRI directed multidisciplinary team pre-operative treatment strategy: the way to eliminate positive circumferential margins? *Colorectal Dis* 2005; 16: 542.

23 Office of the National Statistics Agency. National Service Framework Assessments No1: NHS Cancer Care in England and Wales.

24 Axford AT, Askill C, Jones AJ. Virtual multidisciplinary teams for cancer care. *J Telemed Telecare* 2002; 8: 3–4.

12: Follow-up after colorectal cancer resection

Is it worthwhile?

John Northover and Chris Byrne

Introduction

Follow-up after colorectal cancer surgery is a routine adhered to by most surgeons, but reliable evidence of measurably positive changes in outcome is thin. Despite this, all developed countries spend a considerable proportion of limited health resources on this process. A recent US survey of follow-up regimens showed a wide range of costs for 5 years of follow-up per patient [1]; the cheapest they found was $900, while the most expensive was nearly $27,000. With a million follow-up visits generated by each year's cohort of new US cases, this amounts to billions spent for questionable health gain – and the situation is similar in all industrialized countries.

In this chapter we will examine the origins of post-surgical cancer follow-up, its putative aims, the assumptions made about its utility, and the evidence for its efficacy. Finally, working policies based on evidence will be examined.

How did follow-up start?

As far as can be ascertained, follow-up was not routine in the early years of the twentieth century, at a time when colorectal cancer was becoming more common. Major surgery for this disease was unusual 100 years ago and cure even less common. Indeed, before radical rectal cancer surgery was described by Miles in 1908, it is overwhelmingly likely that almost no patient survived the disease. And as surgery itself was so hazardous (Miles' perioperative mortality was around 40% [2]) reoperative surgery for recurrence was a subtlety which was probably not contemplated.

It should, therefore, be no surprise that follow-up began on a regular basis, not as a means for the early detection of recurrence, but as a tool for research into prognosis after rectal cancer surgery. Cuthbert Dukes' and Percy Lockhart-Mummery, pathologist and surgeon, respectively, at St Mark's Hospital, London, began a program of routine follow-up in the early 1920s aimed specifically at correlating clinical outcome with the pathological anatomy of the disease in resected specimens [2]. Thus the earliest and most palpable result of follow-up was the development of the prognostic Dukes' staging system for rectal cancer.

Certainly, at St Mark's in the middle years of the twentieth century, and in most other institutions dealing with this increasingly prevalent disease, routine follow-up became the norm. In those days it consisted of regular outpatient visits and simple recording of clinical findings. It was only in later decades that technological advancement offered up more sensitive investigations but with little questioning of the health gain secured by their use. By the 1960s and 1970s the natural sense of follow-up was widely assumed. Perpetuation of this assumption is clear in an influential review:

> Early detection of colorectal cancer recurrence can be a daunting and costly task in this era of budget cuts and cost containment, especially since the rewards are few when looked upon in the context of the vast number of patients treated for colorectal cancer every year. However, the rewards are real, and some patients can be cured as a result of diligent follow-up [3].

Such statements beg important questions regarding the cost effectiveness of the process. Do all patients benefit in some way? Might some benefit more if resources were targeted? In short, are the assumptions of the past acceptable today or in the future?

Aims of follow-up

Traditionally, follow-up has been said to have four main aims [3,4]:

1 *Early detection of recurrence or new primary tumor.* Following radical, putatively curative surgery for colorectal cancer, up to 50% of patients will develop recurrent cancer, either locally or in distant organs, and most will die as a direct result [5]. Moreover, up to 8% will develop a new (metachronous) primary malignancy [6–8], and in many more premalignant adenomas will form. Ergo attempts to detect these various threatening lesions at the earliest stage should be made – or so runs the logic of follow-up aimed at their presymptomatic identification.

But does a policy of regular, pro-active follow-up for all lead to more effective management of recurrence compared to investigation at symptom onset? If not, Charles Moertel's reflection on carcinoembryonic antigen

(CEA) monitoring, enunciated 20 years ago – and equally bereft of an evidence base – might be used to describe the whole process of follow-up: "The only outcome for most patients [is] the needless anxiety produced by premature knowledge of the presence of a fatal disease" [9].

2 *Management of post-surgical complications.* Identifying wound problems, providing supportive stoma care, and attending to difficulties with bowel function and neurological deficits after rectal cancer surgery – all these require postoperative outpatient supervision. Most such issues can be resolved, or helped to the limit of possibility, within 1 year of surgery, but by themselves, these issues do not constitute a rationale for 5 years of regular visits.

3 *Reassuring patients.* All senior surgeons have witnessed the wide range of patients' reactions to the experience of having been diagnosed and treated for cancer. At one extreme the patient becomes pathologically attached to the hospital and its staff, preoccupied by the fear of recurrence. Others simply want to put the whole experience behind them and get on with their lives. These attitudes, and all points between, demand different approaches by the medical team; and, in the absence of solid evidence of an oncological imperative for adherence to a particular follow-up regimen, they require different patterns of reassurance through postoperative patient/doctor contact.

4 *Audit and quality control of surgical outcomes.* In the recent past most surgeons would not have seen the need to analyze the outcomes of their cancer surgery. Times and circumstances are changing in ways which may mandate follow-up in order that healthcare purchasers, potential patients, and, indeed, wider society can judge institutional or perhaps individual results.

To this list should be added the process of deciding upon and delivering adjuvant therapy. As evidence for the efficacy of adjuvants in subgroups accumulates, this becomes a more widely applicable reason for continuing contact following surgery, though only initially with the surgeon.

What are the key elements of the follow-up process?

Planning a follow-up program requires decisions about the frequency of surveillance visits and their clinical and investigative content. There is an enormous range of combinations of visit frequencies and investigations that could be included; Kievit and Bruinvels [10] recently computed that there are a mind-boggling $30,000 \times 8^5$ different protocols.

Patient/doctor contact

This can range from symptom-prompted, reactive, contact (i.e. no planned, asymptomatic visits), through the more usual regular interview and physical examination, to frequent and expensive cycles of "high tech" investigation. "History and physical" may reveal the first evidence of recurrence in up to 50% of patients with recurrence [11]. Intervals between visits vary depending on the attitude of the clinician and the time since surgery. As most recurrences become apparent within 2 years [12], most regimens concentrate on this period, with continuing though less frequent visits till 5 years after operation [3]. Each patient can expect to make 12–15 visits in a 5 year program [10]. However, most symptomatic recurrences make themselves apparent to the patient between planned visits, leading either to unplanned urgent visits (making the planned program irrelevant) or to unwarranted delay until the next planned visit [4].

Simple outpatient contact includes routine questioning about symptoms that might indicate either recurrence or functional problems, and physical examination looking for abdominal signs – principally hepatomegaly – and sigmoidoscopic evidence of anastomotic recurrence. The use of various investigations may be prompted either by abnormalities found by this "minimalist" contact or be part of a planned surveillance program.

Certainly the most extreme form of doctor/patient contact after surgery, which predated any of the "high tech" investigative modalities to be discussed below, was the program of second look surgery used by Wangensteen 50 years ago [13]. For him, the case for early diagnosis and treatment of recurrence was sufficiently compelling that he submitted his patients to a "second look" laparotomy 6 months after primary surgery! Any residual cancer found was excised if possible and additional operations were done at intervals of approximately 6 months until one operation was completed at which no more cancer was found. Ultimately it became apparent that the operative mortality outweighed any possible patient benefit, so this extreme modality of follow-up was abandoned.

Serum tumor markers

Serum CEA measurement is used in follow-up very widely and frequently in some parts of the world. In the United States, it has been estimated that 500,000 patients are undergoing regular CEA monitoring at any one time [14], offering the prospect of recurrence detection on average 6 months before the onset of symptoms. There is a large body of evidence that this modality leads to earlier diagnosis and more second look surgery [15], but evidence that this improves the survivability of recurrent disease is controversial.

When CEA was discovered in 1965 [16], it was hailed as the serum marker for colorectal cancer, with an obvious role in mass population screening. It soon became apparent that CEA levels might be raised in other cancers, in nonmalignant bowel diseases, and also in some otherwise normal individuals, particularly associated with changes in smoking or drinking. Moreover, serum CEA was normal in 25% of patients with known bowel cancer. This lack of specificity and sensitivity ruled it out as a mass screening tool. CEA was seen to have a possible role as a prognostic marker when it was found that the risk of recurrent disease within 2 years of primary surgery was more than doubled in those in whom the serum CEA was raised preoperatively [17]. However in recent multivariate analyses, it was not found to be a powerful, independent prognostic [18]. No system of preoperative staging and prognostic prediction has displaced postoperative Dukes'-based pathological systems [18].

Serial measurement of serum markers after primary surgery to predict recurrence, and hence to indicate those who might be candidates for second look surgery, has been studied intensively. Moertel [14] estimated that at any one time 500,000 Americans are being sampled serially in order to predict recurrence prior to the onset of symptoms. In some centers, there has been continuing advocacy of second look surgery based on CEA [19]. So what is the evidence that a policy of second look surgery based on serial CEA follow-up might alter prognosis favorably?

There is no doubt that serum CEA rises in the majority of cases prior to the appearance of symptoms and signs [20]; amongst more than 2000 cases described in series published in the early 1980s, 75% demonstrated a CEA rise as first indicator of recurrent disease [21]. In the mid-1970s, there were several reports that regular monitoring led to early diagnosis of recurrence, up to 30 months before symptoms occurred [18,22–24]. Using historical controls, workers in Columbus, Ohio demonstrated that early re-operation relying on CEA results as the sole indicator for surgery led to macroscopic clearance of recurrence in more patients (63% compared to 27% in the symptom-led second look series [19,25]). Similar conclusions were drawn from other non-randomized studies [26–34], though others have remained unconvinced [35–39]. As a consequence, the Columbus group and others advocated monthly CEA testing to take maximal advantage of lead time [40].

CEA assay has deficiencies in sensitivity and specificity. It indicates the presence of unresectable hepatic recurrence more frequently than potentially curable disease [41], while in 10–25% of patients the raised CEA results in a negative laparotomy [14,42–45]. Conversely a high proportion of patients had incurable disease at surgery [45,46]. Efforts to improve the efficacy of CEA monitoring led to its combination with other tumor markers, but without significantly improved clinical utility [47].

Fletcher pointed out that "Americans have valued cure at almost any cost," while pointing out that society could not be expected to pay for it [40]. In the United Kingdom, a national screening policy in any field is likely to be implemented only after development of convincing evidence of its clinical and economic utility. In the absence of prospective control data it remained impossible to demonstrate any survival advantage from a policy of CEA-led second look surgery. Fletcher suggested that the efficacy of a CEA-based second look policy could only be demonstrated by a randomized trial, but that statistical difficulties precluded any such study [14,40].

Other prognostic serum markers have been developed and used in the same way as CEA; these include tissue polypeptide antigen (TPA), CA 19-9, and CA 50. There have been variable reports of their relative sensitivity and specificity compared to each other, to CEA, and in combination [47,48]. Comparisons are difficult, but Putzki and others [47] have shown no apparent advantage for other antigens or combinations, compared to CEA alone.

In summary, CEA and other serum markers are sensitive, presymptomatic indicators of recurrent disease. Unless more effective methods of treatment can be triggered by a raised marker level, their diagnostic ability offers no more than protracted prior knowledge of a fatal outcome for most patients, as suggested 20 years ago by Charles Moertel [9].

Flexible endoscopy

Fiberoptic large-bowel endoscopy was first reported 30 years ago [49], leading to highly sensitive, minimally invasive diagnosis of primary and recurrent cancer, and to the non-surgical removal of many adenomas. As a technique for follow-up in asymptomatic individuals, the superior sensitivity and therapeutic ability of colonoscopy has made barium enema practically redundant in this task.

In theory, flexible endoscopy can play a part in two aspects of follow-up – detection of metachronous neoplasia, both benign and malignant, and recognition of recurrent cancer.

Detection and removal of metachronous adenomas should diminish the incidence and risk of death due to metachronous cancer [50], which has been reported as having a better outlook than the initial malignancy [51]. Some have found high yields of adenomas, including larger lesions which are more likely to progress to cancer, with lesions found in up to 56% of cases in blanket follow-up [52–54]. Metachronous cancer in the days before colonoscopic surveillance was reported in around 3–4% of postoperative cases [55]. Some modern series quote rates of only 0.2–3.1% [52,53,56]. Conceivably this might reflect a true decrease due to polypectomy during surveillance.

As a method for the detection of recurrent cancer, endoscopy is insensitive as most recurrences begin outside the bowel lumen [1,57]. Audisio's [12] series indicated that colonoscopy yielded the first evidence in less than 1% of cases of recurrent disease, though others have reported a rate of detection up to 3–4% [52,53,55,58].

The natural history of the adenoma–carcinoma sequence would suggest that reexamination in less than 3 years after achievement of a "clean colon" is unlikely to discover significant pathology. However, yearly examination in some hands has found adenomas in more than 14% of patients each year over a 4-year period [56]. This probably reflects the practicality of a follow-up program, with lesions missed at some examinations, rather than truly new pathology. Yearly colonoscopy is advocated by some [58], tailored to the findings at each examination [52]. Nevertheless the evidential case for more frequent investigation than 3 yearly in capable endoscopic hands was not accepted by the group providing guidance for the UK National Health Service [59], who felt, however, that a strong case could be made for establishing a "clean colon" colonoscopically either before surgery or within 6 months of primary treatment [59].

Imaging

Imaging modalities have become increasingly sensitive to the detection of small volumes of recurrent disease and may be applied in follow-up to look for evidence of local or distant recurrence. As most local recurrences begin outside the lumen, modalities which provide information beyond the bowel wall are more useful than endoscopy or luminal contrast studies.

Local recurrence

Endoluminal ultrasound is more informative regarding events within and just beyond the bowel wall, whereas computerized tomography (CT) and magnetic resonance (MR) are more sensitive to disease in the surrounding pelvic cavity. Routinely used, ultrasound may be the only modality to detect local recurrence in a moderate proportion of patients. In two recent series comprising 168 patients in total, ultrasound was the sole indicator of recurrence in 6 of 23 cases [60,61]. Ultrasound, however, is operator dependent and more difficult to measure in serial examinations than axial imaging. A major difficulty in the use of ultrasound, CT, and MR in the diagnosis of local recurrence is the differentiation of post-surgical changes from recurrent cancer. Serial scanning, allowing changes in size, and configuration of abnormal areas to be recognized may be useful in the differential diagnosis of possible recurrence [62]. This requires, however, a delay of typically 12 weeks to assess for changes in size which is less than optimal in the context of cancer. The development of positron emission tomography (PET) scanning combined with CT has allowed functional as well as anatomical definition as a criterion in differential diagnosis of malignant from scar tissue [62,63].

Distant metastases

Despite being considerably cheaper and more portable, ultrasound is able to achieve sensitivity and specificity that compare reasonably well with the other modalities, detecting lesions of over 1 cm diameter in the liver [62]. However, multislice CT scanners with fast acquisition times and high resolution are able to delineate liver and lung lesions of just over 5 mm as well as image nodal stations that are likely sites of metastatic disease [64,65]. The technology is well developed, so the key question becomes clinical utility, in particular the usefulness of presymptomatic diagnosis using these techniques.

Outcome and costs of follow-up programs

Perhaps in an attempt to put objectivity into an argument easily influenced by the subjectivity of the individual surgeon, Kievit and Bruinvels [10] suggested four "conditions of benefice" against which we might measure the usefulness of routine follow-up (Table 12.1). This utilitarian approach provides an appropriate balance between the laudable attempt to identify and help the curable few, a compassionate and sensible approach for the incurable majority, and a realistic eye on the limited contents of the healthcare coffers. Although this list of conditions exhibits manifest sense, it has proven extraordinarily difficult to dissect out the ability of individual tests,

Table 12.1 Conditions of benefice.

1 At least some recurrent disease should be localized and amenable to curative treatment.
   The process of recurrence development should involve two synchronous and counterac-
   tive mechanisms:
   UNDETECTABLE → DETECTABLE PRECLINICAL → SYMPTOMATIC
   CURABLE → PALLIATIVELY RESECTABLE → IRRESECTABLE
   (Present data suggest that curability of recurrent colorectal cancer is not usually a time-
   dependent process)
2 Follow-up should be able to detect curable recurrence, ideally *without bringing forward
   the time of diagnosis of incurable disease*
3 Overall, benefits of follow-up (high quality-adjusted life expectancy, more curative resections) should outweigh non-monetary costs – early detection of incurability, re-operative
   morbidity and mortality, and false positive tests
4 Cost/benefit ratio should be sufficiently favorable to justify routine use

Source: Kievit J, Bruinvels D. *Eur J Cancer* 1995; 31A: 1222–5.

or various combinations in follow-up programs, to live up to these stringent
requirements.

There have been two broad approaches to this debate: the broadly
descriptive review and the more focused randomized comparison. The
former comprises essentially the attempts to describe published programs
in terms of their content, intensity, and cost, and to try to glean evidence of
differences in outcome. Virgo and her colleagues [1] made a recent attempt
to collect, describe, and assess the relative merits of the 11 surveillance strategies in use or being promulgated in the United States. Her main conclusion
was that there is a wide range of cost without any indication that "higher
cost strategies increase survival or quality of life." While cost is easy to
compare between regimens, however (range $910–$26,717, a 28-fold difference), clinical outcome comparison carries all the well-known pitfalls of
non-control comparisons. Perhaps it can be said uncontroversially that the
range of difference in clinical outcome is well short of the cost range. Richard
and McLeod [66] compiled a much larger list of studies and programs by
performing a Medline search spanning 30 years. They differentiated studies and programs according to their statistical and epidemiological quality,
separating cohort studies from the few extant randomized trials. Their comprehensive and presently definitive exploration of this very difficult field
led them to the disappointing and inevitably vague judgment that "there
is inconclusive evidence either to support or to refute the value of follow-up
surveillance programs to detect recurrence of colorectal cancer." They point
out importantly that existing data have not excluded an intensity-related

effect of follow-up on cancer outcomes. These large overviews, necessarily covering a very wide range of programs, patient groups, and clinical environments, both concluded that *large* randomized trials would be necessary to detect any realistic beneficial effect.

Randomized controlled trials

Six published randomized trials have sought to compare the efficacy of different follow-up programs, but have been similarly guarded in their conclusions [67–72]. We should examine these studies in some detail before commenting on what can be drawn from them (Table 12.2). The problem with all these trials is that none of them had sufficient statistical power to detect realistic differences in survival. As the authors of the Swedish trial pointed out, their study could not have detected any difference in overall mortality less than 20% [69]. So, although the trials have not demonstrated an advantage for any particular approach – from no planned program to the most intensive – neither have they excluded that possibility. As the likely maximum overall survival effect is no more than 5% [73], the sample size calculation in these trials was clearly unrealistic.

Meta-analyses of randomized trials

Two independent meta-analyses of five of the above listed randomized controlled trials of various follow-up regimes came to the similar conclusion that a more intensive regime of follow-up resulted in a survival benefit. The first published meta-analysis was the Cochrane publication released in 2001 which pooled 1342 patients from five randomized trials [74]. The authors found the odds ratio for survival by more intensive follow-up to be 0.73 (95% confidence interval of 0.58–0.92) with an absolute survival advantage of 7% less deaths (95% confidence interval from 12% less to 2% less). On sub-analyses, there was a mortality benefit in the groups who underwent "more tests" and/or those who underwent "liver imaging." The authors were, however, guarded in their recommendations about exactly which elements of the follow-up were responsible for this survival advantage. A second independent analysis by Renehan and co-workers from Manchester of the same five trials found similar results but recommended that clinical guidelines needed updating and that a modern regime of more frequent CEA levels and CT imaging was warranted [75]. These assertions, however, were difficult to support from the randomized control trial (RCT) data used in their

Table 12.2 Summary data from randomized trials.

RCT	Number randomized	Comparison intensive vs minimal regimes	Recurrence rate (%)	Number of resections	5-year survival (%) (p)
Swedish [67] Ohlsson et al. 1995	107	HP,LFT,CEA,FOB,Σ,CXR, CT,C vs Zero	33 vs 32	5 vs 3	75 vs 67 (>0.05)
Finnish [68] Makela et al. 1995	106	HP,FBC,CEA,CXR,Σ,BaE C,US,CT,flΣ vs HP,FBC,CEA,CXR,Σ,BaE	42 vs 39	5 vs 3	59 vs 54 (0.5)
Danish [69] Kjeldsen et al. 1997	597	HP,LFT,FBC,CXR,C vs Zero till 5 years	26 vs 26	11 vs 3	70 vs 68 (0.48)
Australian [70] Shoemaker et al. 1998	325	HP,FBC,LFT,CEA,FOB CXR,CT,C vs HP,FBC,LFT,CEA,FOB	33 vs 40	13 vs 14	76 vs 70 (0.2)
Italian [71] Pietra et al. 1998	207	HP,CEA,US,CXR,CT,C vs HP,CEA,US,CXR,C	39 vs 40	17 vs 2	73 vs 58 (0.02)
Italian [72] Secco et al. 2002	358	HP,CEA,US,CXR,Σ (all high frequency) vs HP,CEA,US,CXR,Σ	53 vs 57	31 vs 13	

RCT, randomized control trial; Comparison, investigations in each arm of randomized follow-up programs; Recurrence rate (%), percentage overall recurrence rates; Number of resections (n) (%), "curative" resection rate – total numbers and percentages; 5 year survival % (p), overall percentage 5-year survivals and p value; HP, history and physical examination; LFT, liver function tests; FBC, full blood count; CEA, serum carcinoembryonic antigen; CXR, chest X-ray; Σ, rigid sigmoidoscopy; CT, CT scan; C, colonoscopy; flΣ, flexible sigmoidoscopy.

meta-analysis. For example, in three of four trials using CEA, the frequency of CEA measurement was the same in the intensive as well as the control groups. Nevertheless, it seems logical that the routine use of some test such as CEA or liver imaging that will prompt early identification of resectable metastases should be the major factor in improving survival after primary colorectal cancer resection.

More recently the Manchester group published the results of a cost-effectiveness analysis performed from the perspective of healthcare services [76]. This found that the intensive follow-up patients lived an average of 0.73 to 0.81 years longer over 5 years. The adjusted net cost per patient was £2479 and the cost per life year saved was £3402 which was significantly less than the National Health Service (NHS) threshold of £30,000 for screening programs.

Currently recruiting trials

There are two very large randomized trials currently recruiting. The Italian GILDA (Gruppo Italiano di Lavoro per la Diagnosi Anticipata) study aims to randomize over 1500 patients and to date has recruited over 1000 patients since 1998 into "intensive" and "minimalist" follow-up regimes at 41 centers [77]. The Follow-up After Colorectal Surgery Trial (FACS) in the United Kingdom has randomized over 250 patients in its target of 4900 patients in a 2 × 2 factorial design of "intensive" or "minimalist" follow-up in hospital or community settings [78]. Both of these studies, if successful, will provide better evidence about the impact on not only survival but quality of life, cost, and the impact of advances in surgical techniques, adjuvant therapy, and multidisciplinary teams on cancer follow-up regimes.

What follow-up is appropriate?

A recent review from New York described a follow-up regimen which many would adhere to, though the evidence for many of its elements is lacking (Table 12.3).

Unlike much government-generated advice, the UK NHS has been provided with sensible evidence-based advice on postoperative surveillance after surgery for colorectal cancer [59], as described below. This advice carries an implication of "guilt until proof of innocence," that in the absence of evidence of efficacy, particular investigations or programs should, in general, be omitted rather than included in patient management. Significant caveats

Table 12.3 A suggested follow-up program from Parikh and Attiyeh.

Follow-up	Year 1	Year 2	Year 3	Year 4	>4 years
History and physical	3–4	3–4	2	2	1
Fecal occult blood	3–4	3–4	2	2	1
Sigmoidoscopy*	3–4	3–4	2	2	1
Plasma CEA	3–4	3–4	2	2	1
Colonoscopy or BaE[†]	1	—	—	1	q3 years
Chest X-ray	1	1	1	1	1
CT, MRI, US[‡]	—	—	—	—	—

*For rectal and rectosigmoid cancer patients.
[†]If colon was not cleared preoperatively, then colonoscopy/barium enema should be performed within 6 months postoperatively. If cleared, then every 3 years is sufficient follow-up.
[‡]These tests are only used if there is suspicion of recurrence.
Source: Parikh S, Attiyeh F. *Cancer of the Colon, Rectum and Anus*, 1995: 713–24.

have been placed against perioperative colonoscopy and an 18-month postoperative liver ultrasound scan.

Short term

Follow-up in the weeks after surgery for colorectal cancer should focus on postoperative problems, future planning (including possible use of adjuvant therapy), and stoma management. Patients' needs for emotional and/or practical support should be assessed and appropriate care provided.

Patients who did not undergo complete colonoscopy or barium enema before surgery should be offered colonoscopy within 6 months of discharge. If adenomatous polyps are found, repeat colonoscopy may be appropriate 3 years later. Colonoscopic examination should not be routinely carried out more than once every 3 years.

Longer-term follow-up

There is insufficient reliable evidence on the value of follow-up intended to detect possible recurrence and progression of colorectal cancer after primary treatment. Multi-center clinical trials should therefore be conducted to assess the effectiveness and cost-effectiveness of various types and intensity of follow-up.

Patients and their GPs should be given full information on symptoms which might signify cancer recurrence. They should have rapid access to the colorectal team if they become aware of such symptoms so that treatment can be initiated as quickly as possible. They should be reassured that the risk of recurrence declines rapidly after the first 2 years after treatment, until by year 5, recurrence is very unlikely.

It is thought by some that a yearly ultrasound scan, or an MRI, or CT scan of the liver 18 months after surgery may be appropriate for those patients who might be expected to benefit from early chemotherapy or surgery if they should develop metastatic disease. However, the effectiveness of this practice has not been fully evaluated.

Conclusion

Until evidence suggests to the contrary, in any healthcare system in which major decisions about funding are forced upon providers and consumers, follow-up programs should continue to come below many other priorities aimed at minimizing the morbidity and mortality due to colorectal cancer.

References

1 Virgo K, Vernava A, Longo W *et al.* Cost of patient follow-up after potentially curative colorectal cancer treatment. *JAMA* 1995; 273: 1837–41.

2 Granshaw L. St Mark's Hospital, London. *A Social History of a Specialist Hospital.* King Edward's Hospital Fund for London, King's Fund Historical Series, 1985.

3 Parikh S, Attiyeh F. Rationale for follow-up strategies. In: Coehen A, Winawer S (eds.) *Cancer of the Colon, Rectum and Anus.* New York: McGraw-Hill Inc., 1995: 713–24.

4 Cochrane JP, Williams JT, Faber RG, Slack WW. Value of outpatient follow-up after curative surgery for carcinoma of the large bowel. *Br Med J* 1980; 280: 593–5.

5 Attiyeh F. Guidelines for the follow-up of patients with carcinomas and adenomas of the colon and rectum. In: Stearns M, (ed.) *Neoplasms of the Colon, Rectum and Anus.* New York: Wiley, 1980.

6 Reilly J, Rusin L, Theuerkauf FJ. Colonoscopy: its role in cancer of the colon and rectum. *Dis Colon Rectum* 1982; 25: 532.

7 Ellis H. Recurrent cancer of the large bowel. *Br Med J* 1983; 287: 1741–2.

8 Bulow S, Svendsen L, Mellemgaard A. Metachronous colorectal carcinoma. *Br J Surg* 1990; 77: 502–5.

9 Moertel C, Schutt A, Go V. Carcinoembryonic antigen test for recurrent colorectal cancer. *JAMA* 1978; 78: 1065–6.

10 Kievit J, Bruinvels D. Detection of recurrence after surgery for colorectal cancer. *Eur J Cancer* 1995; 31A: 1222–5.

11 Beart RJ, O'Connell M. Post-operative follow-up of patients with carcinoma of the colon. *Mayo Clin Proc* 1983; 58: 361–3.

12 Audisio R, Setti-Carraro P, Segala M *et al.* Follow-up in colorectal cancer patients: a cost–benefit analysis. *Ann Surg Oncol* 1996; 3: 349–57.

13 Wangensteen O, Lewis F, Arhelger S *et al.* An interim report upon the "second look" procedure for cancer of the stomach, colon, and rectum and for "limited intraperitoneal carcinosis." *Surg Gynecol Obstet* 1954; 99: 257–67.

14 Moertel C, Fleming T, Macdonald J *et al.* An evaluation of the carcinoembryonic antigen (CEA) test for monitoring patients with resected colon cancer. *JAMA* 1993; 270: 943–7.

15 Martin E, Cooperman M, King G *et al.* A retrospective and prospective study of serial CEA determinations in the early detection of recurrent colon cancer. *Am J Surg* 1979; 137: 167–9.

16 Gold P, Freedman S. Demonstration of tumor-specific antigens in human colonic carcinomata by immunological tolerance and absorption techniques. *J Exp Med* 1965; 121: 439–62.

17 Herrera M, Ming T, Holyoke E. Carcinoembryonic antigen (CEA) as a prognostic and monitoring test in clinically complete resection of colorectal carcinoma. *Ann Surg* 1976; 183: 5–9.

18 Reiter W, Stieber P, Reuter C *et al.* Multivariate analysis of the prognostic value of CEA and CA 19-9 serum levels in colorectal cancer. *Anticancer Res* 2000; 20: 5195–8.

19 Martin E, Cooperman M, Carey L, Minton J. Sixty second-look procedures indicated primarily by rise in serial carcinoembryonic antigen. *J Surg Res* 1980; 28: 389–94.

20 Tate H. Plasma CEA in the post-surgical monitoring of colorectal carcinoma. *Br J Cancer* 1982; 46: 323–30.

21 Northover J. Carcinoembryonic antigen and recurrent colorectal cancer. *Gut* 1986; 29: 95–8.

22 Mach J-P, Jaeger P, Bertholet M-M, *et al.* Detection of recurrence of large bowel carcinoma by radioimmunoasssay of circulating carcinoembryonic antigen (CEA). *Lancet* 1974; 535–40.

23 MacKay A, Patel S, Carter S *et al.* Role of serial plasma CEA assays in detection of recurrent and metastatic colorectal carcinomas. *Br Med J* 1974; 4: 382–5.

24 Sorokin J, Sugarbaker P, Zamcheck N *et al.* Serial carcinoembryonic antigen assays. *JAMA* 1974; 228: 49–53.

25 Martin E, Cooperman M, King G *et al.* A retrospective and prospective study of serial CEA determinations in the early detection of recurrent colon cancer. *Am J Surg* 1979; 137: 167–9.

26 Nicholson J, Aust J. Rising carcinoembryonic antigen titers in colorectal carcinoma: an indication for the second-look procedure. *Dis Colon Rectum* 1978; 21: 163–4.

27 Liavag I. Detection and treatment of local recurrence. *Scand J Gastroenterol (Suppl)* 1988; 149: 163–5.

28 Peters K, Grundmann R. The value of tumor markers in colorectal cancer. *Leber Magen Darm* 1989; 19: 18–25.

29 Wanebo H, Llaneras M, Martin T, Kaiser D. Prospective monitoring trial for carcinoma of colon and rectum after surgical resection. *Surg Gynecol Obstet* 1989; 169: 479–87.

30 Ovaska J, Jarvinen H, Mecklin J. The value of a follow up programme after radical surgery for colorectal carcinoma. *Scand J Gastroenterol* 1989; 24: 416–22.

31 Jiang R. Clinical significance of serum CEA determination in the diagnosis of colorectal cancer. *Chung Hua Chung Liu Tsa Chih* 1989; 11: 348–51.

32 Chu D, Erickson C, Russell M *et al.* Prognostic significance of carcinoembryonic antigen in colorectal carcinoma. Serum levels before and after resection and before recurrence. *Arch Surg* 1991; 126: 314–16.

33 Pommier R, Woltering E. Follow up of patients after primary colorectal cancer resection. *Semin Surg Oncol* 1991; 7: 129–32.

34 Himal H. Anastomotic recurrence of carcinoma of the colon and rectum. The value of endoscopy and serum CEA levels. *Am Surg* 1991; 57: 334–7.

35 Fucini C, Tommasi M, Cardona G *et al.* Limitations of CEA monitoring as a guide to second-look surgery in colorectal cancer follow-up. *Tumori* 1983; 69: 359–64.

36 Finlay I, McArdle C. Role of carcinoembryonic antigen in detection of asymptomatic disseminated disease in colorectal carcinoma. *Br Med J* 1983; 286: 1242–4.

37 Tagaki H, Morimoto T, Kato T *et al*. Diagnosis and operation for locally recurrent rectal cancer. *J Surg Oncol* 1985; 28: 290–6.

38 Kagan A, Steckel R. Routine imaging studies for the post treatment surveillance of breast and colorectal carcinoma. *J Clin Oncol* 1991; 9: 837–42.

39 Collopy B. The follow up of patients after resection for large bowel cancer, May 1992. Colorectal Surgical Society of Australia. *Med J Aust* 1992; 157: 633–4.

40 Fletcher R. CEA monitoring after surgery for colorectal cancer. *JAMA* 1993; 270: 987–8.

41 Hine K, Dykes P. Serum CEA testing in the post-operative surveillance of colorectal carcinoma. *Br J Cancer* 1984; 49: 689–93.

42 Carlsson U, Stewenius J, Ekelund G *et al*. Is CEA analysis of value in screening for recurrences after surgery for colorectal carcinoma? *Dis Col Rect* 1983; 26: 369–73.

43 Armitage N, Davidson A, Tsikos D, Wood C. A study of the reliability of carcinoembryonic antigen blood levels in following the course of colorectal cancer. *Clin Oncol* 1984; 10: 141–7.

44 Minton J, Hoehn J, Gerber D *et al*. Results of a 400-patient carcinoembryonic antigen second-look colorectal cancer study. *Cancer* 1984; 55: 1284–90.

45 Wilking N, Petrelli N, Herrera L *et al*. Abdominal exploration for suspected recurrent carcinoma of the colon and rectum based upon elevated carcinoembryonic antigen alone or in combination with other diagnostic methods. *Surg Gynecol Obstet* 1986; 162: 465–8.

46 O'Dwyer P, Mojzisik C, McCabe D *et al*. Reoperation directed by carcinoembryonic antigen level: the importance of thorough preoperative evaluation. *Am J Surg* 1988; 155: 227–31.

47 Putzki H, Reichert B, Heymann H. The tumour markers CEA, CA 19-9 and TPA in colorectal carcinoma. *Theor Surg* 1987; 2: 124–8.

48 Barillari P, Bolognese A, Chirletti P *et al*. Role of CEA, TPA, and CA 19-9 in the early detection of localised and diffuse recurrent rectal cancer. *Dis Colon Rectum* 1992; 35: 471–6.

49 Overholt B. Clinical experience with the fibersigmoidoscope. *Gastrointest Endosc* 1968; 15: 27.

50 Neugut A, Lautenbach E, Abi-Rached B, Forde K. Incidence of adenomas after curative resection for colorectal cancer. *Am J Gastroenterol* 1996; 91: 2096–8.

51 Bekdash B, Harris S, Broughton C *et al*. Outcome after multiple colorectal tumours. *Br J Surg* 1997; 84: 1442–4.

52 Brady P, Straker R, Goldsmid S. Surveillance colonoscopy after resection for colon carcinoma. *South Med J* 1990; 83: 765–8.

53 Granqvist S, Karlsson T. Postoperative follow-up of patients with colorectal carcinoma by colonoscopy. *Eur J Surg* 1992; 158: 307–12.

54 Chen F, Stuart M. Colonoscopic follow-up of colorectal carcinoma. *Dis Colon Rectum* 1994; 37: 568–72.

55 Bussey H, Wallace M, Morson B. Metachronous carcinoma of the large intestine and intestinal polyps. *Proc R Soc Med* 1967; 60: 208.

56 Khoury D, Opelka F, Beck D *et al*. Colon surveillance after colorectal cancer surgery. *Dis Colon Rectum* 1996; 39: 252–6.

57 Galandiuk S, Moertel C, Fitzgibbons R. Patterns of recurrence after curative resection of carcinoma of the colon and rectum. *Surg Gynecol Obstet* 1992; 174: 27–32.

58 Juhl G, Larson G, Mullins R *et al*. Six year results of annual colonoscopy after resection of colorectal cancer. *World J Surg* 1990; 14: 255–60.

59 Haward R. *Improving Outcomes in Colorectal Cancer. The Manual*. NHS [UK National Health Service] Executive,

1997. Guidance on Commissioning Cancer Services.

60 Dresing K, Stock W. Ultrasonic endoluminal examination in the follow-up of colorectal cancer. Initial experience and results. *Int J Colorectal Dis* 1990; 5: 188–94.

61 Rotondano G, Esposito P, Pellechia L *et al.* Early detection of locally recurrent rectal cancer by endosonography. *Br J Radiol* 1997; 70: 567–71.

62 Theoni R. Colorectal cancer. Radiologic staging. *Radiol Clin North Am* 1997; 35: 457–85.

63 Stahl A, Wieder H, Wester HJ *et al.* PET/CT molecular imaging in abdominal oncology. *Abdom Imaging* 2004; 29: 388–97.

64 Pijl ME, Chaoui AS, Wahl RL, van Oostayen JA. Radiology of colorectal cancer. *Eur J Cancer* 2002; 38: 887–98.

65 Beets-Tan RGH, Beets GL. Rectal cancer: review with emphasis on MR imaging. *Radiology* 2004; 232: 335–46.

66 Richard C, McLeod R. Follow-up of patients after resection for colorectal cancer: a position paper of the Canadian Society of Surgical Oncology and the Candian Society of Colon and Rectal Surgeons. *Can J Surg* 1997; 40: 90–100.

67 Ohlsson B, Breland U, Ekberg H *et al.* Follow-up after curative surgery for colorectal carcinoma. Randomised comparison with no follow-up. *Dis Colon Rectum* 1995; 38: 219–26.

68 Makela J, Laitenen S, Kairoluoma M. Five-year follow-up after radical surgery for colorectal cancer. *Arch Surg* 1995; 130: 1062–7.

69 Kjeldsen B, Kronborg O, Fenger C, Jorgensen O. A prospective randomized trial of follow-up after radical surgery for colorectal cancer. *Br J Surg* 1997; 84: 666–9.

70 Schoemaker D, Black R, Giles L, Toouli J. Yearly colonoscopy, liver CT,

and chest radiography do not influence 5-year survival of colorectal cancer patients. *Gastroenterology* 1998; 114: 7–14.

71 Pietra N, Sarli L, Costi R *et al.* Role of follow up in management of local recurrences of colorectal cancer: a prospective, randomized study. *Dis Colon Rectum* 1998; 41: 1127–33.

72 Secco GB, Fardelli R, Gianquinto D *et al.* Efficacy and cost of risk-adapted follow-up in patients after colorectal cancer surgery: a prospective, randomized and controlled trial. *Eur J Surg Oncol* 2002; 28: 418–23.

73 August D, Ottow R, Sugarbaker P. Clinical perspective of human colorectal cancer metastasis. *Cancer Metastasis Rev* 1984; 3: 303–24.

74 Jeffrey GM, Hickey BE, Hider P. Follow-up strategies for patients treated for non-metastatic colorectal cancer. In: Cochrane Library, Issue 1. Oxford: Update Software, 2005. Date of Most Recent Update: November 21, 2003 Accessed June 30, 2005.

75 Renehan AG, Egger M, Saunders MP, O'Dwyer ST. Impact on survival of intensive follow up after curative resection for colorectal cancer: systematic review and meta-analysis of randomised trials. *Br Med J* 2002; 324: 813–6.

76 Renehan AG, O'Dwyer ST, Whynes DK. Cost effectiveness analysis of intensive vs conventional follow up after curative resection for colorectal cancer. *Br Med J* 2004; 328: 81–6.

77 Grossmann EM, Johnson FE, Virgo KS *et al.* Follow-up of colorectal cancer patients after resection with curative intent – the GILDA trial. *Surg Oncol* 2004; 13: 119–24.

78 FACS Website: www.facs.soton.ac.uk/ Information.aspx Accessed June 30, 2005.

13: Chemotherapy of advanced colorectal cancer

Axel Grothey

The last 5–10 years have seen a dramatic expansion of medical therapeutic options in the treatment of advanced colorectal cancer (CRC). After decades of stagnation in which the world of chemotherapy revolved around one single drug, 5-fluorouracil (5-FU), and finding the best way to enhance its efficacy via biomodulation (e.g. with leucovorin – LV) and protracted administration [1], the introduction of irinotecan and oxaliplatin, and, most recently, bevacizumab and cetuximab has completely changed our approach toward metastatic CRC [2]. Response rates (RRs) routinely exceeding 50% and times-to-tumor progression of about 10 months with modern combined chemo-biologic therapy have clearly defined CRC as chemosensitive disease. The abundance of treatment options in the palliative setting, however, comes with the challenge to develop a treatment strategy to maximize outcome for patients (Table 13.1).

Deciding on a specific therapy for patients with advanced CRC is a complex process which takes into account various patient-, tumor-, and treatment-related factors as well as non-medical issues such as reimbursement issues and financial burden to the individual and society (Fig. 13.1).

The most pertinent challenges in the medical management of advanced CRC that need to be addressed for each individual patient are

- What is the best sequence of chemotherapy options?
- Can oral 5-FU prodrugs serve as a substitute for infusional 5-FU in modern combination regimens?
- Should a biologic agent be added upfront?
- How long should first-line treatment be continued?
- Can patients with metastatic disease be candidates for a curative approach?

Table 13.1 Agents with proof-of-efficacy in advanced colorectal cancer.

Conventional chemotherapy
- Fluoropyrimidines
  - 5-fluorouracil (5-FU) (+folinic acid/leucovorin [LV])
  - Capecitabine
  - UFT (+LV)
  - S1
- Raltitrexed
- Pemetrexed
- Mitomycin
- Irinotecan
- Oxaliplatin

Targeted therapy
- VEGF-inhibition
  - Bevacizumab
- EGF-receptor inhibition
  - Cetuximab
  - Panitumumab
  - Matuzumab

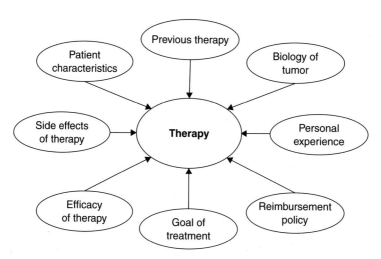

Fig. 13.1 Factors influencing choice of therapy.

What is the best sequence of chemotherapy options?

In the first few years of the twenty-first century, a total of six phase III trials clearly demonstrated that combination regimens using irinotecan or

Table 13.2 Irinotecan- or oxaliplatin-based combination protocols as first-line therapy compared with 5-FU/LV in advanced CRC, results of phase III trials.

Author	Protocol	RR (%)	PFS (mos)	OS (mos)
Saltz *et al.* [8]	Bolus FU/LV (Mayo)	21	4.3	12.6
N = 457 (2 arms)	Bolus FU/LV + CPT-11 (IFL)	39	7.0	14.8
	p value	<0.001	0.004	0.04
Douillard *et al.* [4]	Inf./bolus FU/LV	31	4.4	14.1
N = 338	Inf./bolus FU/LV + CPT-11	49	6.7	17.4
	p value	<0.001	<0.001	0.031
Kohne *et al.* [7]	Inf. FU/LV	34.4	6.4	16.9
N = 430	Inf. FU/LV + CPT-11	62.2	8.5	20.1
	p value	<0.0001	<0.0001	n.s.
De Gramont *et al.* [3]	Inf./bolus FU/LV	22.3	6.2	14.7
N = 420	Inf./bolus FU/LV + Oxaliplatin (FOLFOX4)	50.7	9.0	16.2
	p value	0.0001	<0.0001	n.s.
Grothey *et al.* [6]	Bolus FU/LV (Mayo)	22.6	5.3	16.1
N = 252	Inf. FU/LV + Oxaliplatin (FUFOX)	49.1	7.8	19.7
	p value	<0.0001	0.0001	n.s.

RR, response rate; PFS, progression-free survival; OS, overall survival.

oxaliplatin plus 5-FU/LV (preferentially administered as infusional 5-FU) are superior to 5-FU/LV alone (Table 13.2) [3–8]. This superior efficacy manifested itself in increased RR and prolonged progression-free survival (PFS), but did not necessarily translate into a significant improvement in overall survival (OS), conceivably due to the confounding effects of cross-over and subsequent second- and third-line therapies. While the ill-fated – and now obsolete – IFL regimen (weekly bolus 5-FU/LV/irinotecan) claimed the status of standard of care in the United States from April 2000 to April 2002, the results of Intergroup trial N9741 clearly showed that FOLFOX4 (bolus/infusional 5-FU/LV plus oxaliplatin) is superior to IFL in terms of toxicity and efficacy (Table 13.3) [9]. Inevitable imbalances in second-line therapies at the time when irinotecan, but not oxaliplatin, was readily available for patients on study conceivably contributed to the fact that the difference in OS was perhaps more pronounced than expected from the results on PFS and RR. However, this does not negate the fact that FOLFOX established itself as superior to IFL. Since IFL and FOLFOX use different

Table 13.3 Phase III comparison of combination therapies as first-line treatment in advanced CRC.

Author	Protocol	RR (%)	PFS (mos)	OS (mos)
Goldberg et al. [9]	IFL	31	6.9	15.0
N = 531 (2 arms)	FOLFOX4	45	8.7	19.5
	p value	0.002	0.0014	0.0001
Tournigand et al. [10]	Inf./bolus FU/LV + CPT-11 (FOLFIRI)	56	8.5	21.5
N = 226	FOLFOX6	54	8.1	20.6
	p value	n.s.	n.s.	n.s.
Colucci et al. [11]	Inf./bolus FU/LV + CPT-11 (Douillard)	31	7.0	14
N = 336	FOLFOX4	34	7.0	15
	p value	n.s.	n.s.	n.s.

RR, response rate; PFS, progression-free survival; OS, overall survival.

5-FU/LV backbones, a fairer comparison between optimized oxaliplatin- and irinotecan-based combination regimens can be seen in the trial conducted by Tournigand et al. [10]. In this unfortunately relatively small trial, 220 evaluable patients with advanced CRC were randomized to either FOLFOX6 or FOLFIRI (FOLinic acid, 5-Fluorouracil, IRInotecan) with a planned crossover option on progression (Table 13.3). The key result of this trial was that all pertinent efficacy parameters (RR, PFS, and OS) revealed no appreciable difference between these two arms. These findings were recently confirmed by a slightly larger Italian phase III trial [11]. Thus, the key criteria to choose between FOLFOX and FOLFIRI as the most suitable first-line therapy are the differences in expected toxicities that are associated with each regimen. In this regard, irinotecan's problem is the induction of severe diarrhea in about 15% of patients, a subgroup that could at least partially be characterized by the presence of certain pharmacogenomic polymorphisms of the UGT1A1 enzyme system [12,13]. Patients who tolerate irinotecan normally do not experience cumulative, dose-limiting side effects, meaning irinotecan-based therapy can be continued until tumor progression. In contrast, the acute tolerability of FOLFOX is excellent and side effects mainly relate to the 5-FU/LV component of therapy – with the notable exception of acute, cold-triggered neuropathies induced by oxaliplatin which, however, are rarely dose-limiting [14]. Prolonged treatment with oxaliplatin almost inevitably leads to cumulative, chronic neurotoxicity, the dose-limiting toxicity of oxaliplatin. On the other hand, hepatic insufficiency and elevated bilirubin are relative contraindications for irinotecan while these patients can receive oxaliplatin at full dose [15,16].

The value of using a combination regimen upfront has recently been questioned by results of the large MRC FOCUS (5-Fluorouracil Oxaliplatin, CPT-11 Use and Sequencing) trial conducted in the United Kingdom and Cyprus [17]. This trial tested five different sequences of chemotherapy options in the management of patients with advanced CRC. A total of 2135 patients were randomized to receive either bolus + infusional 5-FU/LV followed by irinotecan, FOLFIRI or FOLFOX on progression, or FOLFIRI or FOLFOX as initial therapy. As expected, combination regimens showed increased RRs and longer PFS compared with 5-FU/LV alone. In terms of OS, however, only a trend toward inferiority of the first option, 5-FU/LV, followed by single agent irinotecan was observed; the survival curves of all five arms were almost superimposable. Unfortunately, only a minority of patients (arm-dependent 12–27%) received all three active chemotherapy agents (5-FU, irinotecan, and oxaliplatin) in the course of their treatment. This factor, together with the fact that patients with potentially resectable liver metastases were reimbursable for FOLFOX therapy and therefore not entered in the trial, resulted in a shorter than anticipated duration of survival (13.9–16.3 months).

The message that making all three drugs available to all patients is more important than starting with a chemotherapy doublet was recently highlighted in a meta-analysis of 21 treatment arms of 11 published phase III trials with 5768 patients [18]. At the trial-arm level, the percentage of patients receiving all three drugs in the course of their treatment was significantly correlated with the reported OS for that arm (median OS (months) $= 13.2 + (\%$pts with three drugs $\times 0.1$); $p = 0.0001$). This correlation remained unchanged when study arms which used single agent 5-FU/LV as first-line treatment were included in the model. In multivariate analysis only exposure to three drugs ($p = 0.0001$), but not use of a doublet first-line ($p = 0.69$), was significantly associated with OS. Nevertheless, patients who receive chemotherapy doublets first-line have a greater chance to receive all three active agents in the course of their therapy, as consistently and approximately only 50–60% of patients starting a line of therapy receive a next-line therapy. Thus, this meta-analysis and even the results of the FOCUS trial eventually confirm that in clinical practice combination therapy should remain the standard of care for first-line treatment of patients with advanced CRC.

Can oral 5-FU prodrugs serve as substitute for infusional 5-FU in modern combination regimens?

It is well established that the anti-tumor activity of 5-FU can be enhanced by protracted intravenous administration which requires the use of catheter devices and portable pumps to allow treatment in an outpatient setting. Oral formulations of fluoropyrimidines could mimic the protracted delivery of 5-FU in a convenient way while maintaining clinical efficacy. Since the bioavailability of oral 5-FU shows substantial inter-individual variability, only 5-FU prodrugs which are readily absorbed and subsequently activated to 5-FU are able to generate predictable serum levels of 5-FU. Several 5-FU prodrugs with proof-of-efficacy in advanced CRC have been developed (Table 13.1).

UFT is uracil/tegafur in a fixed molar ratio of 4 to 1. While tegafur is the actual 5-FU prodrug which is rapidly and completely absorbed after oral administration, uracil competes with 5-FU for binding to dihydropyrimidine dehydrogenase (DPD), the most important enzyme in the degradation cascade of 5-FU. Two randomized trials of 816 and 380 patients compared UFT/LV with bolus 5-FU/LV (Mayo Clinic regimen) [19,20]. While RR were comparable and UFT was found to be more tolerable than bolus 5-FU/LV, PFS in the larger trial was significantly inferior for UFT/LV so that UFT was not approved by the US Food and Drug Administration (FDA). It is, however, available in most European countries and Japan. The lack of FDA approval has clearly limited the further development of UFT as a potential component of modern combination regimens. The oral fluoropyrimidine most commonly used in clinical trials with modern conventional chemotherapies and targeted agents is capecitabine.

Capecitabine is an oral fluoropyrimidines carbamate which requires a three-step enzymatic activation to 5-FU. Two phase-III trials with a total of 1207 patients demonstrated that capecitabine is at least as effective and less toxic than bolus 5-FU/LV (Mayo Clinic regimen) [21–23]. In fact, while PFS was identical, RRs for capecitabine were found to be superior compared with the Mayo Clinic regimen.

The question whether capecitabine can serve as an equipotent and more convenient substitute for infusional 5-FU in combination regimens with oxaliplatin and irinotecan is currently being addressed in several phase-III trials. Results from single-arm phase-II trials are particularly encouraging for the combination of capecitabine with oxaliplatin [24]. First results of a capecitabine-based combination regimen as first-line therapy in CRC on phase III evidence level were recently presented at American Society of Clinical Oncology (ASCO) 2005 and compared the weekly infusional 5-FU/LV plus oxaliplatin regimen FUFOX with a capecitabine/oxaliplatin (CAPOX) combination [25]. This trial enrolled 476 patients and saw no statistically significant difference in the primary endpoint, PFS, although a numeric difference was notable in favor of FUFOX (PFS 8.0 vs 7.0 months, $p = 0.11$). No significant difference in RR was observed (FUFOX 49%, CAPOX 47%). While it is unlikely that this difference in PFS will translate into meaningful differences in OS, the results of larger phase-III trials have to be awaited until capecitabine can truly be regarded as effective as the protracted administration of 5-FU in combination regimens with oxaliplatin.

Capecitabine/irinotecan combinations suffer from overlapping toxicity with regard to diarrhea and have thus been less enthusiastically embraced [26]. In fact, a recent European phase-III trial comparing capecitabine/irinotecan (CAPIRI) with FOLFIRI was prematurely closed in view of unacceptable toxicity associated with CAPIRI [27]. Some phase-II trials, however, have shown good tolerability of this combination when the dose of capecitabine was reduced for elderly patients [28,29].

Should a biologic agent be added upfront?

Talking about biologic agents with proof-of-efficacy in CRC in 2005 means talking about monoclonal antibodies against the epidermal-growth-factor receptor (EGFR – cetuximab and panitumumab) and against vascular endothelial growth factor (VEGF – bevacizumab).

Cetuximab and bevacizumab were both FDA-approved for use in patients with advanced CRC in February 2004, but with very different indications. Based on the results of three phase-II trials – only one of which, the BOND-1 trial, was randomized (Table 13.4) – in patients who had failed irinotecan-based therapy [30–32], cetuximab was approved as salvage therapy for patients pretreated with irinotecan. Since even in tumors refractory to irinotecan the combination of cetuximab with irinotecan was found to be superior to cetuximab alone in RR and TTP (time-to-tumor progression), cetuximab plus irinotecan has emerged as one of the standard salvage options in CRC. Cetuximab does contain significant single-agent activity with confirmed RR of slightly over 10% after irinotecan failure, a rate also found with FOLFOX second-line [33]. So far, however, the designs of the

Table 13.4 Results of randomized trials of cetuximab in metastatic CRC.

Regimen	Cunningham *et al.* [30] (BOND-1)		Saltz *et al.* [41] (BOND-2)	
	C225	C225 + CPT	C225 + BEV	C225 + CPT + BEV
N patients	111	218	40	41
Previous oxaliplatin (% of patients)	64	62	90	85
RR (%)	11	23	20	37
TTP (mos)	1.5	4.1	5.6	7.9
Med. OS (mos)	6.9	8.6	—	—

CPT, irinotecan; BEV, bevacizumab; RR, response rate; TTP, time-to-tumor progression; OS, overall survival.

cetuximab trials have made it impossible to assess whether cetuximab leads to prolonged OS in advanced CRC. In addition, phase III data on first-line use of cetuximab are currently lacking. Data from several phase II studies using cetuximab in combination with effective conventional combination chemotherapy (FOLFOX or FOLFIRI) have revealed remarkably high RR of up to 81% [34,35]. Several ongoing phase-III trials are trying to confirm these intriguing results and to establish cetuximab's role in front-line therapy of advanced CRC. If the high activity of cetuximab combinations upfront can be confirmed, they could present an effective neoadjuvant therapy for patients in whom a curative surgical option appears feasible after downsizing of liver (and possibly extrahepatic) metastases [36]. To date, however – outside of a clinical trial – cetuximab should be used as salvage therapy. Panitumumab will presumably emerge as a direct competitor of cetuximab, targeting the same antigen on tumor cells, EGFR, and providing the advantage of reduced rate of infusion reactions (cetuximab: mouse–human chimeric antibody; panitumumab: fully human antibody) and two-weekly dosing (cetuximab: weekly) [37]. While the initial FDA label of approval will likely also reserve panitumumab as salvage therapy option, a phase-III trial testing panitumumab as component of first-line therapy in advanced CRC is ongoing.

Bevacizumab is a humanized monoclonal antibody against VEGF-A, a member of a family of VEGF-receptor activating ligands. CRC was the first tumor in which evidence for the efficacy of an anti-angiogenic strategy was obtained on a phase-III level. The pivotal phase-III trial demonstrated

Table 13.5 Results of randomized trials of bevacizumab in metastatic CRC.

Author	Protocol	RR (%)	PFS (mos)	OS (mos)
First-line therapy				
Hurwitz *et al.* [38]	IFL + placebo	35	6.2	15.6
N = 813 (2 arms)	IFL + bevacizumab	45	10.6	20.3
	p value	0.004	<0.001	<0.001
Kabbinavar	Weekly bolus 5-FU/LV	15.2	5.5	12.9
et al. [40]	(Roswell Park) + placebo			
N = 209	Bolus 5-FU/LV +	26.0	9.2	16.6
	bevacizumab			
	p value	0.055	0.0002	0.16
Second-line therapy, bevacizumab-naïve patients				
Giantonio *et al.* [39]	FOLFOX4 + placebo	9.2	4.8	10.8
N = 561 (2 arms)	FOLFOX4 + bevacizumab	21.8	7.2	12.9
	p value	<0.001	<0.001	0.0018

RR, response rate; PFS, progression-free survival; OS, overall survival.

a significant survival benefit when bevacizumab was added to the historic standard-of-care in chemotherapy, IFL (Table 13.5) [38]. The addition of bevacizumab to IFL dramatically increased OS from 15.6 to 20.3 months ($p = 0.00004$). This effect was paralleled by the same incremental increase in PFS (6.2 vs 10.6 months, $p < 0.00001$). Interestingly, in view of the magnitude of benefit observed for OS and PFS, the effect of bevacizumab on RR was rather moderate (35 vs 45%, $p = 0.0036$) in line with a more cytostatic-antiangiogenic effect than direct cytotoxicity.

In further trials, bevacizumab significantly enhanced the activity of other conventional chemotherapy regimens such as weekly bolus 5-FU/LV and in a second-line study FOLFOX4 (Table 13.5) [39,40]. In all studies, an increased RR in the range of 10–15% was noted when bevacizumab was added to chemotherapy, but the clear strength of bevacizumab appeared to be a prolongation of PFS in which adequately powered trials routinely translated into significant gains in OS. Bevacizumab does not only add efficacy to conventional chemotherapy in advanced CRC, but apparently also to tumor-directed, targeted agents such as cetuximab. This point was illustrated by the results of the so-called BOND-2 trial which added bevacizumab to both arms of the BOND-1 study (Table 13.4) [41]. Although a direct, historic comparison between BOND-1 and BOND-2 can only be suboptimal at best, the magnitude of difference observed with the addition of bevacizumab to cetuximab and cetuximab/irinotecan deserves attention. Consistent with all other trials using conventional chemotherapy, the addition of bevacizumab appeared to enhance the efficacy of cetuximab and cetuximab/irinotecan in terms of RR, but more strikingly, in terms of TTP.

While most patients cannot distinguish between placebo and beva-cizumab due to the excellent tolerability of the monoclonal antibody, some side effects that occur in a minority of patients have to be taken very seri-ously. This is clearly true for the consistently reported 1.5–2.0% of patients who experience a gastrointestinal (GI) perforation on treatment with beva-cizumab. So far, no definitive risk factors for GI perforations have been identified, not least due to the small number of patients affected by this complication, which makes the identification of a clinical pattern difficult. Another serious complication was recently identified and described as "arte-rial thrombotic events" (ATEs), clinical symptoms caused by ischemic events in the arterial system such as angina, myocardial infarction, and stroke [42]. While the exact definition of ATEs might still be vague, it has to be rec-ognized that the use of bevacizumab is associated with an approximately 2-fold increase in ATEs. In patients with an already higher risk for ATEs at baseline (over 65 years, prior history of ATE), the rate of ATE on beva-cizumab reached almost 18% in a pooled analysis of five trials in three tumor types (CRC, breast, and lung cancer). While this high-risk group of patients clearly deserves special attention and the issue of ATEs needs to be openly discussed (and documented), it is not justified to withhold bevacizumab from this group completely since these patients appear to benefit from the inclu-sion of bevacizumab in their front-line therapy to the same extent as all patients in the pivotal IFL-based phase III study.

Thus, based on these findings, bevacizumab has emerged as the standard component of any first-line therapy in metastatic CRC, which is exactly according to its FDA-approved label. The pertinent question has moved from: "who should receive bevacizumab?" to "who should not receive it?"

How long should first-line treatment be continued?

Traditionally, palliative chemotherapy in CRC was continued until progres-sion or toxicity – which in clinical practice meant that until about 10 years ago with 5-FU as the only available agent with efficacy in this disease, patients were kept on 5-FU or 5-FU/LV with a median TTP of 4–6 months after which treatment was discontinued and best supportive care (BSC) was pursued. This resulted in median OS of around 12 months, a very consistent result in all phase-III trials in the pre-irinotecan/pre-oxaliplatin era [2]. At that time, a UK trial investigated whether patients who showed response or at least stable disease to 5-FU or raltitrexed first-line therapy benefited from further continuation of therapy or if a chemotherapy-free interval was permissive [43]. This trial showed no detrimental effect of intermittent vs continuous therapy in terms of OS with less toxicity observed in the intermittent arm. However, OS was rather short compared with current standards (10.8 and 11.3 months for the respective treatment arms), reflecting the limited therapeutic options available at that time.

The introduction of irinotecan and oxaliplatin and more recently bevacizumab and cetuximab have completely changed this picture. Nowadays CRC is regarded as a chemosensitive disease and patients with stage IV CRC routinely live longer than 2 years. The increase in OS creates specific challenges which can be summarized in the goal of all palliative treatment: to keep patients alive as long as possible while maintaining optimal quality of life on therapy. It is obvious that the more effective but also more toxic modern chemotherapy regimens, which allow several lines of treatment, require different therapeutic strategies and a different approach compared with single agent 5-FU followed by BSC. For instance, one of the most commonly used treatment regimens in advanced CRC, FOLFOX plus bevacizumab, contains a regimen-inherent challenge: the cumulative toxicity of oxaliplatin combined with an agent whose hallmark is delaying TTP leads to an inevitable conflict. In fact, even without the addition of a cytostatic biologic agent, more patients have been reported to get off oxaliplatin due to toxicity than due to progressive disease. A detailed analysis of the FOLFOX arm in N9741 showed a significant difference between TTP (9.3 months) and time-to-treatment failure (TTF – 5.8 months) [44]. This problem was further illustrated in the preliminary results of the sequential TREE-1 and TREE-2 trials in which the addition of bevacizumab to three different oxaliplatin-based treatment regimens first-line did increase RR, but not TTF [45]. In this trial – as in N9741 – median TTF in all arms was in the range of 5.8 months. Data on PFS are not available yet. Thus, it is easy to see that the use of FOLFOX plus bevacizumab as first-line therapy in advanced CRC requires the implementation of a strategy to maximize benefit of therapy (primary goals: prolonged PFS and OS) and reduce toxicity. A practical solution is the use of a stop-and-go approach for oxaliplatin as demonstrated in the OPTIMOX-1 trial [46]. In the OPTIMOX approach, commonly termed "stop-and-go," patients are given an induction regimen of oxaliplatin plus 5-FU/LV until either a predetermined "time to best response" or the beginning of the development of neurotoxicity. They are then maintained on a 5-FU/LV regimen in the absence of oxaliplatin to give any accumulated neurotoxic damage a chance to resolve. Then, oxaliplatin is reintroduced to maximize the potential benefit of the combination regimen. This strategy has been evaluated in a phase-III trial including 526 patients. The results showed a decrease in the severity of the neurotoxicity (grade 3 13 vs 19%) and neutropenia compared with continued FOLFOX4 without compromising efficacy in the OPTIMOX-arm. Studies are ongoing to further test this treatment approach for FOLFOX plus bevacizumab combination regimens.

A rational approach in clinical practice could be to start palliative chemotherapy for advanced CRC with FOLFOX plus bevacizumab and continue until "best response," which is normally achieved within 4 months. If treatment duration of FOLFOX is limited to 4 months, that is, 8 administrations with a cumulative oxaliplatin-dose of 640 mg/m^2, only a very small percentage of patients (3–4%) should have developed severe neurotoxicity. Depending on the aggressiveness of the tumor biology, oxaliplatin can then be paused and the treatment continued with just infusional 5-FU/LV (or capecitabine) plus bevacizumab. In select patients with aggressive tumors an irinotecan-based regimen might be preferable. In case of tumor progression, oxaliplatin can then be reintroduced to prolong time of tumor control. Eventually, all five active agents in CRC, 5-FU (or capecitabine), irinotecan, oxaliplatin, bevacizumab, and cetuximab (or perhaps in future panitumumab) should be used in the course of treatment to maximize the treatment benefit on OS for patients [18,47].

Can patients with metastatic disease be candidates for a curative approach?

The liver is the most common site of metastasis of advanced CRC, at least in part due to hematogenos spread via the portal vein system. In about one-third of patients with metastatic disease the liver will be the only site of metastasis. Untreated hepatic metastasis has a poor prognosis with historic data indicating a median survival of 6–12 months. The value of surgical resection of liver metastasis of CRC was initially demonstrated in 1984 by Wagner et al. [48] who found a 25% 5-year survival of 116 resected patients compared with only 2% in 70 potentially resectable patients who did not undergo surgery. Until recently resection of liver metastasis was deemed feasible in only a small subset of patients with advanced disease and only about 10–15% of patients with liver-only disease were amendable to upfront resection. Major advances in the medical treatment of CRC with significant increase in the quantity and quality of responses, as well as better patient selection, advances in surgical methods, and the emergence of non-surgical tumor ablation techniques have significantly changed the modern approach toward liver-limited metastatic CRC. Using a multimodality neoadjuvant strategy involving medical oncologists, liver surgeons, and interventional radiologists, the number of patients rendered free of metastatic disease as a prerequisite for a curative chance will substantially increase in the future. The main predictor of whether or not a given chemotherapy regimen is able to lead to increased resectability rates in liver-limited disease is the direct anti-tumor activity of the regimen measured by its RR [36]. It is thus easy to understand that these neoadjuvant approaches only emerged with the advent of chemotherapies that reliably induced RRs around or above 50%, much higher than the 15–20% RR associated with systemic biomodulated 5-FU alone. In the era of 5-FU, locoregional approaches using hepatic arterial infusion (HAI) with 5-FUDR combined with systemic 5-FU/LV were applied to maximize response. In fact, several phase-II trials documented RRs of 22–62% (overview Kelly [49]), but toxicities related to 5-FUDR (biliary sclerosis) and catheter-related complications which can conceivably interfere with a subsequent surgical approach have so far precluded HAI from becoming standard-of-care for neoadjuvant treatment of unresectable liver metastases. In addition, modern systemic chemotherapy regimens achieve RRs in the same range as or exceeding HAI.

Oxaliplatin-based regimens have so far been most widely studied as neoadjuvant therapy in patients with initially unresectable liver metastases. Studies presented in the mid-1990s by French investigators established the concept of downsizing unresectable liver metastases with systemic 5-FU/oxaliplatin to obtain surgical resectability when they could demonstrate that the long-term prognosis of these patients did not differ from historic controls with initially resectable metastases [50,51]. In fact, to date several countries have only approved oxaliplatin as part of a neoadjuvant strategy as first-line therapy for advanced CRC. The capability of a certain chemotherapy regimen to downsize metastasis in a neoadjuvant setting is most closely related to the reported overall RR obtained with the given regimen. Given the improved anti-tumor activity of conventional chemotherapy regimens in combination with targeted agents such as bevacizumab [38,39] and cetuximab [30,52] it is conceivable that those novel combination protocols will further increase the number of patients with metastatic CRC eligible for a curative approach. Prospective trials using this approach are underway.

Summary and conclusion

In conclusion, the dramatic advances in the treatment of metastatic CRC have turned this tumor into a "chronic" disease with OS exceeding 2 years for most patients in clinical reality. However, these advances come with the challenge to develop a rational treatment strategy to make use of all available treatment options in an optimized approach (Fig. 13.2). The initial question in the management of patients with metastatic CRC should be if they could potentially be candidates for a neoadjuvant approach with curative intent.

For most patients the answer to this question will be "no." For these patients an appropriate palliative strategy will aim at prolonging OS with minimized toxicity and maintained quality of life. Bevacizumab should be continued until tumor progression and an induction–maintenance–reinduction approach for oxaliplatin is preferable if FOLFOX (or capecitabine/oxaliplatin) is used first-line. In the course of therapy patients

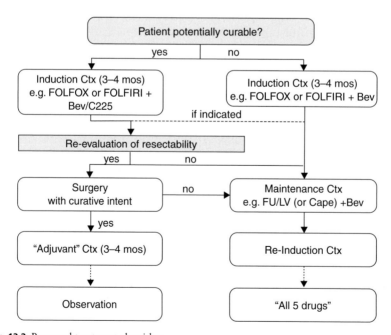

Fig. 13.2 Proposed treatment algorithm.

should receive all five active drug classes (fluoropyrimidine, oxaliplatin, irinotecan, bevacizumab, anti-EGFR-receptor antibodies) and cetuximab can be reserved as salvage therapy.

For patients considered candidates for a neoadjuvant approach, the initial therapy aims at maximizing tumor shrinkage. It is conceivable that in this scenario the upfront use of anti-EGFR-antibodies in combination with cytotoxic doublets plus bevacizumab can enhance the anti-tumor efficacy and thus increase the rate of potentially curative metastasectomies.

References

1 Schmoll HJ, Buchele T, Grothey A et al. Where do we stand with 5-fluorouracil? Semin Oncol 1999, 26: 589–605.

2 Grothey A, Schmoll HJ. New chemotherapy approaches in colorectal cancer. Curr Opin Oncol 2001; 13: 275–86.

3 de Gramont A, Figer A, Seymour M et al. Leucovorin and fluorouracil with or without oxaliplatin as first-line treatment in advanced colorectal cancer. J Clin Oncol 2000; 18: 2938–47.

4 Douillard JY, Cunningham D, Roth AD et al. Irinotecan combined with fluorouracil compared with fluorouracil alone as first-line treatment for metastatic colorectal cancer: a multicentre randomised trial. Lancet 2000; 355: 1041–7.

5 Giacchetti S, Perpoint B, Zidani R et al. Phase III multicenter randomized trial of oxaliplatin added to chronomodulated fluorouracil–leucovorin as first-line treatment of metastatic colorectal cancer. J Clin Oncol 2000; 18: 136–47.

6 Grothey A, Deschler B, Kroening H et al. Phase III study of bolus 5-fluorouracil (5-FU)/folinic acid (FA) (Mayo) vs weekly high-dose 24 h 5-FU infusion/FA + oxaliplatin (OXA) in advanced colorectal cancer (ACRC). Proc Am Soc Clin Oncol 2002; 21: 512.

7 Kohne CH, van Cutsem E, Wils J et al. Phase III study of weekly high-dose infusional fluorouracil plus folinic acid with or without irinotecan in patients with metastatic colorectal cancer:

European Organisation for Research and Treatment of Cancer Gastrointestinal Group Study 40986. J Clin Oncol 2005; 23: 4856–65.

8 Saltz LB, Cox JV, Blanke C et al. Irinotecan plus fluorouracil and leucovorin for metastatic colorectal cancer. Irinotecan Study Group. N Engl J Med 2000; 343: 905–14.

9 Goldberg RM, Sargent DJ, Morton RF et al. A randomized controlled trial of fluorouracil plus leucovorin, irinotecan, and oxaliplatin combinations in patients with previously untreated metastatic colorectal cancer. J Clin Oncol 2004; 22: 23–30.

10 Tournigand C, Andre T, Achille E et al. FOLFIRI followed by FOLFOX6 or the reverse sequence in advanced colorectal cancer: a randomized GERCOR study. J Clin Oncol 2004; 22: 229–37.

11 Colucci G, Gebbia V, Paoletti G et al. Phase III randomized trial of FOLFIRI versus FOLFOX4 in the treatment of advanced colorectal cancer: a multicenter study of the Gruppo Oncologico Dell'Italia Meridionale. J Clin Oncol 2005; 23: 4866–75.

12 Innocenti F, Undevia SD, Iyer L et al. Genetic variants in the UDP-glucuronosyltransferase 1A1 gene predict the risk of severe neutropenia of irinotecan. J Clin Oncol 2004.

13 Innocenti F, Ratain MJ. Update on pharmacogenetics in cancer chemotherapy. Eur J Cancer 2002; 38: 639–44.

14 Grothey A. Clinical management of oxaliplatin-associated neurotoxicity. *Clin Colorectal Cancer* 2005; 5: S38–46.

15 Takimoto CH, Remick SC, Sharma S *et al.* Dose-escalating and pharmacological study of oxaliplatin in adult cancer patients with impaired renal function: a National Cancer Institute Organ Dysfunction Working Group Study. *J Clin Oncol* 2003; 21: 2664–72.

16 Doroshow JH, Synold TW, Gandara D *et al.* Pharmacology of oxaliplatin in solid tumor patients with hepatic dysfunction: a preliminary report of the National Cancer Institute Organ Dysfunction Working Group. *Semin Oncol* 2003; 30: 14–19.

17 Seymour MT, NCRI colorectal group. Fluorouracil, oxaliplatin and CPT-11 (irinotecan), use and sequencing (MRC FOCUS): A 2135-patient randomized trial in advanced colorectal cancer (ACRC). *J Clin Oncol* (Meeting Abstracts) 2005; 23: 3518.

18 Grothey A, Sargent D. Overall survival of patients with advanced colorectal cancer correlates with availability of fluorouracil, irinotecan, and oxaliplatin regardless of whether doublet or single-agent therapy is used first line. *J Clin Oncol* 2005; 23: 9441–2.

19 Carmichael J, Popiela T, Radstone D *et al.* Randomized comparative study of tegafur/uracil and oral leucovorin versus parenteral fluorouracil and leucovorin in patients with previously untreated metastatic colorectal cancer. *J Clin Oncol* 2002; 20: 3617–27.

20 Douillard JY, Hoff PM, Skillings JR *et al.* Multicenter phase III study of uracil/tegafur and oral leucovorin versus fluorouracil and leucovorin in patients with previously untreated metastatic colorectal cancer. *J Clin Oncol* 2002; 20: 3605–16.

21 Hoff PM, Ansari R, Batist G *et al.* Comparison of oral capecitabine versus intravenous fluorouracil plus leucovorin as first-line treatment in 605 patients with metastatic colorectal cancer: results

of a randomized phase III study. *J Clin Oncol* 2001; 19: 2282–92.

22 Van Cutsem E, Twelves C, Cassidy J *et al.* Oral capecitabine compared with intravenous fluorouracil plus leucovorin in patients with metastatic colorectal cancer: results of a large phase III study. *J Clin Oncol* 2001; 19: 4097–106.

23 Cassidy J, Twelves C, Van Cutsem E *et al.* First-line oral capecitabine therapy in metastatic colorectal cancer: a favorable safety profile compared with intravenous 5-fluorouracil/leucovorin. *Ann Oncol* 2002; 13: 566–75.

24 Cassidy J, Tabernero J, Twelves C *et al.* XELOX (capecitabine plus oxaliplatin): active first-line therapy for patients with metastatic colorectal cancer. *J Clin Oncol* 2004; 22: 2084–91.

25 Arkenau HT, Schmoll H, Kubicka S *et al.* Infusional 5-fluorouracil/folinic acid plus oxaliplatin (FUFOX) versus capecitabine plus oxaliplatin (CAPOX) as first line treatment of metastatic colorectal cancer (MCRC): results of the safety and efficacy analysis. *J Clin Oncol* (Meeting Abstracts) 2005; 23: 3507.

26 Grothey A, Goetz MP. Oxaliplatin plus oral fluoropyrimidines in colorectal cancer. *Clin Colorectal Cancer* 2004; 4: S37–42.

27 Kohne CH, de Greve J, Bokemeyer C *et al.* Capecitabine plus irinotecan versus 5-FU/FA/irinotecan +/− celecoxib in first line treatment of metastatic colorectal cancer. Safety results of the prospective multicenter EORTC phase III study 40015. *J Clin Oncol* (Meeting Abstracts) 2005; 23: 3525.

28 Borner MM, Dietrich D, Stupp R *et al.* Phase II study of capecitabine and oxaliplatin in first- and second-line treatment of advanced or metastatic colorectal cancer. *J Clin Oncol* 2002; 20: 1759–66.

29 Cartwright T, Lopez T, Vukelja SJ *et al.* Results of a phase II open-label study of capecitabine in combination with irinotecan as first-line treatment for metastatic colorectal cancer. *Clin Colorectal Cancer* 2005; 5: 50–6.

30 Cunningham D, Humblet Y, Siena S *et al*. Cetuximab monotherapy and cetuximab plus irinotecan in irinotecan-refractory metastatic colorectal cancer. *N Engl J Med* 2004; 351: 337–45.

31 Saltz LB, Meropol NJ, Loehrer PJ, Sr *et al*. Phase II trial of cetuximab in patients with refractory colorectal cancer that expresses the epidermal growth factor receptor. *J Clin Oncol* 2004; 22: 1201–8.

32 Saltz LB, Rubin M, Hochster H *et al*. Cetuximab (IMC-C225) plus irinotecan (CPT-11) is active in CPT-11-refractory colorectal cancer (CRC) that expresses epidermal growth factor receptor (EGFR). *Proc Am Soc Clin Oncol* 2001; 20: 7.

33 Rothenberg ML, Oza AM, Bigelow RH *et al*. Superiority of oxaliplatin and fluorouracil–leucovorin compared with either therapy alone in patients with progressive colorectal cancer after irinotecan and fluorouracil–leucovorin: interim results of a phase III trial. *J Clin Oncol* 2003; 21: 2059–69.

34 Diaz Rubio E, Tabernero J, van Cutsem E *et al*. Cetuximab in combination with oxaliplatin/ 5-fluorouracil (5-FU)/folinic acid (FA) (FOLFOX-4) in the first-line treatment of patients with epidermal growth factor receptor (EGFR)-expressing metastatic colorectal cancer: An international phase II study. *J Clin Oncol* (Meeting Abstracts) 2005; 23: 3535.

35 Seufferlein T, Dittrich C, Riemann J *et al*. A phase I/II study of cetuximab in combination with 5-fluorouracil (5-FU)/folinic acid (FA) plus weekly oxaliplatin (L-OHP) (FUFOX) in the first-line treatment of patients with metastatic colorectal cancer (mCRC) expressing epidermal growth factor receptor (EGFR). Preliminary results. *J Clin Oncol* (Meeting Abstracts) 2005; 23: 3644.

36 Folprecht G, Grothey A, Alberts S *et al*. Neoadjuvant treatment of unresectable colorectal liver metastases: correlation between tumour response and resection rates. *Ann Oncol* 2005; 16: 1311–19.

37 Malik I, Hecht JR, Patnaik A *et al*. Safety and efficacy of panitumumab monotherapy in patients with metastatic colorectal cancer (mCRC). *J Clin Oncol* (Meeting Abstracts) 2005; 23: 3520.

38 Hurwitz H, Fehrenbacher L, Novotny W *et al*. Bevacizumab plus irinotecan, fluorouracil, and leucovorin for metastatic colorectal cancer. *N Engl J Med* 2004; 350: 2335–42.

39 Giantonio B, Catalano D, Meropol NJ *et al*. High-dose bevacizumab improves survival when combined with FOLFOX4 in previously treated advanced colorectal cancer: results from the Eastern Cooperative Oncology Group (ECOG) study E3200. *J Clin Oncol* 2005; 23: 2.

40 Kabbinavar FF, Schulz J, McCleod M *et al*. Addition of bevacizumab to bolus fluorouracil and leucovorin in first-line metastatic colorectal cancer: results of a randomized phase II trial. *J Clin Oncol* 2005; 23: 3697–705.

41 Saltz LB, Lenz HJ, Hochster H *et al*. Randomized phase II trial of cetuximab/bevacizumab/irinotecan (CBI) versus cetuximab/bevacizumab (CB) in irinotecan-refractory colorectal cancer. *J Clin Oncol* 2005; 23: 3508.

42 Skillings JR, Johnson DH, Miller K *et al*. Arterial thromboembolic events (ATEs) in a pooled analysis of 5 randomized, controlled trials (RCTs) of bevacizumab (BV) with chemotherapy. *J Clin Oncol* (Meeting Abstracts) 2005; 23: 3019.

43 Maughan TS, James RD, Kerr DJ *et al*. Comparison of intermittent and continuous palliative chemotherapy for advanced colorectal cancer: a multicentre randomised trial. *Lancet* 2003; 361: 457–64.

44 Green E, Sargent D, Goldberg R *et al*. Detailed analysis of oxaliplatin-associated neurotoxicity in Intergroup trial N9741, 2005 Gastrointestinal Cancers Symposium – GI ASCO. Hollywood, FL, 2005, p 175, abstr. 182.

45 Hochster HS, Welles L, Hart L *et al*. Safety and efficacy of bevacizumab (Bev) when added to oxaliplatin/ fluoropyrimidine (O/F) regimens as

first-line treatment of metastatic colorectal cancer (mCRC): TREE 1 & 2 Studies. *J Clin Oncol* (Meeting Abstracts) 2005; 23: 3515.

46 de Gramont A, Cervantes A, Andre T *et al*. OPTIMOX study: FOLFOX7/LV5FU2 compared to FOLFOX4 in patients with advanced colorectal cancer. *J Clin Oncol* 22, 14S (July 15 Suppl): 3525, 2004.

47 Grothey A, Sargent D, Goldberg RM *et al*. Survival of patients with advanced colorectal cancer improves with the availability of fluorouracil–leucovorin, irinotecan, and oxaliplatin in the course of treatment. *J Clin Oncol* 2004; 22: 1209–14.

48 Wagner JS, Adson MA, Van Heerden JA *et al*. The natural history of hepatic metastases from colorectal cancer. A comparison with resective treatment. *Ann Surg* 1984; 199: 502–8.

49 Kelly RJ, Kemeny NE, Leonard GD. Current strategies using hepatic arterial infusion chemotherapy for the treatment of colorectal cancer. *Clin Colorectal Cancer* 2005; 5: 166–74.

50 Adam R, Avisar E, Ariche A *et al*. Five-year survival following hepatic resection after neoadjuvant therapy for nonresectable colorectal. *Ann Surg Oncol* 2001; 8: 347–53.

51 Bismuth H, Adam R, Levi F *et al*. Resection of nonresectable liver metastases from colorectal cancer after neoadjuvant chemotherapy. *Ann Surg* 1996; 224: 509–20; discussion 520–2.

52 Díaz Rubio E, Tabernero J, van Cutsem E *et al*. Cetuximab in combination with oxaliplatin/ 5-fluorouracil (5-FU)/folinic acid (FA) (FOLFOX-4) in the first-line treatment of patients with epidermal growth factor receptor (EGFR)-expressing metastatic colorectal cancer: an international phase II study. *J Clin Oncol* 2005; 23: 254s (suppl, abstr 3535).

14: Surgery for metastatic disease in colorectal cancer

Timothy G. John and Myrddin Rees

Introduction

The liver is the most common site of metastasis in patients with colorectal cancer. Following hematogenous dissemination through the portal venous system, the liver is thought to present as the first and only target site for overt metastatic spread in 30–40% of cases [1]. Up to 25% of colorectal cancer patients present with synchronous liver metastases at the time of diagnosis, and approximately 50% of all patients who undergo radical resection for primary colorectal cancer may be affected by isolated metastatic disease confined to the liver, usually within the first 2 years [2–4]. It is now recognized that for selected patients with colorectal liver metastases, hepatic resectional surgery is unique in offering the prospect of cure and has become a paradigm in the management of some such patients with "advanced" disease.

The proportion of patients with colorectal liver metastases eligible for hepatic resection with curative intent has been estimated at 20–30% [5]. While this may vary between centers and depends on prevailing selection policies, the general adoption of less restrictive selection criteria continues to broaden the limits of resectability as further advances in hepatobiliary surgical practice and multimodality treatments become established. Conversely, colorectal liver metastases do not usually cause symptoms and no role for palliative hepatic resection has been established. Also, the benefits of essentially palliative surgical therapies such as implantation devices for hepatic arterial chemotherapy remain unclear and shall not be considered further herein.

The evidence for hepatic resection

It is recognized that the majority of patients with colorectal liver metastases left untreated will die from carcinomatosis within 9–12 months and that survival at 5 years is exceptional [5]. Although significant advances in treatment with systemic chemotherapy have been achieved in recent years, conventional non-surgical treatment alone has shown only modest survival benefits with no significant survival beyond 3 years [6]. In contrast, hepatic resection offers the prospect of long-term disease-free survival and may potentially be curative. It is therefore very unlikely that randomized controlled trials of liver resection in patients with colorectal metastases will ever be conducted because of ethical considerations in pursuing comparative data on non-surgical treatment in patients with resectable disease.

Evidence for the effectiveness of hepatic resection must, by necessity, be based on published case series and reviews, while available control data is historical. Wagner and colleagues [7] reported that, left untreated, patients with potentially resectable, unilobar disease had a median survival of less than 2 years. Similarly, Wood and co-workers [8] cited a median survival of only 17 months in 15 untreated patients with solitary colorectal liver metatases.

A recent evidence-based cost-effectiveness analysis was conducted by Beard and colleagues to address any uncertainty among UK healthcare purchasers regarding the role of liver resection for colorectal liver metastases [6]. From the very large body of literature reporting the results of hepatic metastasectomy, they considered 19 independent case series representing distinct cohorts of at least 100 patients and cited overall 5-year survival rates of 21–44%. A modeled health economic evaluation also supported hepatic resection as highly cost effective with significant marginal survival benefits compared with "conventional" non-surgical treatments in the contemporary UK healthcare setting [6]. Hepatic resection has thus come of age and is established as "best practice" for selected patients with colorectal liver metastases.

Indications for hepatic resection

The traditional view that liver resection yields best results in young fit patients with small solitary colorectal liver metastases has evolved to accept a much wider definition of resectability. However, there is no doubt that resection of solitary colorectal liver metastases has been associated with beneficial

5-year survival rates of 30–47% in several large series [4,9–11], while those highly selected patients with metastases that are solitary, small (<4 cm), and metachronous may fare even better [12].

The concept of the clinical risk score (CRS), as a basis for patient selection for surgery and for subgroup analysis for clinical studies, has been developed and popularized by Fong and co-workers [13]. The CRS is calculated assigning one point for each of five criteria, all independent predictors of poor long-term outcome [4,9,10], and include lymph-node positive primary-tumor, disease-free interval (<12 months), number of hepatic tumors (>1), serum carcino embryonic antigen level (>200 ng/ml), and size of largest hepatic tumor (>5 cm diameter). Thus, "low risk" patients with CRS 0–2 were found to have better outcomes (47% 5-year survival/median survival of 56 months) compared with those with CRS 3–4 (24% 5-year survival/median survival of 32 months) [13].

Broadly similar findings were reported on 1818 patients in a retrospective multicenter study by the French Association of Surgery [14], although no significant difference in outcomes was evident between those undergoing unilobar and bilobar hepatic resections as long as radical resection margins were achieved.

Although liver resection may still be expected to offer the best chance of prolonged survival, and the opportunity should certainly not be denied those in this group, it may be that the management of such "high risk" patients can be modified. This may involve a "test of time," with or without further systemic chemotherapy, additional imaging such as positron emission tomography-computed tomography (PET-CT) and/or staging laparoscopy and/or more aggressive treatment with adjuvant systemic chemotherapy following liver resection.

In straightforward terms, liver resection is indicated in any patient with colorectal liver metastases where the procedure can be performed safely and effectively, preserving adequate hepatic function and achieving a radical tumor-free margin. These criteria may be satisfied irrespective of a variety of seemingly unfavorable tumor-related factors such as bilobar distribution, multiple metastases, larger size, synchronous presentation, unfavorable primary pathology and, in some cases, extrahepatic disease.

Extrahepatic disease

Five subgroups of patients with extrahepatic disease can be identified – lung metastases, hilar lymph node metastases, peritoneal carcinomatosis, locoregional primary colorectal cancer recurrence (including retroperitoneal nodes), and a miscellaneous group comprising those with metastases to the ovaries, adrenals, body wall, and other extra-abdominal sites. A slightly separate group comprises those colorectal liver metastases extending locally to invade adjacent viscera such as the diaphragm or right adrenal in which en bloc resection is usually performed.

It is now widely accepted that colorectal pulmonary metastases suitable for resection (or ablation) should not necessarily be regarded a contraindication to liver resection as 5-year survival rates up to 50% have been reported following sequential liver and lung resections in patients with resectable hepatic and pulmonary colorectal metastases [4,15–17].

Also, the traditional view that intra-abdominal extrahepatic tumor represents an absolute contraindication to resection in patients with otherwise potentially resectable colorectal liver metastases has been challenged. Elias and colleagues [18] reported simultaneous hepatic and extrahepatic resections in 111 (30%) out of 376 patients for overall 3- and 5-year survival rates of 38 and 20%, respectively. They observe that these results surpass those associated historically with a non-surgical/chemotherapy-based approach [5] and suggest that the impact of cytoreductive surgery in combination with host immune factors and chemotherapy on a systemic disease process, rather than one which is purely regionalized, may explain these surprisingly good outcomes. Nevertheless, patients with more than five colorectal liver metastases in whom extrahepatic disease was discovered incidentally at laparotomy fared particularly badly and it seems that this particular pattern of disease continues to contraindicate attempts at resectional surgery. Also, poorer outcomes were observed in patients with peritoneal carcinomatosis and in those with extrahepatic disease at multiple sites [18].

While it is generally agreed that there is no rationale to support systematic routine en bloc hilar lymphadenectomy, anecdotal success stories support regional lymphadenectomy in selected individuals with limited hilar lymphatic involvement in favorable circumstances [18].

Synchronous colorectal liver metastases and the timing of liver resection

Decisions regarding the timing of hepatic resection relative to both primary colorectal resection and subsequent systemic chemotherapy require careful consideration for those with potentially resectable synchronous hepatic metastases. It is certainly feasible to perform simultaneous bowel resection (with anastamosis) and hepatic metastasectomy safely [19]. However, there are good reasons for preferring separate staged operations in the majority of cases. A staged approach to hepatic resection allows proper interval liver-specific imaging, may improve surgical access through a more appropriate abdominal incision and avoids the risk of complications, such as anastamotic leakage, which may be poorly tolerated in the patient also recovering from a major hepatic resection. Planned limited hepatic resections for previously defined accessible small metastases are the main exception.

Decisions regarding the appropriateness of adjuvant chemotherapy vs hepatic resection as the next step following radical primary colorectal cancer resection will depend on individual patients' circumstances. This mandates discussion between the multidisciplinary colorectal and hepatobiliary teams at an early stage, as hepatic metastasectomy may be preferred before empirical chemotherapy. In many patients, an attempt at complete tumor cytoreduction before chemotherapy may offer the best chance of cure. Also, a "window of opportunity" for hepatic resection may be lost among the approximately 50% of patients who fail to respond to chemotherapy, where metastases encroach upon vital vascular structures with potentially tight resection margins.

Conversely, systemic chemotherapy as a prelude to surgery may be beneficial to other patients. This particularly applies to those with unfavorable primary pathology and an increased risk of locoregional recurrence (such as perforated primary tumor or extensive regional malignant lymphadenopathy). Also, patients in whom the resectability of liver lesions is considered questionable, particularly those with multiple bilobar disease, or where evidence for extrahepatic disease is indeterminate, may benefit from systemic chemotherapy followed by re-staging investigations, typically after 3 months.

In this way, the concept of the "test of time" is well established as an appropriate strategy for improving patient selection for liver resection. Concerns regarding the possibility of metastases themselves metastasising during the period of observation (to the lungs, intrahepatic satellite nodules, and hilar lymph nodes especially) must be offset by the advantages of avoiding inappropriate surgery in those patients in whom further (unresectable) metastatic disease declares itself during this interval. This was studied by Lambert *et al.* [20] who identified no survival disadvantage following such interval reevaluation. Indeed, unnecessary surgery was avoided in approximately one-third of their patients due to the appearance of distant or additional metastases.

Furthermore, for patients with synchronous and potentially resectable colorectal liver metastases, the importance of a response to neoadjuvant chemotherapy has recently been highlighted in retrospective studies. Allen *et al.* [21] observed significant improvements in outcome following liver resection in patients who had responded to neoadjuvant chemotherapy compared with those who had received none. Similarly, Adam and colleagues reported a substantial benefit following tumor control with neoadjuvant chemotherapy as a prelude to resection in those with multiple (≥ 4) colorectal liver metastases [22]. Chemotherapy non-responders fared significantly worse following curative liver resection leading to suggestions that "escape" from chemotherapy may represent a relative contraindication to metastasectomy.

The results of randomized controlled trials (such as the EORTC study) are needed to define the exact role of neoadjuvant chemotherapy before performing liver resection in patients with synchronous colorectal liver metastases and to address concerns that routine "pre-treatment" in patients with resectable disease might compromise the chance of cure.

Staging investigations

Although the role of routine intensive follow-up after curative primary colorectal cancer resection remains controversial, there is no doubt that a proportion of patients found to have liver metastases will benefit from prompt and appropriate treatment [23]. Interval CT (computed tomography) scanning and serial serum carcinoembryonic antigen (CEA) estimations are probably the "best buy" and have superseded the more basic and less sensitive traditional approach of clinical examination, liver function testing, and transbdominal ultrasonography. Ideally, chest CT is performed in search of pulmonary metastases, and colonoscopy (or barium enema or CT pneumocolon) is performed to confirm a "clean colon" having excluded local recurrence or metachronous primary disease. Thus, CT chest, abdomen, and pelvis will typically have been performed in the patient referred for consideration of liver resection. Further liver-specific imaging using more refined CT and/or MRI (magnetic resonance imaging) techniques in liaison with the hepatobiliary surgical team are the mainstay of the staging algorithm and are usually performed before final decisions regarding resectability can be made (Fig. 14.1).

The highly sensitive, but invasive, technique of CT angioportography (CTAP) has now been superseded by thin slice (≤ 5 mm collimation) portal

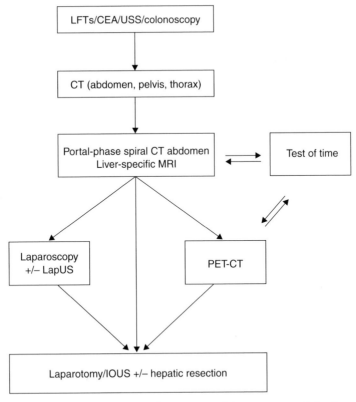

Fig. 14.1 Investigative/staging algorithm for patients with liver metastases following radical resection of primary colorectal cancer.

venous-phase spiral CT, or MRI performed with intravenous gadolinium and liver-specific contrast agents, to maximize tumor conspicuity and diagnostic specificity. It is important that these staging investigations are performed before the commencement of systemic chemotherapy. Tumor imaging characteristics may change significantly during chemotherapy and good quality baseline imaging may be especially important where a good response to chemotherapy results in disappearance of metastases.

The importance of restraint in the biopsy of potentially resectable liver metastases should be emphasised (whether by radiological-guided needle biopsy, or surgical wedge biopsy during primary bowel resection). Although a histological diagnosis may be desirable in the palliative management of patients with unresectable disease, it is almost always unnecessary for diagnosis in those under consideration for liver resection, and it carries the well-documented risk of malignant needle-track seeding [24] and is associated with a significant reduction in long-term survival even when following curative liver resection [25]. In the authors' experience, the rate of inadvertent liver resection for benign disease in patients not biopsied in this way was 1.2% which is considered acceptable within the context of modern, low morbidity surgery.

Staging laparoscopy remains an option in the investigation of some patients with colorectal liver metastases although its exact role continues to be debated. Interest in the technique as a means of improving patient selection arose following concerns regarding the apparent fallibility of conventional cross-sectional imaging in understaging disease in as many as 21% of patients [26]. The negative effects of such unnecessary operations are self-evident and include physical (postoperative pain, immunosupression, potential complications), psychological (anxiety, false hope), health economic factors, and delays in commencing palliative chemotherapy. While it seems likely that the yield of laparoscopy is too low to justify as a routine procedure, it may nevertheless be useful in selected "high-risk" patients with multiple bilobar metastases, unfavorable primary pathology and/or indeterminate imaging. The authors' experience with selective laparoscopic staging following modern staging investigations indicates a 21% yield in detecting factors precluding curative resection, with a resectability rate of 88% in the remainder. However, it seems likely the technique will continue to be practiced only on a selective basis, with problem solving in high-risk patients increasingly deferred to the novel technique of PET-CT (Fig. 14.1).

Positron emission tomography with the glucose analog (18F) fluoro-2-deoxy-D-glucose images tumors based on their increased uptake of glucose and represents a significant advance in the investigation of patients with potentially resectable colorectal liver metastases. Meta-analysis of PET scanning in the detection of recurrent colorectal cancer has reported an overall sensitivity and specificity of 97 and 76%, respectively, and occult intrahepatic and extrahepatic metastases may be apparent in approximately 25% of patients previously studied with standard investigations [27]. Recently, Fernandez and co-workers [28] reported a superior 5-year overall survival rate of 58% following hepatic resection for colorectal liver metastases in 100 patients, all of whom had been selected on the basis of favorable PET scans. They suggest that improved patient selection with flurodeoxyglucose-positron emission tomography (FDG-PET) may have been primarily responsible for defining a new cohort of patients with a substantially improved prognosis following hepatic resection.

However, where less liberal access to PET scanning is available, its role may remain restricted to problem solving, confirming, or refuting the presence of extrahepatic intra-abdominal disease in patients with indeterminate imaging in particular (Fig. 14.1). Recognized pitfalls associated with PET scanning include poor sensitivity in detecting smaller liver metastases in patients on chemotherapy. The fusion of contrast-enhanced CT and PET scanning (PET-CT) represents an important refinement in technique. Selzner et al. [29] recently reported improved diagnostic sensitivity for PET-CT compared with conventional contrast-enhanced CT in the detection of locoregional recurrence and other extrahepatic disease, as well as the detection of intrahepatic recurrence during follow-up in the aftermath of hepatic resection.

Technical considerations in hepatic resection

The majority of liver resections are performed via upper abdominal incisions without resort to thoracotomy. Fixed costal margin retraction and careful mobilization of the liver by division of its retroperitoneal ligamentous attachments usually provide adequate access. Extensive adhesiolysis may be required following previous colorectal resection and a thorough inspection, palpation, and intraoperative ultrasound examination of the liver and extrahepatic tissues are performed before arriving at a final decision regarding resectability. Many hepatobiliary surgeons regard intraoperative ultrasonography as indispensable, and it has been estimated that it alone may be responsible for changing the operative plan in a proportion of patients [30].

The aims of hepatic resection are to achieve radical oncological (RO) clearance with tumor-free resection margins on the one hand, while preserving sufficient functioning hepatic parenchyma to avert postoperative hepatic failure on the other. Resections must preserve vital inflow (hepatic artery and portal vein) and outflow (hepatic vein and bile duct) structures, and an understanding of the hepatic segmental anatomy and intrahepatic vascular "watersheds" is fundamental. Couinaud's seminal classification of the hepatic segmental anatomy [31] has been updated and the nomenclature standardized by the IHPBA Brisbane 2000 committee [32]. In this way, the vascular inflow to "hemilivers," "sections," and/or "segments" may be controlled selectively by extrahepatic dissection, or intrahepatically following parenchymal transection, and it forms the basis for precise resections "à la carte." Liver resections are classified as major (≥3 hepatic segments), minor (<3 hepatic segments), or atypical wedge resections.

Although the traditional view held that tumor-free margins of ≥1 cm should be achieved to minimize the risk of oncological relapse, it is now recognized that the width of negative surgical margins does not necessarily affect the risk of recurrence and that RO resections may be achieved with very tight resection margins contingent on the preservation of the tumor pseudocapsule [33–37]. Similarly, although major hepatectomies sacrifice larger volumes of liver, perhaps ensuring generous margins and removing occult intrahepatic metastases or satellite lesions, a trend toward "tailored," segment-orientated, parenchyma-sparing resections has emerged in recent years with the belief that this does not disadvantage patients oncologically and may facilitate re-resection in the event of intrahepatic recurrence.

Substantial falls in the perioperative mortality rates associated with major liver resection for colorectal liver metastases to 1–4% have been documented in recent years [6,33]. Perioperative blood loss requiring transfusion has been identified as the dominant risk factor for adverse outcome after liver resection [38], and the importance of minimizing blood loss during the dissection, parenchymal transection, and revascularization phases of hepatic resection has led to the concept of bloodless major liver surgery [33]. In this regard, the practice of low central venous pressure (0–4 cm H_2O) anesthesia is critical in minimizing hepatic venous bleeding. Also, meticulous parenchymal transection technique using technology such as the cavitron ultrasonic surgical aspirator (CUSA Ex, Valleylab Inc., Amersham, Bucks, UK), and argon beam coagulation, have helped achieve a mean operative blood loss of 360 ml during hepatic resection. Indeed, the practice of perioperative blood transfusion is now regarded as exceptional in the authors' practice [33] and by many others.

The liver's unique regenerative properties, functional reserve, and tolerance of extended warm ischaemia permit extensive parenchymal resections to be performed utilizing intermittent portal triad inflow clamping (the "Pringle maneuver"), another important technique in the pursuit of bloodless liver surgery. However, more advanced clamping techniques such as hepatic vascular exclusion (portal triad occlusion plus suprahepatic and infrahepatic inferior vena cava (IVC) clamping) have been associated with increased hemodynamic intolerance and postoperative morbidity [39] and tend to be restricted to more complex resections involving the hepatic veins and IVC.

Liver related morbidity, such as bile leaks, hemorrhage, and mild hepatic insufficiency, as well as relatively minor complications such as right-sided pleural effusion, occur in 10–15% of patients and are usually managed successfully by conservative means.

Liver failure is now recognized as the main mode of postoperative death and is directly related to both the extent of resection and the presence of background liver disease. Estimation of an acceptable residual functioning liver volume, and the prediction of hepatic dysfunction following resection, can be difficult. Although objective tests such as CT volumetry and indocyanine green clearance studies are available, in practice it is generally accepted that a subjective estimate of approximately one-third the standard liver volume or the equivalent of a minimum of two normal liver segments is usually sufficient.

In this regard, a growing concern which merits consideration is the risk of post chemotherapy hepatotoxicity and its impact on the ability to perform major liver resection safely, specifically with the newer chemotherapeutic agents such as irinotecan and oxaliplatin. Fernandez and colleagues [40] recently reported that treatment with irinotecan and/or oxaliplatin, especially in obese patients, presented a risk for the development of severe steatohepatitis, and highlighted the concomitant risk of liver failure following major liver resection.

Subsequent suggestions included consideration of preoperative liver biopsy in patients considered at risk and delay of chemotherapy until after liver resection where possible. The authors' own experience with liver resection for colorectal metastases following neoadjuvant chemotherapy of all types identifies no measurable excess morbidity or mortality in such patients. However, there appears to be evidence of an increased risk of complications when the duration of chemotherapy is prolonged beyond 3 months. This underlines the importance of the early involvement of specialist hepatobiliary surgeons in the multidisciplinary management of patients with metastatic colorectal cancer.

Follow up and hepatic re-resection

Following radical liver resection for colorectal metastases, up to 60% of patients may subsequently develop recurrent disease. Of these, approximately 20–30% may have metastases isolated to the liver and potentially amenable to hepatic re-resection. Repeat hepatic resection can present a daunting technical challenge, and the oncological rationale for re-resection of recurrent colorectal liver metastases may seem counterintuitive. Indeed, such concerns have stimulated interest in alternative minimal access techniques such as percutaneous radiofrequency ablation (RFA) [41].

Nevertheless, favorable accounts of hepatic re-resection for patients with recurrent colorectal liver metastases have reported 5-year survival rates of 26–41% [42–44], and it seems appropriate to treat such patients in the same way as those first presenting with colorectal liver metastases.

Despite the technical demands presented by dense intra-abdominal adhesions and variations in hepatobiliary anatomy in the hypertrophied regenerated liver remnant, concerns regarding excess morbidity and mortality associated with repeat hepatic resection have not been borne out. In the authors' own experience of 71 repeat hepatic resections in 66 patients with recurrent colorectal liver metastases, there were no postoperative deaths and the low morbidity rate of 11% compared favorably with that experienced following index hepatectomy [45]. Furthermore, beneficial 1-, 3-, and 5-year actuarial survival rates of 94, 68, and 44% were observed following repeat hepatic resection which exceeded those of all patients following a first hepatectomy for colorectal liver metastases.

It therefore seems appropriate to follow-up patients who have undergone hepatic resection for colorectal liver metastases. This is usually performed for a period of 5 years using CT of the chest and liver and serial serum CEA estimations in an attempt to identify those patients who may benefit from further intervention.

Laparoscopic liver resection

Though feasible, laparoscopic liver resection for patients with colorectal liver metastases is controversial and remains at an early stage of development. Thus far, most surgeons have focused on the more accessible small lesions in hepatic segments 2/3 and the caudal aspect of segments 4, 5, and 6. More adventurous procedures including right hepatectomy have been performed in highly selected cases and usually mandate a hand-assisted technique. While effective strategies for dealing with the risks of intraoperative hemorrhage, gas embolism, and bile leaks continue to evolve, the immediate benefits compared with conventional open surgery remain unclear.

Extending the limits of resectability

In recent years, the development of novel strategies and advanced techniques has dramatically extended the boundaries of resectability, permitting radical liver resections to be performed in patients who would formerly have been regarded as unresectable. It is important to emphasize that it is often a combination of the following techniques which are required to tackle colorectal liver metastases which have reached an advanced stage [36] (Fig. 14.2).

Neoadjuvant chemotherapy

The concept of downstaging neoadjuvant chemotherapy for otherwise unresectable colorectal liver metastases, first introduced 10 years ago [46], has reproducibly been shown to offer the chance of curative liver resection to 16–23% of such patients with reported 5-years survival rates of up to 40% [36].

Interestingly, the possibility that patients presenting with colorectal liver metastases initially deemed unresectable might be downstaged by oxaliplatin-based chemotherapy to become resectable comprised the sole recommendation for the provision of oxaliplatin-based chemotherapy in the UK National Institute for Clinical Excellence (NICE) 2002 guidance.

However, the success of downstaging chemotherapy in achieving a dramatic response, typically in patients with initially unresectable or indeterminate multiple bilateral metastases, can result in the disappearance of lesions from the imaging study. Thus, the dilemma presented in treating definitively the "missing metastasis" is increasingly encountered and reemphasizes the importance of pursuing good quality baseline staging investigations before commencing chemotherapy. Intuitively, "disappeared" metastases might be expected to eventually reappear as only a small minority of resected lesions demonstrate complete necrosis at histopathology [36]. Ideally, liver resections should target the parenchyma harboring the original lesion, but intraoperative localization can be problematic. Referral of such patients to the hepatobiliary team is therefore recommended before a "complete response" is necessarily achieved by their colleagues in Medical Oncology. Elias and co-workers [47] recently reported a subgroup of 11 patients identified as having "missing metastases," none of which could be identified or resected, and eight (73%) of which remained quiescent during a median 31-month follow-up period.

Portal vein embolization

Some patients may be denied a technically feasible liver resection because of concerns that an insufficient future remnant liver volume may risk severe

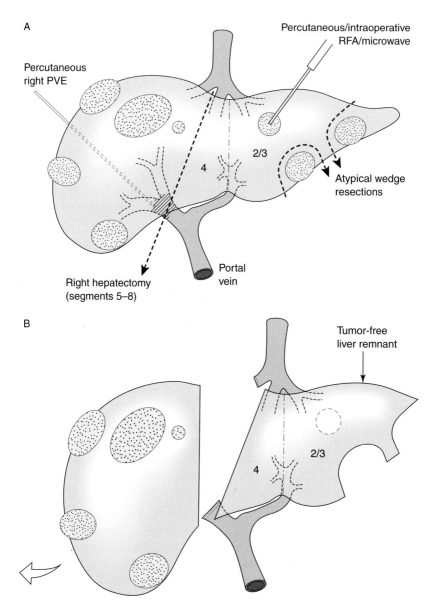

Fig. 14.2 Combined advanced techniques used to extend the limits of resectability to patients with multiple bilobar colorectal liver metastases. A. Percutaneous right portal vein embolization (PVE), staged or simultaneous ablation and wedge resection of contralateral lesions with subsequent right hemihepatectomy (hepatic segments 5–8). B. The aims of this approach are to achieve a viable tumor-free functional hepatic remnant (in this example based on an hypertrophied left hemiliver [hepatic segments 2–4]).

postoperative hepatic failure. Preoperative percutaneous selective portal vein embolization (PVE) may be performed in an attempt to induce hypertrophy of the future liver remnant (estimated volume ≤25%) and appears to be especially useful where there are concerns regarding background liver disease or following prolonged chemotherapy (estimated liver remnant volume ≤40%). Typically, right PVE is performed with a view to right hepatectomy or extended right hepatectomy a month later in the patient with small hepatic segment 2/3 volume, and subsequent 5-year survival rates have been reported as comparable to those resected without PVE [48]. Such has been the acceptance of PVE in this role that the prospect of randomized trials of its efficacy is no longer regarded as ethical.

Interestingly, there is evidence that right PVE is not beneficial for patients with normal liver in whom a straightforward right hepatectomy is planned [49], nor is embolization of segment 4 in addition to right PVE thought to be necessary [50]. Disadvantages associated with the PVE/hepatic resection approach include a local and systemic inflammatory response which is usually mild, a slightly higher perioperative mortality rate, the possibility that liver resection will not be achieved following PVE, and the rapid growth of occult metastases found out with the embolization zone [48].

Staged liver resections

Two-stage liver resections involve a preliminary non-curative procedure followed by a second resection of residual hepatic metastases. This aggressive surgical approach may facilitate compensatory hypertrophy of a tumor-free residual liver remnant, with or without interim PVE, in patients with multiple bilobar metastases. Subsequent major resection of the contralateral embolized liver has been reported to yield long-term survival rates similar to those associated with initially resectable patients [51].

Combinations of resection and ablative techniques

Percutaneous interstitial ablative techniques include cryotherapy, ethanol injection, laser hyperthermia, microwave thermotherapy, and RFA whose dominant role remains the palliative treatment of surgically unfit patients or those with unresectable disease. These procedures performed intraoperatively, particularly RFA, have been used to treat deep-seated metastases within the future liver remnant in combination with major hepatectomy, staged resections, chemotherapy, and/or PVE to extend further the boundaries of resectability in an attempt to offer the best chance of cure to patients in an otherwise hopeless situation [52] (Fig. 14.2).

Conclusions

Liver resection offers the only chance of long-term survival, or cure, to selected patients with colorectal liver metastases. Major hepatic resection can be performed with negligible mortality in well-staged patients by experienced hepatobiliary surgical teams paying meticulous attention to bloodless surgery and the balance between hepatic functional reserve and oncological clearance. The basic risks compare favorably with those of other elective abdominal procedures such that perioperative mortality will become redundant as the main endpoint in favor of alternative measures such as quality of life and cost-effectiveness.

Intensive follow-up identifies patients with recurrence suitable for re-resection which may be performed safely and with expectations not dissimilar to those of the index liver resection. The substantial improvements in long-term survival offered by liver resection for colorectal liver metastases may have attained a plateau, perhaps because the indications for resection have widened as hepatobiliary specialists continue to embrace increasing numbers of ever more difficult and advanced cases. However, it may be that a phase has been reached where surgical ingenuity alone is unlikely to significantly improve further the resectability or survival rates. Rather, the combination of hepatic resectional surgery with more efficient adjuvant and neoadjuvant therapy and/or interventional ablation techniques may offer the hope of further progress.

For patients treated with more powerful forms of chemotherapy, the timing of referral for hepatic resection may be critical. Some patients with synchronous disease may benefit from immediate hepatic resection and the results of current trials of neoadjuvant chemotherapy may help address this. For others, potentially disadvantageous effects of prolonged chemotherapy on hepatic functional reserve and precise tumor localization justify early involvement of hepatobiliary specialists in decision making. Indeed, such have the limits of resectability been extended that each and every fit patient with colorectal liver metastases, even those with apparently irresectable disease, deserves assessment by a hepatobiliary surgical team.

References

1 Weiss E, Grundmann L, Torhorst J et al. Haematogenous metastatic patterns in colonic carcinoma: an analysis of 1541 necropsies. *J Pathol* 1986; 150: 195–203.

2 Scheele J, Stangl R, Altendorf-Hofman A. Hepatic metastases from colorectal cancer: impact of surgical resection on the natural history. *Br J Surg* 1990; 77: 1241–6.

3 Sugarbaker PH. Surgical decision making for large bowel cancer metastatic to the liver. *Radiology* 1990; 174: 621–6.

4 Scheele J, Stangl R, Altendorf-Hofman A, Paul M. Resection of colorectal liver metastases. *World J Surg* 1995; 19: 59–71.

5 Stangl R, Altendorf-Hofman A, Charnley R, Scheele J. Factors influencing the natural history of colorectal liver metastases. *Lancet* 1994; 343: 1405–10.

6 Beard SM, Holmes M, Price C, Majeed AW. Hepatic resection for colorectal liver metastases: a cost-effectiveness analysis. *Ann Surg* 2000; 232: 763–76.

7 Wagner J, Adson M, Van Heerdan J, Ilstrup D. The natural history of hepatic metastases from colorectal cancer. A comparison with resective treatment. *Ann Surg* 1984; 199: 502–8.

8 Wood CB, Gillis CR, Blumgart LH. A retrospctive study of the natural history of patients with liver metastases from colorectal cancer. *Clin Oncol* 1976; 2: 285–8.

9 Rosen CB, Nagorney DM, Taswell HF et al. Perioperative blood transfusion and determinants of survival after liver resection for metastatic colorectal carcinoma. *Ann Surg* 1992; 216: 493–505.

10 Fong Y, Cohen AM, Fortner J et al. Liver resection for colorectal metastases. *J Clin Oncol* 1997; 15: 938–46.

11 Taylor M, Forster J, Langer B et al. A study of prognostic factors for hepatic resection for colorectal liver metastases. *Am J Surg* 1997; 173: 467–71.

12 Nuzzo G, Giuliante F, Giovannini I et al. Resection of hepatic metastases from colorectal cancer. *Hepatogastroenterology* 1997; 44: 751–9.

13 Fong Y, Fortner J, Sun RL et al. Clinical score for predicting recurrence after hepatic resection for metastatic colorectal cancer: analysis of 1001 consecutive cases. *Ann Surg* 1999; 230: 309–18.

14 Nordlinger B, Jaeck D, Guiguet M et al. Surgical resection of hepatic metastases. Multicentric retrospective study by the French Association of Surgery. In: Nordlinger B, Jaeck D, eds. *Treatment of Hepatic Metastases of Colorectal Cancer.* Paris: Springer-Verlag, 1992: 129–61.

15 McAfee MK, Allen MS, Trastek VF. Colorectal lung metastases: results of surgical excision. *Ann Thorac Surg* 1992; 53: 780–6.

16 Murata S, Moriya Y, Akasu T et al. Resection of both hepatic and pulmonary metastases in patients with colorectal carcinoma. *Cancer* 1998; 83: 1086–93.

17 Ike H, Shimada H, Togo S et al. Sequential resection of lung metastasis following partial hepatectomy for colorectal cancer. *Br J Surg* 2002; 89: 1164–8.

18 Elias D, Ouellet J-F, Bellon N et al. Extrahepatic disease does not contraindicate hepatectomy for colorectal liver metastases. *Br J Surg* 2003; 90: 567–74.

19 Elias D, Detroz B, Lasser P et al. Is simultaneous hepatectomy and intestinal anastamosis safe? *Am J Surg* 1995; 169: 254–60.

20 Lambert LA, Colacchio TA, Barth RJ. Interval hepatic resection of colorectal metastases improves patient selection. *Br J Surg* 2000; 135: 473–80.

21 Allen PJ, Kemeny N, Jarnagin W et al. Importance of response to neoadjuvant chemotherapy in patients undergoing resection of synchronous colorectal liver metastases. *J Gastrointest Surg* 2003; 7: 109–15.

22 Adam R, Pascal G, Castaing D et al. Tumor progression while on chemotherapy: a contraindication to liver

resection for multiple colorectal metastases? *Ann Surg* 2004; 240: 1052–64.

23 Jeffrey GM, Hickey BE, Hider P. Follow-up strategies for patients treated for non-metastatic colorectal cancer. *Cochrane Database Syst Rev* 2002.

24 John TG, Garden OJ. Needle track seeding of primary and secondary liver carcinoma after percutaneous liver biopsy. *HPB Surg* 1993; 6: 199–204.

25 Jones OM, Rees M, John TG *et al.* Biopsy of resectable colorectal liver metastases causes tumour dissemination and adversely affects survival after liver resection. *Br J Surg* 2005; 92: 1165–8.

26 Jarnagin WR, Fong Y, Ky A *et al.* Liver resection for metastatic colorectal cancer: assessing the risk of occult irresectable disease. *J Am Coll Surg* 1999; 188: 33–42.

27 Huebner RH, Park KC, Shepherd JE *et al.* A meta-analysis of the literature for whole-body FDG PET detection of recurrent colorectal cancer. *J Nucl Med* 2000; 41: 1177–89.

28 Fernandez FG, Drebin JA, Linehan DC *et al.* Five-year survival after resection of hepatic metastases from colorectal cancer in patients screened by positron emission tomography with F-18 fluorodeoxyglucose (FDG-PET). *Ann Surg* 2004; 200: 438–50.

29 Selzner M, Hany TF, Widbrett P *et al.* Does the novel PET/CT imaging modality impact on the treatment of patients with metastatic colorectal cancer of the liver. *Ann Surg* 2004; 240: 1027–36.

30 Jarnagin WR, Bach AM, Winston CB *et al.* What is the yield of intraoperative ultrasonography during partial hepatectomy for malignant disease? *J Am Coll Surg* 2001; 192: 577–83.

31 Couinaud C. Le foie: études anatomiques et chirurgicales. Paris: Masson; 1957.

32 Strasberg SM, Belghiti J, Clavien PA *et al.* Terminology of liver anatomy and resections. *HPB* 2000; 2: 333–9.

33 Rees M, Plant G, Wells J, Bygrave S. One hundred and fifty hepatic resections: the evolution of technique towards bloodless

surgery. *Br J Surg* 1996; 83: 1526–9.

34 Rees M, Plant G, Bygrave S. Late results justify resection for multiple hepatic metastases from colorectal cancer. *Br J Surg* 1997; 84: 1136–40.

35 Yamamoto J, Sugihara K, Kosuge T *et al.* Pathologic support for limited hepatectomy in the treatment of liver metastases from colorectal cancer. *Ann Surg* 1995; 221: 74–8.

36 Adam R, Delvart V, Pascal G *et al.* Rescue surgery for unresectable colorectal liver metastases downstaged by chemotherapy. A model to predict long-term survival. *Ann Surg* 2004; 240: 644–58.

37 Pawlik TM, Scoggins CR, Zorzi D *et al.* Effect of surgical margin status on survival and site of recurrence after hepatic resection for colorectal metastases. *Ann Surg* 2005; 241: 715–22.

38 Kooby DA, Stockman J, Ben-Portat L *et al.* Influence of transfusions on perioperative and long-term outcome in patients following hepatic resection for colorectal metastases. *Ann Surg* 2003; 237: 860–70.

39 Belghiti J, Noun R, Zante E *et al.* Portal triad clamping or hepatic vascular exclusion for major liver resection. A controlled study. *Ann Surg* 1996; 224: 155–61.

40 Fernandez FG, Ritter J, Goodwin JW *et al.* Effect of steatohepatitis associated with irinotecan or oxaliplatin pretreatment on resectability of hepatic colorectal metastases. *J Am Coll Surg* 2004; 200: 845–53.

41 Elias D, DeBaere T, Smayra T *et al.* Percutaneous radiofrequency thermoablation as an alternative to surgery for treatment of liver tumour recurrence after hepatectomy. *Br J Surg* 2002; 89: 752–6.

42 Neeleman N, Andersson R. Repeated liver resection for recurrent liver cancer. *Br J Surg* 1996; 83: 893–901.

43 Petrowsky H, Gonen M, Jarnagin W *et al.* Second liver resections are safe and effective treatment for recurrent hepatic metastases from colorectal cancer: a

bi-institutional analysis. *Ann Surg* 2002; 235: 863–71.

44 Adam R, Huguet E, Azoulay D *et al.* Hepatic resection after down-staging of unresectable hepatic colorectal metastases. *Surg Oncol Clin N Am* 2003; 12: 211–20.

45 Shaw IM, Rees M, Welsh F *et al.* Repeat hepatic resection for recurrent colorectal liver metastases is associated with favourable long term survival. *Br J Surg* 2006; (in press).

46 Bismuth H, Adam R, Lévi F *et al.* Resection of nonresectable liver metastases from colorectal cancer after neoadjuvant chemotherapy. *Ann Surg* 1996; 224: 509–22.

47 Elias D, Youssef O, Sideris L *et al.* Evolution of missing colorectal liver metastases following inductive chemotherapy and hepatectomy. *J Surg Oncol* 2004; 86: 4–9.

48 Elias D, Ouellet J-F, de Baère T *et al.* Preoperative selective portal vein embolization before hepatectomy for liver metastases: long-term results and impact on survival. *Surgery* 2002; 131: 294–9.

49 Farges O, Belghiti J, Kianmanesh R *et al.* Portal vein embolization before right hepatectomy: prospective clinical trial. *Ann Surg* 2003; 237: 208–17.

50 Capussotti L, Muratore A, Ferrero A *et al.* Extension of right portal vein embolization to segment 4 portal branches. *Arch Surg* 2005; 140: 1100–3.

51 Jaeck D, Oussoultzoglou E, Greget M *et al.* A two-stage hepatectomy procedure combined with portal vein embolization to achieve curative resection for initially unresectable multiple and bilobar colorectal liver metastases. *Ann Surg* 2004; 240: 1037–49.

52 Elias D, Baton O, Sideris L *et al.* Hepatectomy plus intraoperative radiofrequency ablation and chemotherapy to treat technically unresectable multiple colorectal liver metastases. *J Surg Oncol* 2005; 90: 36–42.

15: Palliative care of the colorectal cancer patient

Melanie Jefferson and Ilora Finlay

Introduction

Palliative care has been defined by the World Health Organization (WHO) as the

> active total care of patients whose disease is not responsive to curative treatment. Control of pain and other symptoms, and of psychological, social and spiritual problems, is paramount. The goal of palliative care is achievement of the best quality of life for patients and their families [1].

Many aspects of palliative care also apply earlier in an illness, in conjunction with anticancer treatments, and there is a place for palliative care for patients, including those with potentially curable disease (Fig. 15.1).

Palliative care is not synonymous with terminal care, and may be applicable to some degree at any stage in a patient's illness [2]. Research has shown that, in addition to receiving the best possible treatment, patients want and expect [3]:

1 to know that their physical symptoms will be managed to a degree that is acceptable to them throughout their illness;

2 to receive emotional support from professionals who are prepared to listen to them;

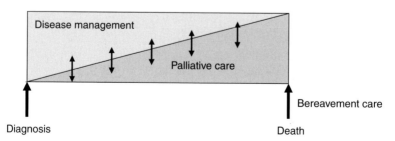

Fig. 15.1 The relationship of palliative care and interventions against the disease process.

232

3 to receive support to enable them to explore spiritual issues; and
4 to die in the place of their choice.

Specialist palliative care, although a separate specialty, can advise and manage more complex situations, but the generalist is still expected to apply the "palliative care approach" as part of their clinical management.

Patients with cancer have multifaceted problems. Good clinical management includes assessing these holistic needs and addressing them with the assistance of the multidisciplinary team. Such assessment and discussion of these needs is crucial at key points (such as diagnosis, commencement, during, and at the end of treatment; at relapse; and when death is approaching) [2].

Ethical issues may also be raised and this chapter aims to offer some guidance on some of these holistic and ethical problems.

Physical problems common in colorectal cancer

How prevalent is pain and can it be effectively managed?

Twenty to fifty percent of cancer patients have pain at the time of diagnosis and the prevalence increases with advancing disease. The mean prevalence of pain in advanced colorectal cancer recorded in 1990 [4] was 70% (range 47–95); the better use of analgesics would be expected to have improved through the intervention of palliative care teams [5]. Adequate pain management depends on careful assessment to identify the likely cause of the pain and then appropriate treatment. This short case-history illustrates the unnecessary suffering for patients that may result from inadequate pain assessment.

> *Case history*
> A 70-year old lady who was known to have rectal cancer and liver metastases was admitted to the hospice with a 4-week history of intractable rectal pain. She had been commenced on strong opioids in increasing doses to little benefit, and codanthramer as a laxative to prevent constipation. When admitted she was sleepy and hallucinating due to opioid toxicity and clearly distressed. Full history and examination, including rectal examination, revealed severe perianal skin burns secondary to codanthramer and her symptoms were relieved by change of laxative, barrier creams and a significant reduction in opioids.

About two-thirds of patients have more than one pain [6] and thus assessment requires categorization of each co-existing pain in turn. The mnemonic PQRST (see below) is useful in the history taking.

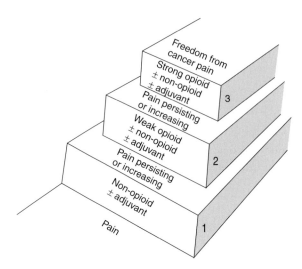

Fig. 15.2 WHO analgesic ladder for the management of cancer pain (1986).

Pain assessment should include the following:
- Description for each site of pain:
  - precipitating and relieving factors (P)
  - quality (Q)
  - radiation (R)
  - severity (S)
  - temporal pattern (T) of pain
- Associated symptoms and signs
- Impact on the patient's quality of life
- Effect of previous treatments
- Relevant physical examination
- Review of relevant investigations
- Patient's wishes and health beliefs.

A simple scheme such as the WHO analgesic ladder (Fig. 15.2) can give good pain relief in up to 90% of patients [7], with drugs being given orally, regularly, and the dose titrated in a stepwise fashion according to response. Adjuvant drugs such as drugs for neuropathic pain, laxatives, antiemetics, and sedatives are also often needed.

Analgesic ladder

The three main types of pain commonly encountered in patients with colorectal cancer (visceral, somatic, and neuropathic pain) are individually considered, although many patients will have a combination of them.

Visceral pain

This is due to compression or infiltration of a viscus by the tumor, for example with liver or peritoneal metastases, resulting usually in constant dull aching pain which is often poorly localized. This responds well to the step-wise use of analgesics moving from paracetamol to weak opioids and strong opioids as required. The European Association of Palliative Care (EAPC) [8] recommends the following key guidelines regarding the safe use of oral morphine.

- The opioid of first choice for moderate to severe cancer pain is morphine, initially given as normal release morphine every 4 h with additional "rescue" doses as required up to hourly.
- Patients who have taken full dose step-2 weak opioids should be started on 10 mg normal release morphine, whereas if step 2 of analgesic ladder is omitted 5 mg every 4 h it may still suffice.
- The opioid requirements should be reassessed within 12–24 h depending on severity of pain and dose of 4-h morphine titrated up according to use of regular and rescue doses. For example, if 30 mg of morphine has been used as breakthrough medication in addition to 60 mg of regular morphine, the regular dose should be increased to 15 mg every 4 h.
- The patient should be converted to sustained release preparations once the analgesic requirements are stable and normal release morphine continued as needed for breakthrough pain.

Most patients will require a laxative to be started with the morphine to prevent constipation and an antiemetic should be available if needed as 30% of patients experience nausea when starting morphine.

What is the best treatment for intestinal colic and tenesmus?

Colic is very distressing. It may be due to potentially reversal causes such as constipation or bowel obstruction, but occasionally the patient is too unwell or definitive treatment is not possible.

Standard management [9] would be:
- Stop stimulant laxative.
- Immediate treatment: hyoscine butylbromide 20 mg stat sc (subcutaneous) or glycopyrronium 0.1–0.2 mg stat sc.

• Continued treatment: glycopyrronium 0.2–0.6 mg/24 h or hyoscine butylbromide 40–160 mg/24 h via continuous subcutaneous infusion (CSCI).

• Antispasmodics such as mebeverine or peppermint may have a limited role. Although a short review of 31 papers [10] on the use of buscopan (hyoscine butylbromide) in abdominal colic (all causes) in emergency medicine found no benefit compared to standard analgesics, the clinical impression in advanced colorectal cancer is that antispasmodics can be helpful.

Tenesmoid pain (a painful sensation of rectal fullness) is usually related to local tumor in the unresected rectum, or to involvement of the presacral plexus by recurrent tumor or occasionally presents as a phantom phenomenon after rectal excision. This distressing symptom can give the need to defecate up to 20 times a day and may be associated with offensive rectal discharge. Patients describe a constant feeling of fullness or a severe spasmodic or shearing pain [11] making it difficult to distinguish from lumbosacral plexus neuropathic pain [12]. The continuous pressure is usually due to an enlarging tumor which causes local pressure on stretch receptors in the rectum. The intermittent shearing pain is possibly due to direct tumor invasion of levator ani and coccygeal muscles or the anal sphincter resulting in muscle spasm.

A 5-year follow-up study of 177 patients found perineal pain after rectal amputation was caused by local tumor recurrence or deafferentation pain following section of the pudendal nerve; the late development of symptoms were a significant indicator of recurrent disease [13].

Treatment depends on the use of the following [14]:

• Antitumor treatments where possible, including laser treatment of tumor [15].

• Analgesics according to analgesic ladder which decreases the continuous pressure sensation [16].

• Adjuvants – for neuropathic pain (see below), corticosteroids to reduce peritumoral oedema [17], antispasmodics such as nifedipine 10–20 mg bd [18], and local treatments such as rectal instillations of lidocaine [19] or morphine [20].

• Anaesthetic procedures may be required for intractable pain: lumbar sympathectomy has been reported to improve symptoms in 10 out of 12 patients and well tolerated [21].

• There are also reports of successful use of cryoanalgesia and spinal infusions [22].

The incidence of rectal pain has not been documented but a fall in the incidence of local recurrence has made this distressing symptom less common.

Somatic pain (musculoskeletal)

In colorectal cancer patients somatic pain is commonly due to either bone infiltration or metastases, or musculoskeletal pain; the latter may pre-exist but is exacerbated by weakness and weight loss. Treatment of musculoskeletal pain involves the use of nonsteroidal anti-inflammatory drugs (NSAIDs), which may be used topically with effect [23] if systemic NSAIDs are contraindicated, together with non-drug treatments such as Transcutaneous Electrical Nerve Stimulation (TENS), acupuncture, and physiotherapy. Complementary therapies are used by about half of all cancer patients, suggesting many patients derive great benefits from their concurrent use.

Colorectal cancer sometimes metastasises to bone and may also cause sacral pain due to bony infiltration from local recurrence. Single-dose palliative radiotherapy provides good sustained pain relief in over 80% of patients [24] and early referral is warranted. Although studies [25,26] have failed to confirm a benefit, many patients seem to benefit from NSAIDs, particularly whilst awaiting radiotherapy. There may be benefit from the concurrent use of opioids [16], corticosteroids [17], and, in intractable cases, bisphosphonates [27,28]. Local sacral infiltration often associated with neuropathic pain may require a caudal block, spinal infusion, or cryoanalgesia [22].

Neuropathic pain

Neuropathic pain contributes to up to 40% of cancer-related pain [29] and remains the most challenging pain to treat, often requiring combined use of opioids, adjuvant analgesics, and anesthetic interventions. Neuropathic pain caused by compression or destruction of neural structures results in aberrant somatosensory nerve transmission, so the patient experiences intermittent stabbing and burning pain often associated with hyperalgesia and allodynia. In colorectal cancer patients it is most commonly as a result of direct invasion of the lumbosacral plexus, presenting as pain in the buttocks or leg in 93% of patients [30] progressing to numbness, paresthesia, and weakness. Some authors [31] have classified the plexopathy according to whether it involves the upper, lower, or whole plexus which influences the sensory and motor changes according to which nerve roots are principally involved, and may guide choice of appropriate anesthetic procedure, for example epidural vs caudal block.

It is now generally accepted that opioids are effective in malignant neuro-pathic pain [32] and opioids alone have been found to control neuropathic pain in one-third of patients [33]. If opioids titrated to maximum tolerated dose are insufficient, the addition of an adjuvant analgesic is required. The choice of adjuvant is guided by concomitant symptoms and possible side effects as there is no clear evidence that one treatment is better than another.

Antidepressants

Low dose antidepressants in non-malignant and to a lesser degree, malig-nant neuropathic pain are co-analgesics. Tricyclic antidepressants such as amitryptyline are the most effective but some evidence suggests newer antide-pressants such as Selective Serotonin Reuptake Inhibitors (SSRIs) may also have a weak effect [34]. Amitryptyline should be started in low doses of 10–25 mg nocte (to be given at night) according to the clinical condition of the patient and the dose increased after 5–7 days if not beneficial up to 100 mg/day. If this is not effective or cannot be tolerated, change to a different adjuvant should be considered.

Anticonvulsants

Most anticonvulsants such as carbamazepine or sodium valproate are of benefit in neuropathic pain [35]; this benefit is comparable to that seen with antidepressants. Recently gabapentin has become the anticonvulsant of choice for neuropathic pain as it is effective, well tolerated, and with-out known drug interactions [36]. The usual starting dose is 300 mg nocte increasing up to 300 mg tds over 3–7 days depending on the condition of the patient. Some patients may require up to 2400 mg/day for maximal analgesic effect.

Corticosteroids

Corticosteroids may help alleviating neuropathic pain [37], possibly by reducing perineural oedema or their anti-inflammatory action. Some authors [9] suggest a high initial dose such as 8 mg/day for up to 3 days for rapid results and then reducing dexamethasone to a minimum, for exam-ple 2 mg/day, with regular review to prevent long-term side effects. If there is no benefit at all after 5 days on steroids, they should not be continued as side effects can occur rapidly, particularly emotional liability.

Suggested scheme for management of neuropathic pain

1 Would antitumor treatment (e.g. radiotherapy) help?

2 Commence weak/strong opioid according to WHO analgesic ladder.

3 If the above scheme is unsuccessful, consider use of any of the most appropriate adjuvant as given below:
- Start amitryptyline 10–25 mg nocte if patient is not sleeping well and does not suffer from dry mouth or medical contraindications such as cardiac arrhythmias.
- Commence gabapentin 300 mg increasing to tds if patient has dry mouth, urinary problems, or glaucoma.
- Commence corticosteroids if the patient has associated symptoms such as nausea, anorexia, and liver capsule pain.

4 Increase adjuvant and consider using two adjuvant drugs concurrently if pain not responding.

5 If pain not promptly responding, refer urgently to specialist palliative care for further advice on other specialist interventions such as a ketamine infusion.

Management of anorexia, nausea, and vomiting

Anorexia, nausea, and vomiting affects 40–70% of patients [38] but are often poorly managed [39]. Initial assessment depends on clarifying if the patient has anorexia, nausea, or vomiting as many patients will describe the former two as sickness and will diagnosing the underlying cause of the symptom to effective target treatment.

It is important to:
- distinguish between vomiting, expectoration, and regurgitation;
- note the content of the vomitus – for example undigested food, bile, feculent;
- separately evaluate nausea and vomiting;
- enquire whether nausea is absent or persistent for prolonged periods after vomiting;
- ask about diurnal variation;
- review the drug regimen;
- examine the mouth, pharynx, and abdomen;
- check for papilledema (although its absence does not exclude raised intracranial pressure);
- exclude uremia, hypercalcemia, and digoxin toxicity;

• consider radiological investigations if there is still major doubt about the cause [40];

If symptoms persist after reversible causes have been treated, the use of one or two of these first-line antiemetics is recommended [40].

Prokinetic antiemetics. For gastritis, gastric stasis, and functional bowel obstruction use *metoclopramide 10 mg qds orally/subcutaneously or 40–100 mg/24 h by continuous subcutaneous infusion.*

Antiemetic acting principally in area postrema. For most chemical causes of vomiting – for example morphine, hypercalcemia, and renal failure use *haloperidol 1–2 mg nocte orally or 1–2 mg bd orally or 5 mg/24 h by continuous subcutaneous infusion.*

Antiemetic acting principally in the vomiting center. For mechanical bowel obstruction, raised intracranial pressure, and motion sickness use *cyclizine 50 mg tds orally or 150 mg/24 h by subcutaneous infusion.*

It may be helpful to use a combination of cyclizine and haloperidol by subcutaneous infusion until drugs can be absorbed orally. Intractable symptoms may require the use of dexamethasone, levomepromazine, or ondansetron and advice from specialist palliative care should be sought.

Anorexia often points to underlying nausea. Oropharyngeal pathology, or a cancer-induced anorexia-cachexia syndrome. Corticosteroids such as dexamethasone 2–4 mg/day give a short-term improvement in appetite in some patients [41], but their benefit is often outweighed by troublesome side effects such as emotional lability, insomnia, ankle edema and weakness from proximal myopathy.

Medical management of intestinal obstruction

Ten to twenty-eight percent of patients with colorectal cancer [42] develop obstruction. For single site, large-bowel obstruction, surgical treatment is appropriate, but those with the following are unlikely to benefit from surgery (abridged from [43]):
• Diffuse peritoneal disease
• Frailty and cachexia
• Multiple partial bowel obstruction
• Previous radiotherapy to abdomen or pelvis

- Distant metastatic disease
- Previous laparotomy confirming widespread disease
- Ascites.

The medical management depends upon the level of obstruction as well as condition of the patient although in practice it is not always clear or possible to elucidate the level of the intestinal obstruction. Radiographic evaluation following history and clinical examination may be helpful and studies suggest that the plain abdominal X-ray can diagnose small-bowel obstruction with an accuracy of 30% [44]. Small-bowel contrast studies have an accuracy of 70–100% in locating small-bowel obstruction [45] but these are probably useful mainly in patients who are to be considered for surgery. Barium/gastrograffin enemas are useful to clarify the site of colonic obstruction particularly if placement of a colonic stent is being considered. Many consider the use of CT to be the gold standard in diagnosing bowel obstruction as it has a high sensitivity and specificity [46]. The appropriateness of investigations should be determined by comparing the benefits vs the burdens of each intervention to the patient.

Decompression of the proximal bowel through the use of either a nasogastric tube or venting gastrostomy may sometimes give rapid relief, although the former can be very uncomfortable in the long term [46]. Venting gastrostomy is more acceptable to decompress in the medium-long term as the patient can continue oral intake without the discomfort and aesthetic problems associated with long-term nasogastric tube use and the patient can be concurrently fed via jejunostomy, allowing home care [47,48].

Self-expanding metal stents are increasingly used when a single narrowing involves the gastric outlet, proximal small bowel, or colon. A duodenal stent can be inserted endoscopically [49] and stents are increasingly used to relieve colorectal obstruction [50,51].

Pharmacological treatment of inoperable malignant bowel obstruction

The relief of nausea and vomiting, pain, and other symptoms using antiemetics, antisecretory drugs, and analgesics, pioneered by Dr Mary Baines [52], has enabled patients to be treated in hospitals, hospices, or at home; recommendations have been published by the *EAPC* [53]. In our practice we recommend the following drugs parenterally, preferably via a subcutaneous infusion:

- Antiemetic options

  1 Metoclopramide 1–2 mg/kg body weight/day for partial occlusion without colic, or

  2 Levomepromazine 6.25–25 mg/day for complete obstruction, or

  3 Haloperidol 2.5–5 mg/day with cyclizine 150–200 mg/day for complete obstruction.

- Antisecretory drugs can be given concomitantly

  1 Hyoscine butylbromide 40–120 mg/day or hyoscine hydrobromide 0.8–2.0 mg/day or glycopyrronium 0.2–0.4 mg/day

  2 Octreotide 0.2–0.8 mg/day.

Steroids

Steroids may relieve obstruction by reducing peri-tumoral oedema; the cochrane review shows a trend for evidence that intravenous dexamethasone (6–16 mg/day) may ameliorate bowel obstruction and suggests a 4–5 day trial [54].

Analgesics

Most patients are on strong opioids which should be converted to parenteral preparations and titrated as appropriate. Hyoscine can be added to relieve persisting colic.

Symptomatic management of constipation

Constipation, defined as the passage of small hard feces infrequently and with difficulty [55], is a very frequent and often debilitating symptom. The causes of constipation may be due to

- the cancer directly
- the treatment of the cancer (drugs, chemotherapy, surgery, radiotherapy)
- general effects of the cancer (poor dietary and fluid intake, immobility, depression)
- preexisting or unrelated conditions (hemorrhoids, rectal prolapse, diabetes mellitus, etc.).

Diagnosing the underlying cause of constipation requires a full history, examination including rectal examination, and if necessary abdominal X-ray to guide best treatment. Subacute or potential bowel obstruction must be excluded.

Ideally, constipation should be prevented by regular monitoring, dietary advice, and early use of laxatives, particularly when prescribing strong analgesics. However up to 80% of patients with advanced cancer often experience troubling constipation, despite regular laxative use [56]. Most patients require a combination of laxatives to soften the stool and stimulate peristalsis, which is more effective and better tolerated than when each given individually [57]; they must be continued long term to prevent further problems such as fecal impaction.

Suggested plan for management of constipation:

• Explore possibility of non-drug interventions, for example diet, privacy, mobility.

• Start prophylactic laxatives with weak and strong opioids.

• Use combination of softener with stimulant such as senna liquid/ magnesium hydroxide 10/10 ml od–bd or codanthramer capsules 2–4 a day (note codanthramer is only licensed in the United Kingdom for use in very elderly and palliative care patients).

• For resistant problems consider use of polyethylene glycol [58].

• If there is stool in the rectum consider concurrent use of microlax/phosphate enema.

• For severe fecal impaction a manual evacuation with caudal analgesia or sedation and analgesia may be required.

• If rectum is empty and stool palpable in colon on abdominal examination consider high arachnis-oil retention enema overnight and repeat until stool palpable in rectum.

Symptomatic management of diarrhea

Diarrhea, the passage of frequent loose stools with urgency [55], is a less frequent symptom that is usually due to the cancer itself or as a result of its treatment (surgery, radiotherapy, or chemotherapy), but overflow from intestinal obstruction or fecal impaction (commonly), or malabsorption diarrhea must be excluded.

Opioids are widely used in palliative care patients because of their efficacy and palatability. Loperamide is significantly more effective than codeine or diphenoxylate (the relative specificity for antidiarrheal effects being 5.52, 5.24, and 23.7, respectively) and can be used in doses up to 54 mg/day without adverse effects [55]. As loperamide acts mainly on the colon [59] it can be combined with codeine or morphine in intractable diarrhea. Octreotide has shown to be useful in refractory diarrhoea secondary to ileostomy or colectomy [60].

Symptomatic management of rectal bleeding and discharge

In advanced colorectal cancer local tumor bleeding is common, but treatable causes such as hemorrhoids, postradiation proctitis, or clotting disorders must be excluded. Radiotherapy has been shown to reduce or stop bleeding or discharge in 85% of patients with 10 fractions of external beam treatment [61], but increasingly intraluminal brachytherapy is used to deliver a high dose locally as a single treatment.

A trial of tranexamic acid 1 g tds for a week should be considered, which can be discontinued if not effective or reduced to 500 mg tds if effective but bleeding recurs [62]. There are also reports of the use of rectal tranexamic acid [63] and alum solution [64] for control of hemorrhage. Patients with good performance status and at risk of major hemorrhage should be considered for arterial embolization [65].

A persistent offensive discharge warrants microbiological investigation. Usually, metronidazole suppositories will decrease swell without the side effects from systemic treatment. Gentle rectal washout with saline or iodine solutions can also reduce discharge and smell on a temporary basis.

Ascites

Ascites, usually associated with disseminated disease, causes abdominal distension and discomfort, dyspnoea, nausea, dyspepsia, and constipation. For rapid relief of tense ascites large volume paracentesis (up to 5 l/day) is generally well tolerated [66] and this may be repeated in patients with a short prognosis of less than 4 weeks. For moderate ascites or patients with longer prognosis, a trial of diuretic therapy can be considered, although the evidence of efficacy is in patients with cirrhosis and it may take up to 28 days for maximum effect.

For persistent recurring ascites in good performance patients a peritoneovenous shunt should be considered [67].

Psychosocial problems common in colorectal cancer patients

The importance of psychosocial care at every stage of disease and the benefits of interventions on the incidence of anxiety, depression, and mood [68], and emotional and functional adjustment [69] are well recognized. The NICE guidelines on care of the dying are based on this vast area of research [2].

Maguire *et al.* [70] studied the physical and psychological needs of 61 patients with terminal colorectal cancer, their carers, and GPs. They found little concordance between patients and carers regarding their concerns: Patients were most concerned about their illness, physical symptoms and their inability to do things, whilst carers were most concerned. About the illness, the future, and the emotional demands placed on them. Twenty-two percent of the patients had a major mood disorder (depression, anxiety, or adjustment disorder) usually unrecognized by medical staff, and 33% of carers reported a mood disorder. This concurs with findings in other patient groups [2], emphasizing the need for regular review as the patients' and carers' needs change rapidly.

Every effort should be made to fulfill patients' wishes about where they wish to die [71]. Regardless of place of death, an integrated care pathway for the last days of life has been shown to improve care for patients and carers, ensuring patients receive the high quality holistic care they expect [2]. Determining the point when active measures which control the disease should be reduced can be difficult. There are some core ethical principles underlying such decision making.

Autonomy depends on the patient's ability to make realistic informed choices about the options available to them, so without presenting appropriate choices to the patient their autonomy is undermined. Information needs to be clear, accurate, and sensitively given. The principles of beneficence and nonmaleficence require that there is a constant ongoing assessment of the benefits of an intervention to the patient as a person, weighed against the risks and the burdens. This constant reassessment is essential so that as the patient's condition changes those interventions which have become futile are abandoned and others are instigated. The sudden switch from one type of management to another can be traumatic to the patient and usually does not result in good care. The sensitive delivery of comfort measures, the careful withdrawal of treatments that clearly are not benefiting the patient, and the avoidance of interventions that carry a risk can effect a smooth transition as patients near the end of their lives.

The principle of justice requires that patients have the right to the best treatment within the resources available, as well as an equitable distribution of resources; thus those who may benefit should be referred for advice from the palliative care team. No patient should be denied morphine or other suitable symptom relief through ignorance or fear on the part of the doctor.

Drugs titrated up to attain symptom control do not shorten life and indeed may prolong good quality life as patients do not become exhausted.

Feeding and hydration have become vexed topics. Although interventions to provide nutrition may be futile, subcutaneous fluids can sometimes have a helpful role. As patients near the end of their lives, there can be very important moments of deep spiritual meaning in conversations with family members; past disagreements can be resolved and it is an important time for the family to express their love verbally and through caring. Children in the family must be prepared for the bereavement that they will face. Young parents who are dying can find it helpful to create a memory box of photographs, memorabilia, and letters for the child to have in the years ahead. When children are bereaved, they should be included as much as they want in the processes of the funeral; some children find it helpful to be able to visit the body of their dead parent several times, perhaps taking a flower or drawing a picture to go in the coffin.

As patients near the last days of their life, it is essential that the family is told quite explicitly that they are now dying. Unnecessary medication should be stopped. Medication that might be needed, such as breakthrough doses of morphine, a small dose of midazolam subcutaneously for restlessness, and hyoscine for the bubbly chest that causes a death rattle have become standard drugs on the care of the dying pathway to ensure good symptom control in the last 48 h of life. Family may wish to organize a rota to sit at the bedside and they should be told how death is anticipated, with a slow decreasing level of consciousness and gently failing respiratory efforts; many families value being told that nothing sudden is expected to happen but that the person will gently slip into a coma and die from a coma. When children are present, it is very important that the terms "going to sleep" and other euphemisms are avoided because the child may then become frightened that when their surviving parent goes to sleep they also may die. Children cope well with very clear simple explanations of what is and what is not happening.

After the death, the family may wish to help with washing and laying out the body and many of the different religions will have their own traditions that they wish to follow. In the few days prior to death, it is important to ascertain from the family which traditions they wish to practice so that no offence is caused around the time of death. Some patients wish to die at home, and rapid transfer to home, even in the last hours, may be extremely important and greatly valued by patient and family if that is the patient's clear informed wish.

Good care at the end of life is expected; bad care is a legacy that lives on in the bereaved, causing problems often many years later with a higher psychosocial morbidity in the bereaved and a loss of confidence in the healthcare system itself.

Patients with colorectal cancer have palliative care needs at different stages of their illness which often may be addressed by the attending clinical team. If there are complex or intractable problems early referral to Specialist Palliative Care may be helpful so that issues may be addressed holistically by the multidisciplinary team.

References

1 Technical Report Series 804. Cancer Pain Relief and Palliative Care. Geneva: World Health Organization 1990.

2 National Institiute for Clinical Excellence. Improving Supportive and Palliative care for Adults with Cancer 2004 NHS UK.

3 Cancerlink. Cancer Supportive Care Services Strategy: users priorities and perspectives. London: July 2000.

4 Bonica JJ. Cancer pain: current status and future needs. In: Bonica JJ, ed. *The Management of Pain*, 2nd edn. Philadelphia: Lea & Febiger, 1990: 400–5.

5 McQuillar R, Finlay I, Roberts D *et al.* The provision of a palliative care service in a teaching hospital and subsequent evaluation of that service. *Palliat Med* 1996; 10: 231–40.

6 Grond S, Zech D, Diefenbach C *et al.* Assessment of cancer pain: a prospective evaluation in 2266 cancer patients referred to a pain service. *Pain* 1996; 64: 107–14.

7 Zech DFJ, Grond S, Lynch J *et al.* Validation of World Health Organisation guidelines for cancer pain relief. A 10-year prospective study. *Pain* 1995; 63: 65–76.

8 Hanks GW, Conno F, Cherny N *et al.* Morphine and alternative opioids in cancer pain: the EAPC recommendations. *Br J Cancer* 2001; 84: 587–93.

9 Back IN. *Palliative Medicine Handbook*, 3rd edn. BPM Books, 2001.

10 Mackway-Jones K, Teece S. Towards evidence based emergency medicine: best BETs from the Manchester Royal Infirmary. Buscopan (hoscine butylbromide) in abdominal colic. *Emerg Med J* 2003; 20: 267.

11 Baines M, Kirkham SR. Cancer pain. In: Wall PD, Melzack R, eds. *Textbook of Pain*, 2nd edn. Edinburgh: Churchill Livingstone, 1989: 590–7.

12 Hagen NA. Sharp, shooting neuropathic pain in the rectum or genitals: pudendal neuralgia (editorial). *J Pain Symptom Manage* 1993; 8: 496.

13 Boas RA, Schug SA, Acland RH. Perineal pain after rectal amputation: a 5-year follow-up. *Pain* 1993; 52: 67–70.

14 Portenoy RK, Forbes K, Lussier D, Hanks G. Difficult pain problems: an integrated approach. *Oxford Textbook of Palliative Care*, 3rd edn. Oxford: Oxford University Press, 2004.

15 Kimmey MB. Endoscopic methods (other than stents) for palliation of rectal carcinoma. *J Gastrointest Surg* 2004; 8: 270–3.

16 Hanks GW. Opioid-responsive and non-responsive pain in cancer. *Br Med Bull* 1991; 47: 718–31.

17 McQuay H. Pharmacological treatment of neuralgic and neuropathic pain. *Cancer Surv* 1998; 7: 141–59.

18 McLoughlin R, McQuillar R. Using nifedipine to treat tenesmus. *Palliat Med* 1997; 11: 419–20.

19 Hunt RW. The palliation of tenesmus. *Palliat Med* 1991; 5: 352–3.

20 Krajnik M, Zylicz Z, Finlay I *et al.* Potential use of topical opioids in palliative care-report of 6 cases. *Pain* 1999; 80: 121–5.

21 Bristow A, Foster JMG. Lumbar sympathectomy in the management of rectal tenesmoid pain. *Ann R Coll Surg Engl* 1998; 70: 38–9.

22 Rich A, Ellershaw JE. Tenesmus/rectal pain – how is it best managed? *CME Bull Palliat Med* 2000; 2: 41–4.

23 Moore RA, Tramer MR, Carroll D *et al.* Quantitative systematic review of topically applied non-steroidal anti-inflammatory drugs. *Br Med J* 1998; 316: 333–8.

24 Bone Pain Trial Working Party. 8 Gy single fraction radiotherapy for the treatment of metastatic skeletal pain: randomized comparison with a multifraction schedule over 12 months of patient follow-up. *Radiother Oncol* 1999; 52: 111–21.

25 Shah S, Hardy J. Non-steroidal anti-inflammatory drugs in cancer pain: a review of the literature as relevant to palliative care. *Prog Pall Care* 2001; 9: 3–7.

26 Mercadante S, Casuccio A, Agnello A *et al.* Analgesic effects of nonsteroidal anti-inflammatory drugs in cancer due to somatic or visceral mechanisms. *J Pain Symptom Manage* 1999; 17: 351–6.

27 Mannix K, Ahmedzai SH, Anderson H *et al.* Using bisphosphonates to control the pain of bony metastases: evidence based guidelines for palliative care *Palliat Med* 2000; 14: 455–61.

28 Wong R, Wiffen PJ. Bisphosphonates for the relief of pain secondary to bone metastases. *Cochrane Database Syst Rev* 2002; (2): CD002068.

29 Caraceni A, Portenoy RK. An international survey of cancer pain characteristics and syndromes. *Pain* 1999; 82: 263–74.

30 Thomas JE, Cascino TL, Earl JD. Differential diagnosis between radiation and tumor plexopathy of the pelvis. *Neurology* 1985; 35: 1–7.

31 Jaeckle KA, Young DF, Foley KM. The natural history of lumbosacral plexopathy in cancer. *Neurology* 1985; 35: 8–15.

32 Dellemijn P. Are opioids effective in relieving neuropathic pain? *Pain* 1999; 80: 453062.

33 McQuay HJ, Jadad AR, Carroll D *et al.* Opioid sensitivity of chronic pain; A patient-controlled analgesia method. *Anaesthesia* 1992; 47: 757–67.

34 McQuay HJ. A systematic review of antidepressants in neuropathic pain. *Pain* 1996; 68: 217–27.

35 McQuay HJ, Carroll D, Jadad AR *et al.* Anticonvulsant drugs for the management of pain; a systematic review. *Br Med J* 1995; 311: 1047–52.

36 Chandler A, Williams JE. Gabapentin an adjuvant treatment for neuropathic pain in a cancer hospital. *J Pain Symptom Manage* 2000; 20: 82–6.

37 Wantanabe S, Bruera E. Corticosteroids as adjuvant analgesics. *J Pain Symptom Manage* 1994; 9: 442–5.

38 Dunlop GM. A study of the relative frequency and importance of gastrointestinal symptoms, and weakness in patients with far advanced cancer. *Palliat Med* 1989; 4: 37–43.

39 Bruera E, Seifert L, Watanabe S *et al.* Chronic nausea in advanced cancer patients: a retrospective assessment of a metoclopramide-based antiemetic regimen. *J Pain Symptom Manage* 1996; 11: 147–53.

40 Twycross R, Back IN. Nausea and vomiting in advanced cancer. *Eur J Palliat Care* 1998; 5: 39–45.

41 Bruera E, Koca E, Cedaro L *et al.* Action of oral methylprednisolone in terminal cancer patients: a prospective randomized double-blind trial. *Cancer Treat Rep* 1985; 69: 751–4.

42 Davis MP, Nouneh D. Modern management of cancer-related intestinal obstruction. *Curr Pain Headache Rep* 2001; 5: 257–64.

43 Ripamonti C, Mercadante S. Pathophysiology and management of malignant bowel obstruction. In: Doyle D, Hanks GW, McDonald N, and Cherny N, eds. *Oxford Textbook of Palliative Medicine*, 3rd edn. New York: Oxford University Press, 2004.

44 Daneshmand S, Hedley CG, Stain SC. The utility and reliability of computed tomography scan in the diagnosis of small bowel obstruction. *Am J Surg* 1999; 65: 922–6.

45 Ericksen AS, Krasna MJ, Mast BA et al. Use of gastrointestinal contrast studies in obstruction of the small and large bowel. *Dis Colon Rectum* 1990; 33: 56–64.

46 Krouse RS, McCahill LE, Easson AM, Dunn GP. When the sun can set on an unoperated bowel obstruction: management of malignant bowel obstruction. *J Am Coll Surg* 2002; 195: 117–27.

47 Scheidbach H, Horbach T, Groitl H, Hohenberger W. Percutaneous endoscopic gastrostomy/jejunostomy (PEG/PEJ) for decompression in the upper gastrointestinal tract. *Surg Endosc* 1999; 13: 1103–5.

48 Gemlo B, Rayner AA, Lewis B et al. Home support of patients with end-stage malignant bowel obstruction using hydration and venting gastrostomy. *Am J Surg* 1986; 152: 100–4.

49 Park HS, Do YS, Suh SW et al. Upper gastrointestinal tract malignant obstruction: initial results of palliation with a flexible stent. *Radiology* 1999; 210; 865–70.

50 Law WL, Choi HK, Lee YM, Chu KW. Palliation for advanced malignant colorectal obstruction by self-expanding metallic stents: prospective evaluation of outcomes. *Dis Colon Rectum* 2004; 47: 39–43.

51 Khot UP, Lang AW, Murali K, Parker MC. Systematic review of the efficacy and safety of colorectal stents. *Br J Surg* 2002; 89: 1096–102.

52 Baines M, Oliver DJ, Carte RL. Medical management of intestinal obstruction in patients with advanced malignant disease. *Lancet* 1985; 2: 990–93.

53 Ripamonti C, Twycross R, Baines M et al. Clinical-practice recommendations for the management of bowel obstruction in patients with end-stage cancer. *Support Care Cancer* 2001; 9: 223–33.

54 Cochrane Review, Use of Corticosteroids in Intestinal Obstruction. *Cochrane Review Library*, UK, 2002.

55 Sykes N. Constipation and Diarrhoea. *Oxford Textbook of Palliative Medicine*, 3rd edn. Oxford: Oxford University Press, 2004.

56 Sykes NP. The relationship between opioid use and laxative use in terminally ill cancer patients. *Palliat Med* 1998; 12; 375–82.

57 Sykes NP. A volunteer model for the comparison of laxatives in opioid-induced constipation. *J Pain Symptom Manage* 1997; 11: 363–9.

58 Culbert P, Gillett H, Ferguson A. Highly effective new oral therapy for faecal impaction. *Br J Gen Pract* 1998; 48: 1599–600.

59 Oooms LA, Degryse AD, Janssen PA. Mechanisms of action of loperamide. *Scand J Gastroenterol* 1984; 96: 145–55.

60 Kornblau S, Benson AB, Catalano R et al. Management of cancer treatment-related diarrhoea. Issues and therapeutic strategies. *J Pain Symptom Manage* 2000; 19: 118–29.

61 Taylor RE, Kerr GR, Arnott SJ. External beam radiotherapy for rectal adenocarcinoma. *Br J Surg* 1987; 74: 455–9.

62 Dean A, Tuffin P. Fibrinolytic inhibitors for cancer-associated bleeding problems. *J Pain Symptom Manage* 1997; 13: 20–4.

63 McElligott E, Quigley C, Hanks GW. Tranexamic acid and rectal bleeding (letter). *Lancet* 1991; 337: 431–2.

64 Paes TRF. Alum solution in the control of intractable haemorrhage from advanced rectal cancer. *Br J Surg* 1986; 73: 192.

65 Phillips-Hughes J. The role of embolisation in the treating of bleeding tumors. *Palliat Care Today* 1997; 5: 50–2.

66 Kao HW, Rakov NE, Savage E, Reynolds TB. The effect of large volume paracentesis on plasma volume-a cause of hypovolaemia? *Hepatology* 1985; 5: 403–7.

67 Schumacher DL, Saclarides TJ, Staren ED. Peritoneovenous shunts for palliation of the patient with malignant ascites. *Ann Surg Oncol* 1994; 1: 378–81.

68 Devine E, Westlake S. The effects of psychoeducational care provided to adults with cancer:meta-analysis of 116 studies. *Oncol Nurs Forum* 1995; 22: 1369.

69 Meyer TJ, Mark MM. Effects of psychosocial interventions with adult cancer patients: a meta-analysis of randomized experiments. *Health Psychol* 1995; 14: 101–8.

70 Maguire P, Walsh S, Jeacock J, Kingston R. Physical and psychological needs of patients dying from colorectal cancer. *Palliat Med* 1999; 13: 45–50.

71 Dunlop RJ, Davies RJ, Hockley JM. Prefered versus actual place of death: a hospital palliative care support team study. *Palliat Med* 1989; 3: 197–201.

72 Hoskin PJ, de Canha SM, Bownes P *et al.* High dose rate after loading intraluminal brachytherapy for advanced inoperable rectal carcinoma. *Radiother Oncol* 2004; 73(2): 195–8.

16: Future directions in the oncological treatment of colorectal cancer

Anthony El-Khoueiry and Heinz-Josef Lenz

The treatment of colorectal cancer (CRC) has witnessed significant advances over the last 5 years. Patients with metastatic colorectal cancer (MCRC) have benefited from a significant improvement in overall survival (OS) which is largely due to the adoption of combination chemotherapy regimens that include oxaliplatin or irinotecan in front-line therapy [1]. Novel targeted agents such as bevacizumab (Vascular Endothelial Growth Factor (VEGF) antibody) and cetuximab (Endothelial Growth Factor Receptor Antibody) have contributed to the improved efficacy of chemotherapy in patients with MCRC [2,3]. In the adjuvant setting, two trials have confirmed the positive impact of the combination of oxaliplatin with 5-flurururacil and leucovorin (5-FU/LV – FOLFOX) on disease-free survival (DFS) [4,5]. A significant amount of effort has been invested into the identification of molecular markers that predict response to therapy and others that may influence prognosis. These advances, and many others not specifically noted in this introduction, have influenced the treatment paradigm of patients with CRC. As we move into the future, cure remains the ultimate goal of patients and oncologists alike. This goal requires the oncology community to build on the current achievements by refining them and by adopting new approaches to therapy that may transform cure from an elusive target into a tangible reality. In this chapter, as we discuss the future of the treatment of CRC, we will focus on future directions in chemotherapy and on the application of predictive and prognostic molecular markers to the treatment of patients with CRC (Fig. 16.1).

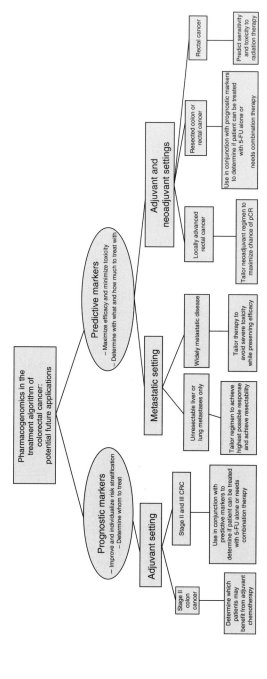

Fig. 16.1 Pharmacogenomics in the treatment algorithm of colorectal cancer: potential future applications.

The future of adjuvant chemotherapy

A brief overview of the current reality

The oxaliplatin-based combination regimen (FOLFOX) has demonstrated superiority over 5-FU/LV in the adjuvant treatment of resected stage II and III colon cancer [4,5]. Both the MOSAIC (Multicenter International Study of Oxaliplatin/5-Fluorouracil/Leucovorin in the Adjuvant Treatment of Colon Cancer) and the NSABP C-07 (National Surgical Adjuvant Breast and Bowel Project) trials showed superior DFS with FOLFOX at 4 and 3 years, respectively. While this regimen is safe, it does entail significant toxicity; in the MOSAIC trial, the most common grade 3/4 toxicities were neutropenia (41%), diarrhea (10.8%), and vomiting (5.9%). Grade 3 peripheral neuropathy was reported in 12.4% of patients, and one-third of the patients had some degree of residual peripheral neurotoxicity 1 year after the completion of therapy [6]. In the NSABP C-07 trial, 85% of patients had some degree of neuropathy during treatment and 29% had greater than or equal to grade 1 neuropathy at 12 months. Irinotecan in combination with 5-FU and LV has been evaluated in the adjuvant setting but has not achieved similar results. Intergroup C89803, ACCORD, and PETACC-3 (Pan-European Trials in Alimentary Tract Cancer) compared different schedules of FU/LV with or without irinotecan [7–9]. None of them revealed a statistically significant survival difference with the addition of irinotecan to adjuvant 5-FU/LV for patients with stage II and III colon cancer.

Despite the impact of oxaliplatin, the adjuvant treatment of patients with stage II colon cancer continues to present a challenge. Three large analyses have led to conflicting conclusions about the benefit of adjuvant chemotherapy with 5-FU [10–12]. In the MOSAIC trial, patients with stage II disease achieved a 20% risk reduction, but the 95% confidence intervals (CIs) overlapped [13]. As a consequence, some patients are "over-treated" and subjected to toxicity that could have been avoided.

Given this reality, objectives for the future of adjuvant chemotherapy include the improvement of the current degree of risk reduction (RR) as well as the determination of subsets of patients with the most benefit from a specific therapy.

New adjuvant regimens: the incorporation of targeted agents

The first objective of improving the current degree of RR entails the usage of more effective chemotherapeutic regimens that would improve survival and lead to more cures. Such an improvement may come from the incorporation of targeted agents such as bevacizumab or cetuximab into adjuvant regimens. Bevacizumab is a humanized antibody directed at VEGF [14], which is highly expressed in colorectal cancer. The rationale for the usage of bevacizumab is based on the fact that angiogenesis has an influence on the metastatic potential of tumors [15]. VEGF expression by IHC (immunohistochemistry) has been found to be correlated with outcome and survival in patients with Dukes' B colon cancer [16]. Turning off the "angiogenic switch" may lead to an early inhibition of micrometastases and potentially add to the current benefit of adjuvant FOLFOX. Ongoing NSABP C-08 trial is designed to evaluate the benefit of adding 12 months of bevacizumab therapy to 6 months of FOLFOX.

Cetuximab is a chimeric immunoglobulin G1 monoclonal antibody that targets the EGFR, inhibits its phosphorylation, and consequently prevents the initiation of several intracellular events related to angiogenesis, apoptosis, proliferation, and invasion [17]. It has single-agent activity in patients with metastatic disease who have failed 2 or 3 lines of therapy [18] and has also resulted in higher RR when combined with FOLFOX [19]. EGFR polymorphisms in codon 497 as well as in intron 1 have been associated with an increased risk of local recurrence in patients with rectal cancer treated with adjuvant or neoadjuvant chemoradiotherapy [20]. As a result, cetuximab may play a role in the eradication of micrometastases in the adjuvant setting. The planned intergroup study N0147 may shed some light on the effect of the addition of cetuximab to adjuvant FOLFOX in stage II and III colon cancer patients.

The relevance of molecular prognostic and predictive markers

The second future objective noted above is the determination of subsets of patients who would benefit most from adjuvant therapy and of subsets of patients who would respond better to one regimen vs another. Prognostic molecular markers that help predict tumor behavior as well as host/tumor interactions could be helpful in risk stratification and in restriction of treatment to patients who would derive the most benefit from it [21].

There are several examples of identified genes that are thought to be prognostic indicators of recurrence. They include microsatellite instability (MSI), Deleted in Colon Cancer (DCC), thymidilate synthase (TS), transforming growth factor-β (TGF-β), p53, p27, K-ras, and others. Due to the general topic of this chapter, we will restrict our discussion to MSI, DCC,

TS, and TGF-β as examples of prognostic markers that may play a role in determining subgroups of patients with benefit from adjuvant chemotherapy. MSI is present in about 15% of CRCs and reflects the inactivation of mismatch repair (MMR) genes. Analysis of pooled data from published studies by Popat *et al.* reveals that CRCs with MSI have a better prognosis (hazard ratio [HR]) 0.65, 95% CI, 0.59 to 0.71). MSI tumors appeared to derive no benefit from adjuvant 5-FU but the data are limited with HR of 1.24 and a 95% CI of 0.72 to 2.14 [22]. Deletions in chromosome 18q, termed DCC, has been shown to be a negative predictor of prognosis in colon cancer [23]. In a retrospective study, Gal *et al.* [24] showed that positive expression of DCC by immunohistochemistry identified patients who respond favorably to adjuvant 5-FU-based chemotherapy. These data highlight the prognostic significance of MSI and DCC but do not provide a definite answer as to their relevance in determining benefit from adjuvant chemotherapy. Prospective validation of the role of these markers in determining when and who to treat is needed. E5202 is a planned prospective randomized trial that assigns patients with stage II colon cancer to a high- or low-risk category based on the presence of 18q deletion and MSI. Patients with high-risk features are randomized to FOLFOX with or without bevacizumab. Low-risk patients are assigned to an observation group. This type of clinical trial will shed a more definite light on the role of MSI and 18q deletion in determining prognosis and response to adjuvant chemotherapy.

Thymidilate synthase is the target of fluoropyrimidines like 5-FU. TS inhibition prevents the cell from its sole de novo source of thymidilate, which is essential for DNA replication and repair. TS expression has been shown to have prognostic value with low intratumoral levels predicting longer survival [25,26]. More recently, low TS expression assessed by immunohistochemistry in tumors from 1326 patients with stage II and III CRC was found to be a statistically valid independent prognostic factor [27]. While the prognostic value of TS has been established, its role in predicting benefit from adjuvant 5-FU-based chemotherapy has been somewhat controversial, likely secondary to the small patient numbers and the difference in the methodology used to assess the expression level (IHC vs RT-PCR) [28]. TS deserves prospective validation like MSI and 18q.

The TGF-β signaling pathway has a complex role in tumorigenesis [29]; for example, it stimulates the growth of colon cancer cells through a Ras-dependent mechanism, induces angiogenesis, and promotes invasiveness and metastases. TGF-β1 serum levels have been found to be predictive of liver metastases after surgery for colon cancer (CC) [30]. The CC genotype poly-morphism of TGF-β1, which is associated with higher TGF-β1 serum levels, was found to be associated with a higher risk of recurrence in patients with stage II and III colon cancer [31].

As more prognostic molecular makers are identified, one needs to note that the survival of patients with stage II and III colorectal cancer as well as their response to adjuvant therapy is influenced by multiple genes and pathways. In addition to incorporating other potential prognostic markers, such as TS and TGF-β, into prospective randomized clinical trials, there is a clear need for technological advances that would define a more compre-hensive molecular fingerprint that would serve as the basis of the decision to treat or not to treat. Microarray technology is quickly emerging as a tool to obtain a comprehensive and global profile of a tumor's gene expression characteristics. Using Affymetrix U133a gene chip (Affymetrix, Santa Clara, Ca), Wang *et al.* [32] reported a 23-gene signature that predicted recurrence in Dukes' B colon cancer patients. Despite the small sample size of 74 and the retrospective nature of the clinical information, this provocative data, if validated, could serve as a way to "upstage" some patients with Dukes' B colon cancer to receive adjuvant chemotherapy.

The future of locally advanced rectal cancer therapy

The incorporation of new drugs in neoadjuvant regimens

Preoperative chemoradiotherapy for T3, T4, or node positive rectal cancer has been adopted by most centers based on improved local control and reduced toxicity results compared to postoperative chemoradiotherapy [33]. Another reason for the increasing interest in neoadjuvant chemoradiother-apy is to enhance sphincter-conserving surgeries for distal rectal cancers [34]. Pathologic complete response (PCR) is thought to be a good surrogate marker for long-term outcome in rectal cancer as it may predict improved overall survival [35]. The incorporation of oxaliplatin and irinotecan into neoadjuvant chemoradiotherapy regimens is undergoing evaluation with the hope of increasing the rate of sphincter preservation and of PCR, thereby improving OS [36]. For example, the SOCRATES phase I/II study has determined the safety of capecitabine in combination with oxaliplatin and preoperative radiation therapy; PCR was noted in 18% of patients and 80% had radical oncological (RO) resection [37]. Neoadjuvant irinotecan with continuous infusion 5-FU and radiation have resulted in 22% PCR rate and

80% RO resections [38]. These PCR rates appear favorable with histor-ical rates of up to 10% with 5-FU or 5-FU/LV [33]. It is important that future endeavors include randomized clinical trials that compare intensified neoadjuvant treatment regimens with oxaliplatin or irinotecan and radia-tion to 5-FU and radiation. We are awaiting the results of RTOG 0012, a randomized phase II study that assigned patients with T3-T4 rectal cancer to radiation with 5-FU and irinotecan vs radiation and 5-FU. An ongo-ing German trial (CAO/ARO/AIO-05) is randomizing patients to 5-FU and radiation vs XELOX and radiation.

Targeted agents such as bevacizumab and cetuximab are undergoing evaluation in combination with chemoradiotherapy for rectal cancer. This approach is based on the radiosensitizing properties of these agents and on the positive impact that they have had on efficacy of chemotherapy [36]. For example, a German phase I/II study is evaluating preoperative XELOX with cetuximab and radiation therapy.

Maximizing the benefit of the preoperative approach: tailored therapy

Molecular predictors of response to 5-FU, oxaliplatin, and irinotecan have been the subject of intensive translational research over the last several years [39]. The ultimate goal of the identification of these predictors is to assign patients to the most effective, and least toxic, therapy. This approach would be highly significant in the setting of neoadjuvant chemoradiother-apy for rectal cancer because it would potentially improve the PCR rate and potentially prolong survival. Future directions in the neoadjuvant treatment of rectal cancer need to focus on PCR as an endpoint and to utilize pharma-cogenomics to guide the treating oncologist in choosing the most effective drug combination for the individual patient.

Since most of the current data about predictive markers of response are retrospective, efforts are under way to assess these markers prospectively with the hope of better understanding their role and paving the way for randomized pharmacogenomics trials. In this context, an ongoing study by Mcleod et al. [40] uses TS genotype polymorphisms to assign patients with T3/T4 rectal cancer to neoadjuvant 5-FU and radiotherapy vs 5-FU, irinote-can, and radiotherapy. Patients who are homozygous for the triple repeat (3R) of a 28-base pair sequence in the promoter region of TS are treated with the irinotecan containing combination based on the knowledge that they have higher TS levels [41] and on the fact that they have a lower rate of downstaging with 5-FU based neoadjuvant therapy [42]. Patients with the genotypes 2R/2R and 2R/3R are considered "good risk" patients and receive 5-FU alone. It is important to note that this is not a randomized trial but a combination of two distinct phase II trials directed by the TS genotype. Preliminary results reported at American Society of Clinical Oncology (ASCO) 2005 revealed a higher than historically observed rate of downstaging in the "good risk" group, presumably due to the selection of the patients based on their genotype. Only 13 "bad risk" patients had been enrolled and treated with the more aggressive combination containing irinotecan; interestingly, they achieved an 85% rate of downstaging, which is higher than anticipated. Despite the potential criticisms of these preliminary results, they do establish the feasibility of genotype-guided neoadjuvant therapy. Along the same lines, the Southwest Oncology Group (SWOG) has initiated the first prospective multicenter feasibility study aimed at assigning patients with T3/T4 rectal cancer to a specific neoadjuvant chemotherapy combination based on their tumors' molecular profile. SWOG 0304 will use the gene expression levels of TS, DPD, and ERCC-1 to determine whether patients receive induction chemotherapy with FOLFIRI (high ERCC 1 group) vs FOLFOX (low TS, DPD, and ERCC 1 group) vs IROX (low ERCC 1, high TS, and DPD group); induction chemotherapy will be followed by capecitabine and concurrent radiation therapy.

In addition to predictive markers of response, prognostic markers may become relevant in determining which patients to treat with intensified combination chemotherapy and radiation vs 5-FU and radiation.

The future approach to the treatment of metastatic colorectal cancer

The overall survival of patients with mCRC has surpassed 20 months when they receive the oxaliplatin-based combination (FOLFOX) followed by the irinotecan-based combination (FOLFIRI) upon progression or the reverse sequence [1]. This impressive survival reaches 25 months when patients are exposed to bevacizumab in addition to oxaliplatin and irinotecan [43]. The new hope derived from this improvement in survival is not without challenges. The first challenge for the future is to continue to enhance the effectiveness of chemotherapy while minimizing toxicity and while not causing unjustified increases in healthcare cost. The second challenge is to make cure a feasible reality for select patients with mCRC, especially ones with metastases limited to the liver or lung.

The sequencing of regimens and the integration of targeted agents

Bevacizumab and cetuximab are the two approved targeted agents for the treatment of mCRC. The former has been shown to improve the RR and survival of patients treated with irinotecan in combination with bolus 5-FU/LV in first line [2] as well as patients treated with FOLFOX in second line [44]. The latter allows patients who have failed irinotecan-based therapy to respond to the combination of irinotecan and cetuximab with a prolongation of their time to progression [3]. Currently, both bevacizumab and cetuximab are being evaluated for their role in front-line therapy with oxaliplatin- or irinotecan-based combinations with RRs ranging between 57 and 72% [19,45,46]. Furthermore, the novel concept of combining the two targeted agents has resulted in a significant degree of efficacy, even as third-line therapy. Cetuximab and bevacizumab with irinotecan (CBI) in patients with irinotecan failure as well as oxaliplatin failure in 85% of cases has a RR of 37% and median time to progression of 7.3 months. Cetuximab and bevacizumab given together (CB) in the same setting have a RR of 20% with TTP (time to progression) of 5.6 months [47]. Based on these data, it is currently difficult to define the exact place of targeted agents in the sequencing order of the different regimens. Future studies are needed to answer several questions:

1 Do all patients need to receive combination chemotherapy in front line?

2 Should all patients receive a targeted agent along with first-line chemotherapy?

3 Should patients receive a combination of targeted agents with first-line chemotherapy?

4 Is there a rationale to continue the administration of a targeted agent, such as bevacizumab, once patients have experienced progression of disease on a certain chemotherapy regimen given in combination with bevacizumab?

Answering these questions requires the design of appropriate clinical trials as well as the identification of patient sub-populations who would benefit from aggressive front-line chemotherapy vs others who would not. It seems reasonable to adopt the combination regimen with the highest RR as front-line therapy for patients with a potential for cure (i.e. potentially resectable metastatic disease), patients with a poor prognostic profile, and patients with significant symptoms related to their disease burden. However, other patients may be adequately treated with 5-FU as a single agent followed by a combination of 5-FU with oxaliplatin and irinotecan. This approach was evaluated in the FOCUS trial which showed higher RR and PFS with front-line combination therapy but similar OS in patients who received single agent 5-FU followed by combination therapy upon progression. The advantage of such an approach is a lower degree of unnecessary toxicity [48].

The question in regards to the continuation of a targeted agent after progression of disease with a combination of the same targeted agent plus chemotherapy remains unanswered. The planned BOND 2.5 trial will contribute to this answer by evaluating the efficacy of cetuximab/bevacizumab/irinotecan (CBI) after bevacizumab failure.

Minimizing toxicity

The improved efficacy of combination chemotherapy regimens results in longer exposure time and consequently, a higher risk of significant cumulative toxicity. Minimizing toxicity may be achieved in the future through clinical innovation related to the dosing and administration schedule of drugs. For example, peripheral neuropathy, acute and chronic, is one of the most common toxicities associated with oxaliplatin administration [49]. Chronic neuropathy is cumulative with grade 3 toxicity being present in 50% of patients who reach doses over 1000 mg/m^2 [50]. Several medical interventions including the administration of calcium and magnesium salts, gapapentin, carbamazepine, celecoxib, and amifostime have been evaluated with no definite conclusion due to conflicting results and small patient numbers in most studies [49]. Another method to counteract the cumulative character of the neuropathy is through "oxaliplatin holidays." The OPTIMOX-1 study design serves as an example of the "stop and go" strategy whereby patients receive FOLFOX first, followed by 5-FU/LV, and subsequently FOLFOX reintroduction upon progression [51]. Alternating FOLFOX and FOLFIRI prior to progression of disease may be another alternative which reduces the cumulative dose of oxaliplatin [52]. As the newer targeted agents are incorporated into front-line regimens, they may play a useful role in allowing for reduction in the dose intensity of oxaliplatin and in the introduction of drug holidays without compromising efficacy.

The search for molecular predictors of toxicity has been an active area of research. Ultimately, the goal is to resort to the patient's molecular fingerprint to assess the risk of toxicity with a specific drug or combination and weight it against the expected benefit. In the case of oxaliplatin, there is limited knowledge in regard to genotype variations that are associated with toxicity. Recently, Glutathione S-transferase P1 I105V polymorphism was found to be associated with early onset of oxaliplatin-induced neurotoxicity [53]. More data related to the influence of variations in drug metabolism and transport genes on irinotecan toxicity has been accumulated. UDP-glucoronosyltransferase (UGT1A1) is known to glucoronidate SN-38, the active metabolite of irinotecan, to become an inactive product. The UGT1A1 7/7 variant has been shown to be associated with the risk of neutropenia [54]. Since the drug metabolism pathway of irinotecan is polygenic, it is unlikely that UGT1A1 polymorphisms alone will allow for adequate toxicity risk stratification. Current and future efforts need to identify other relevant genes that may be assessed and analyzed together in order to delineate different risk groups. An example of this approach can be found in a study by Innocenti et al. [55] in which patients were assigned to low, intermediate, and high-risk groups for neutropenia based on polymorphisms in UGT1A1, SLCO1b1 (an organic anion transporter gene expressed in liver), and gender.

In summary, as patients live longer thanks to effective chemotherapeutic and targeted agents, oncologists have to be aware of the effect of drug toxicity on the patient's quality of life. In addition to innovation in the dosing and frequency of drug administration, translational studies are needed to better elucidate molecular predictors of toxicity that can be interpreted in the context of the risk-benefit assessment for each patient.

The aim for cure in the setting of metastatic disease

Chemotherapy administered to patients with metastatic CRC has traditionally been aimed at improving survival and palliating symptoms. However, the advent of effective chemotherapeutic combinations in conjunction with the encouraging results achieved after resection of liver or lung metastases suggest that cure may be a reasonable expectation in select patients. Five-year survival rates between 20 and 45% have been observed historically after surgical resection of liver metastases [56]. These data preceded the current chemotherapeutic combinations. Some of the future goals include improving the rate of resectability as well as the duration of remission. Since it is not the intent of this chapter to present an exhaustive review of surgical resection of metastases from CRC, we will focus our discussion on select chemotherapeutic and molecular advances that may be valuable in achieving the above stated objectives.

Neoadjuvant chemotherapy for patients with mCRC to liver or lung only

Combinations chemotherapy regimens such as 5-fluorouracil (5-FU), leucovorin (LV), and oxaliplatin (FOLFOX) or 5-FU, LV, and irinotecan (FOLFIRI) have achieved response rates of 50–55% in patients with mCRC [1]. Given the high RR achieved, these regimens may allow a higher number of patients to become eligible for surgical resection of metastases and hopefully prolong survival through the control of systemic micrometastases. This approach has been undergoing evaluation with encouraging results. One hundred and thirty nine out of 1400 (13%) initially unresectable patients with mCRC to the liver were able to undergo resection following neoadjuvant treatment with oxaliplatin or irinotecan-based regimens. The overall 5-year survival was 36% [57]. In a North Central Cancer Treatment Group (NCCTG) study, 17 (41%) patients with unresectable liver metastases underwent resection after neoadjuvant FOLFOX4 with a median survival of 31.4 months [58].

The response rates noted with oxaliplatin or irinotecan-based regimens in the setting of metastatic disease have become even higher with the addition of cetuximab or bevacizumab to FOLFOX or FOLFIRI [19,45,46]. For example, FOLFOX in combination with cetuximab as first-line therapy for mCRC has resulted in a RR of 72%, including a 9% rate of complete response (CR) [19]. Capecitabine in combination with oxaliplatin and bevacizumab (Avastin) (XeloxA) administered to previously untreated patients with mCRC has a RR of 57% and disease stability rate of 37% [59]. These data have provided the rationale for the ongoing or planned evaluation of FOLFOX or FOLFIRI in combination with a targeted agent for their role in "downstaging" liver metastases and improving survival after resection.

In summary, improved resectability and survival rates may be achievable in the future if we are able to administer the most appropriate and most effective neoadjuvant regimen to patients with metastases to the liver or lung only. Furthermore, the identification of predictive molecular markers of response to chemotherapy may be a valuable tool in choosing the optimal neoadjuvant combination that would achieve the highest response rate and allow for potentially curative resection.

Molecular predictive markers of response in the metastatic setting

Over the last few years, translational research aimed at defining molecular markers of prognosis and response has rapidly evolved. Different technologies used in the molecular profiling of tumors have been developed. While this chapter is not intended to present an in-depth discussion of this area, it is worthwhile that we address it given its relevance for the future treatment of colorectal cancer. As noted previously, tailored therapy may be useful in the neoadjuvant approach to the treatment of rectal cancer. Similarly, a molecular map may be valuable for patients receiving neoadjuvant chemotherapy with the goals of downstaging liver or lung metastases and eventual curative resection. When treatment is palliative, the potential to avoid failed therapies or excess toxicity can make a marked difference in a patient's quality of life.

Several methods have been used in the identification and evaluation of individual genes involved in specific drug metabolism, DNA repair, angiogenesis, cell cycle control, apoptosis, and others. Immunohistochemistry has been utilized to evaluate the protein expression of a gene. Proteomics examine a specific tissue's entire protein complement [60]. Alternatively, one could look for gene expression at the RNA level using techniques such as reverse transcription polymerase chain reaction (RT-PCR) [61]. Microarrays or "chips" allow the researcher to perform whole-genome expression profiles and potentially derive a molecular signature that is relevant to prognosis or response to a specific therapy [62]. Polymorphisms are variations within a gene, such as repeats of nucleotide sequences or substitutions of one or more nucleotide. When the polymorphism affects the transcription or translation of a gene related to the efficacy of a drug, the polymorphism may be associated with clinical outcome [63].

Below are some examples of genetic markers relevant to colorectal cancer that are likely be relevant to future attempts at tailoring therapy. Thymidilate synthase (TS) gene expression levels have been shown to predict response to treatment with 5-FU and survival [64]. However, taken by itself, TS does not separate all responders from non-responders. Thymidine phosphorylase (TP) and dihydropyrimidine dehydrogenase (DPD) also play a role in 5-FU metabolism and have been shown to correlate with response. When evaluated together, TS, TP, and DPD resulted in a clear separation of patients with response from those with no response; patients with low levels of all three enzymes had significantly better response (11/11 patients, 100%, $p = 0.0001$) than patients with higher levels of all three enzymes (0/22 patients) [65]. Excision repair complementation group 1 (ERCC1) gene family is thought to prevent DNA injury and mutations via the nucleotide excision repair pathway. Given the mechanism of action of oxaliplatin which forms bulky DNA adducts, ERCC1 has been evaluated for its role in predicting outcome with oxaliplatin. Stoehlmacher *et al.* evaluated tumors of patients treated with 5-FU/oxaliplatin for the mRNA expression of TS and ERCC-1. Both TS and ERCC-1 mRNA expression levels had a statistically significant association with survival in these patients. ERCC1 polymorphisms have also been found to be associated with improved clinical outcome [66].

More recently, attempts at identifying molecular markers to predict the efficacy of targeted agents are under way. For instance, lower mRNA levels of Cox 2, EGFR, and IL-8 were significantly associated with overall survival in a small series of 39 patients treated with cetuximab alone [67].

The challenges for the future include:

1 The validation of the association of molecular markers with clinical outcome in prospective trials. (It is encouraging to note that these efforts are already under way.)

2 The refining of technologies and statistical methods in order to accommodate the complexity of the molecular map that may determine outcome. (In other words, clinical outcome is not dependent on one polymorphism in one gene, or one gene in a pathway, and not even on a single pathway.)

3 The standardization of testing methods and results' interpretation.

4 The adaptation of these findings and methods to everyday practice, especially in the community.

New agents and combinations

Efforts to develop new cytotoxic drugs as well as biologic agents such as antibodies, antisense oligonucleotides, and tyrosine kinase inhibitors are continuing. It is beyond the scope of this chapter to enumerate all the new drugs in development. However, it is worthwhile to highlight some of the targets that play a role in the molecular carcinogenesis of colorectal cancer and that have served as the catalyst for the design of new targeted agents. They include focal adhesion kinase (FAK), insulin growth factor receptor (IGFR), vascular endothelial growth factor receptor (VEGFR), and endothelial growth factor (EGF). Other compounds have been designed to inhibit multiple targets such as SU11248, PTK/ZK, and BAY 43-9006. PTK/ZK is an inhibitor of all three VEGF receptors as well as of platelet derived growth factor receptor (PDGFR) and c-KIT. FOLFOX in combination with PTK/ZK did not result in improved efficacy or prolonged survival when compared to FOLFOX alone [68]. Explanations for this result may be found at the pharmacokinetic, molecular target, and patient selection levels.

In addition to the multitargeted inhibitors, investment into the identification of cross-talk mechanisms between different pathways may guide future directions related to the combination of different targeted agents. For example, the synergism noted clinically between the inhibition of the EGF pathway with cetuximab and the VEGF pathway with bevacizumab [47] can be explained by several interactions at the molecular level between the two pathways through neuropilin and the hypoxia induced factor (HIF1) [69,70]. Other combinations like this may carry the promise of high clinical efficacy and low toxicity.

Molecular markers of response or prognosis, including genomic polymorphisms, may represent appropriate targets for new drug design in the future since the inhibition or the enhanced expression of these markers could influence the molecular behavior of tumors. This novel approach to drug development could be further enhanced through novel phase I designs that incorporate pharmacokinetic and pharmacodynamic modulation in order to determine the dose that achieves the highest degree of target inhibition. In other words, biologic activity may need to replace the concept of maximum tolerated dose (MTD) as an endpoint for certain targeted agents.

Conclusions

Future directions in the treatment of colorectal cancer hold promise for more effective therapies leading to longer survival and higher chances of cure. However, the oncology community faces the challenge of adapting to the rapid pace of drug development and technological advances in order to utilize them appropriately in advancing the field. Recent lessons point to the need to integrate molecular biology, pharmacology, pharmacodynamics, and pharmacogenomics into drug development. Simultaneously, the prospective validation of prognostic and predictive molecular markers as well as the standardization of methods utilized to identify them promise to move us from the era of the "one size fits all" chemotherapy to the era of the individually tailored treatment algorithm.

References

1 Tournigand C, Andre T, Achille E *et al.* FOLFIRI followed by FOLFOX6 or the reverse sequence in advanced colorectal cancer: a randomized GERCOR study. *J Clin Oncol* 2004; 22: 229–37.

2 Hurwitz H, Fehrenbacher L, Novotny W *et al.* Bevacizumab plus irinotecan, fluorouracil, and leucovorin for metastatic colorectal cancer. *N Engl J Med* 2004; 350: 2335–42.

3 Cunningham D, Humblet Y, Siena S *et al.* Cetuximab (C225) alone or in combination with irinotecan (CPT-11) in patients with epidermal growth factor (EGFR) positive, irinotecan refractory metastatic colorectal cancer (MCRC). *39th Annual Meeting of American Society of Clinical Oncology*; May 31–June 23, 2003; Chicago, Ill. (abstr 1012).

4 Wolmark N, Wieand HS, Kuebler JP *et al.* Phase III trial comparing FULV to FULV + oxaliplatin in stage II or III carcinoma of the colon: results of NSABP Protocol C-07. *Am Soc Clin Oncol Annual Meeting* 2005 (abstr LBA 3500).

5 De Gramont A, Boni C, Navarro M *et al.* Oxaliplatin/5FU/LV in the adjuvant treatment of stage II and stage III colon cancer: efficacy results with a median follow-up of 4 years. *Am Soc Clin Oncol Annual Meeting* 2005 (abstr 3501).

6 De Gramont A, Boni C, Navarro M *et al.* Oxaliplatin/5-FU/LV in adjuvant colon cancer: safety results of the international randomized MOSAIC trial. *38th Annual Meeting of American Society of Clinical Oncology* 2002 (abstr 525).

7 Saltz LB, Niedzwiecki D, Hollis D *et al.* Irinotecan plus fluorouracil/leucovorin (IFL) versus fluorouracil/leucovorin alone (FL) in stage III colon cancer (intergroup trial CALGB C89803). *Proc Am Soc Clin Oncol* 22: 2004 (abstr 3500).

8 Van Cutsem E, Labianca R, Hossfeld D *et al.* Randomized phase III trial comparing infused irinotecan/ 5-fluorouracil (5-FU)/folinic acid (IF) versus 5-FU/FA (F) in stage III colon cancer patients (pts) (PETACC 3). *Am Soc Clin Oncol Annual Meeting* 2005 (abstr LBA8).

9 Ychou M, Raoul J, Douillard J *et al.* A phase III randomized trial of LV5FU2+CPT-11 vs. LV5FU2 alone in adjuvant high risk colon cancer (FNCLCC Accord02/FFCD9802). *Am Soc Clin Oncol Annual Meeting* 2005 (abstr 3502).

10 Gill S, Loprinzi CL, Sargent DJ *et al.* Pooled analysis of fluorouracil-based adjuvant therapy for stage II and III colon cancer. Who benefits and by how much? *J Clin Oncol* 2004; 22: 1797–806.

11 Mamounas E, Weiand S, Wolmark N *et al.* Comparative efficacy of adjuvant chemotherapy in patients with Dukes' B versus Dukes' C colon cancer: Results from four National Surgical Adjuvant Breast and Bowel Project adjuvant studies (C-01, C-02, C-03, and C-04). *J Clin Oncol* 2004; 17: 1349–55.

12 Internaltional Multicenter Pooled Analysis of B2 Colon Cancer Trials (IMPACT B2) investigators. Efficacy of adjuvant fluorouracil and folinic acid in B2 colon cancer. *J Clin Oncol* 1999; 17: 1356–63.

13 Andre T, Boni C, Mounedji-Boudiaf L *et al.* for the Multicenter International study of oxaliplatin/5-fluorouracil/ leucovorin in the adjuvant treatment of colon cancer investigators. Oxaliplatin, fluorouracil, and leucovorin as adjuvant treatment for colon cancer. *N Engl J Med* 2004; 350: 2343–51.

14 Presta IG, Chen H, O'Connor SJ *et al.* Humanization of an anti-vascular endothelial growth factor monoclonal antibody for the therapy of solid tumors and other disorders. *Cancer Res* 1997; 57: 4593–99.

15 Takahashi Y, Kitadai Y, Bucana CD *et al.* Expression of vascular endothelial growth factor and its receptor, KDR, correlates with vascularity, metastasis, and proliferation. *Cancer Res* 1995; 55: 3964–8.

16 Boxera GM, Tsiompanoua E, Levineb R *et al.* Immunohistochemical expression of vascular endothelial growth factor and microvessel counting as prognostic indicators in node-negative colorectal cancer. *Tumor Biology* 2005; 26: 1–8.

17 Mendelson J. Targeting the epidermal growth factor receptor for cancer therapy. *J Clin Oncol* 2002; 20: 1s–13s.

18 Lenz H, Mayer RJ, Gold P *et al.* Activity of Erbitux (cetuximab) in patients with colorectal cancer refractory to a fluoropyrimidine, irinotecan, and oxaliplatin. *Am Soc Clin Oncol Annual Meeting* 2005 (abstrt 225).

19 Diaz-Rubio E, Taberbero J,
Van Custem E *et al*. Cetuximab in
combination with oxaliplatin/
5-fluorouracil (5-FU)/folinic acid (FA)
(FOLFOX-4) in the first-line treatment of
patients with epidermal growth factor
receptor (EGFR) – expressing metastatic
colorectal cancer: an international phase
II study. *Am Soc Clin Oncol Annual
Meeting* 2005 (abstr 3535).
20 Zhang W, Park D, Lu B *et al*. Epidermal
growth factor receptor gene
polymorphisms predict pelvic recurrence
in patients with rectal cancer treated with
chemoradiation. *Clin Cancer Res* 2005;
11: 600–5.
21 Lenz HJ. Pharmacogenomics in
colorectal cancer. *Semin Oncol* 2003;
30: 47–53.
22 Popat S, Hubner R, Houlston RS.
Systematic review of microsatellite
instability and colorectal cancer
prognosis. *J Clin Oncol* 2005;
23: 609–17.
23 Jen J, Kim H, Piantadosi S *et al*. Allelic
loss of chromosome 18q and prognosis
in colorectal cancer. *N Engl J Med* 1994;
331: 213–21.
24 Gal R, Sadikov E, Sulkes J *et al*. Deleted
in colorectal cancer protein expression as
a possible predictor of response to
adjuvant chemotherapy in colorectal
cancer patients. *Dis Colon Rectum* 2004;
47: 1216–24.
25 Johnston PG, Fisher ER, Rockette HE
et al. The role of thymidilate synthase
expression in prognosis and outcome of
adjuvant chemotherapy in patients with
rectal cancer. *J Clin Oncol* 1994;
12: 2640–7.
26 Lenz HJ, Danenberg KD, Leichman CG
et al. p53 and thymidilate synthase
expression in untreated stage II colon
cancer: associations with recurrence,
survival, and site. *Clin Cancer Res* 1998;
4: 1227–34.
27 Johnston PG, Benson A, Catalano P *et al*.
The clinical significance of thymidilate
synthase (TS) expression in primary
colorectal cancer: an intergroup
combined analysis. *Am Soc Clin Oncol
Annual Meeting* 2005 (abstr 3510).
28 Popat S, Matakidou A, Houlston RS.
Thymidilate synthase expression and
prognosis in colorectal cancer:
a systematic review and meta-analysis.
J Clin Oncol 2004; 22: 529–36.
29 Elliott R, Blobe G. Role of transforming
growth factor beta in human cancer.
J Clin Oncol 2005; 23: 2078–93.
30 Tsushima H, Ito N, Tamura S *et al*.
Circulating transforming growth factor
beta 1 as a predictor of liver metastasis
after resection in colorectal cancer. *Clin
Cancer Res* 2001; 7: 1258–62.
31 Hendifar A, Zhang W, Yang DY *et al*.
Polymorphisms of transforming growth
factor-beta (TGF-β1) and recurrence in
stage II and III colon cancer. *Am Soc Clin
Oncol Annual Meeting* 2005 (abstr
3634).
32 Wang Y, Jatkoe T, Zhang Y *et al*. Gene
expression profiles and molecular
markers to predict recurrence of Dukes'
B colon cancer. *J Clin Oncol* 2004; 22:
1564–71.
33 Sauer R, Becker H, Hohenberger W *et al*.
Preoperative versus postoperative
chemoradiotherapy for rectal cancer.
N Engl J Med 2004; 351: 1731–40.
34 Zhu A, Willet C. Combined modality
treatment of rectal cancer. *Semin Oncol*
2005; 32: 103–12.
35 Gullem J, Chessin D, Cohen A *et al*.
Long-term oncologic outcome following
preoperative combined modality therapy
and total mesorectal excision of locally
advanced rectal cancer. *Ann Surg* 2005;
241: 829–36.
36 Zhu AX, Willett CG. Chemotherapeutic
and biologic agents as radiosensitizers in
rectal cancer. *Semin Radiat Oncol* 2003;
13: 454–68.
37 Glynne-Jones R, Sebag-Montefiore D,
Samuel L *et al*. Socrates Phase II study
results: capecitabine (CAP) combined
with oxaliplatin (OX) and preoperative
radiation (RT) in patients with locally
advanced rectal cancer. *Am Soc Clin
Oncol Annual Meeting* 2005 (abstr
3527).
38 Klautke G, Feyerherd P, Ludwig K
et al. Intensified concurrent
chemoradiotherapy with 5-fluorouracil

and irinotecan as neoadjuvant treatment in patients with locally advanced rectal cancer. *Br J Cancer* 2005; 92: 1215–20.

39 Iqbal S, Stoehlmacher J, Lenz HJ. Tailored therapy for colorectal cancer: a new approach to therapy. *Cancer Invest* 2004; 22: 762–73.

40 McLeod HL, Tan B, Malyapa R *et al.* Genotype-guided neoadjuvant therapy for colorectal cancer. *Am Soc Clin Oncol Annual Meeting* 2005 (abstr 3024).

41 Pullarkat ST, Stoehlmacher J, Ghaderi V *et al.* Thymidylate synthase gene polymorphism determines response and toxicity of 5-FU based chemotherapy. *Pharmacogenom J* 2001; 1: 65–70.

42 Villafranca E, Okruzhnov Y, Dominguez M *et al.* Polymorphisms of the repeated sequences in the enhancer region of the thymidylate synthase gene promoter may predict downstaging after preoperative chemoradiation in rectal cancer. *J Clin Oncol* 2001; 1: 1779–86.

43 Hedrick E, Hurwitz H, Sarkar S *et al.* Post-progression therapy (PPT) effect on survival in AVF2107, a phase III trial of bevacizumab in first-line treatment of metastatic colorectal cancer (mCRC). *Proc Am Soc Clin Oncol* 22, 2004 (abstr 3517).

44 Giantonio BJ, Catalano PJ, Meropol NJ *et al.* High-dose bevacizumab improves survival when combined with FOLFOX4 in previously treated advanced colorectal cancer: Results from the Eastern Cooperative Oncology Group (ECOG) study E3200. *Am Soc Clin Oncol Annual Meeting* 2005 (abstr 2).

45 Hochster HS, Welles L, Hart L *et al.* Safety and efficacy of bevacizumab (Bev) when added to oxaliplatin/ fluoropyrimidine (O/F) regimens as first-line treatment of metastatic colorectal cancer (mCRC): TREE 1&2 studies. *Am Soc Clin Oncol Annual Meeting* 2005 (abstr 3515).

46 Giantonio BJ, Levy D, O'Dwyer PJ *et al.* Bevacizumab (anti-VEGF) plus IFL (irinotecan, fluorouracil, leucovorin) as front-line therapy for advanced colorectal cancer (advCRC): Updated results from the Eastern Cooperative Oncology Group (ECOG) Study E2200. *Am Soc Clin Oncol Annual Meeting* 2005 (abstr 289).

47 Saltz LB, Lenz H, Hochster H *et al.* Randomized phase II trial of cetuximab/bevacizumab/irinotecan (CBI) versus cetuximab/bevacizumab (CB) in irinotecan-refractory colorectal cancer. *Am Soc Clin Oncol Annual Meeting* 2005 (abstr 3508).

48 Seymour MT, for the UK NCRI colorectal clinical studies group. Fluorouracil, oxaliplatin and CPT-11 (irinotecan), use and sequencing (MRC FOCUS): a 2135-patient randomized trial in advanced colorectal cancer (ACRC). *Am Soc Clin Oncol Annual Meeting* 2005 (abstr 3518).

49 Cersosimo R. Oxaliplatin-associated neuropathy: a review. *Ann Pharmacol* 2005; 39: 128–34.

50 De Gramont A, Figer A, Seymour M *et al.* Leucovorin and fluorouracil with or without oxaliplatin as first-line treatment in advanced colorectal cancer. *J Clin Oncol* 2000; 18: 2938–47.

51 De Gramont A, Cervantes A, Andre T *et al.* OPTIMOX study: FOLFOX7/LV5FU2 compared to FOLFOX4 in patients with advanced colorectal cancer. *Proc Am Soc Clin Oncol* 22: 2004 (abstr 3525).

52 Fernandez-Martos C, Aparicio J, Vicent JM *et al.* Biweekly alternating FOLFOX and FOLFIRI in patients with previously untreated, advanced colorectal cancer: Updated results. *Proc Am Soc Clin Oncol* 22: 2004 (abstr 3563).

53 Grothey A, McLeod HL, Green EM *et al.* Glutathione S-transferase P1 I105V (GSTP1 I105V) polymorphism is associated with early onset of oxaliplatin-induced neurotoxicity. *Am Soc Clin Oncol Annual Meeting* 2005 (abstr 3509).

54 McLeod HL, Sargent DJ, Marsh S *et al.* Pharmacogenetic analysis of systemic toxicity and response after 5-fluorouracil (5FU)/CPT-11, 5FU/oxaliplatin (oxal), or CPT-11/oxal therapy for advanced

colorectal cancer (CRC): results from an intergroup trial. *Proc Am Soc Clin Oncol* 22: 2003 (abstr 1013).

55 Innocenti F, Undevia SD, Rosner GL *et al.* Irinotecan (CPT-11) pharmacokinetics (PK) and neutropenia: interaction among UGT1A1 and transporter genes. *Am Soc Clin Oncol Annual Meeting* 2005 (abstr 2006).

56 Fong Y, Cohen A, Fortner J *et al.* Liver resection for colorectal metastases. *J Clin Oncol* 1997; 15: 938–46.

57 Adam R, Delvart V, Pascal G *et al.* Resection of non resectable liver metastases after chemotherapy: prognostic factors and long term results. *Proc Am Soc Clin Oncol* 22(14S): 2004 (abstr 3550).

58 Alberts SR, Donohue JH, Mahoney MR *et al.* Liver resection after 5-fluorouracil, leucovorin and oxaliplatin for patients with metastatic colorectal cancer (MCRC) limited to the liver: A North Central Cancer Treatment group (NCCTG) phase II study. *Proc Am Soc Clin Oncol* 22: 2003 (abstr 1053).

59 Fernando N, Yu D, Morse M *et al.* A phase II study of oxaliplatin, capecitabine and bevacizumab in the treatment of metastatic colorectal cancer. *Am Soc Clin Oncol Annual Meeting* 2005 (abstr 3556).

60 Posadas EM, Simpkins M, Liotta LA *et al.* Proteomic analysis for the early detection and rational treatment of cancer – realistic hope? *Ann Oncol* 2005; 16: 16–22.

61 Lord RV, Salonga D, Danenberg KD *et al.* Telomerase reverse transcriptase expression is increased early in the Barrett's metaplasia, dysplasia, adenocarcinoma sequence. *J Gastrointest Surg* 2000; 4: 135–42.

62 Kreiner T, Buck KT. Moving toward whole-genome analysis: a technology perspective. *Am J Health-Syst Pharm* 2005; 62: 296–305.

63 Tan B, McLeod H. Pharmacogenetic influences on treatment response and toxicity in colorectal cancer. *Semin Oncol* 2004; 32: 113–19.

64 Leichman CG, Lenz HJ, Leichman L *et al.* Quantitation of intratumoral thymidylate synthase expression predicts for disseminated colorectal cancer response and resistance to protracted-infusion fluorouracil and weekly leucovorin. *J Clin Oncol* 1997; 15: 3223–9.

65 Salonga D, Danenberg KD, Johnson M *et al.* Colorectal tumors responsding to 5-fluorouracil have low gene expression levels of dihydropyrimidine dehydrogenase, thymidylate synthase, and thymidine phosphorylase. *Clin Cancer Res* 2000; 6: 1322–7.

66 Stoehlmacher J, Park DJ, Zhang W *et al.* A multivariate analysis of genomic polymorphisms: prediction of clinical outcome to 5-FU/oxaliplatin combination chemotherapy in refractory colorectal cancer. *Br J Cancer* 2004; 91: 344–54.

67 Zhang W, Vallbohmer D, Yun J *et al.* Pharmacogenetic study of EGFR-positive metastatic colorectal cancer patients treated with epidermal growth factor receptor (EGFR) inhibitor cetuximab (C225). *Am Soc Clin Oncol Annual Meeting* 2005 (abstr 169).

68 Hecht JR, Trarbach T, Jaeger E *et al.* A randomized, double-blind, placebo-controlled, phase III study in patients (Pts) with metastatic adenocarcinoma of the colon or rectum receiving first-line chemotherapy with oxaliplatin/5-fluorouracil/leucovorin and PTK787/ZK 222584 or placebo (CONFIRM-1). *Am Soc Clin Oncol Annual Meeting* 2005 (abstr LBA3).

69 Luwor R, Lu Y, Li X *et al.* The antiepidermal growth factor monoclonal antibody cetuximab/C225 reduces hypoxia-inducible factor-1 alpha, leading to transcriptional inhibition of vascular endothelial growth factor expression. *Oncogene Advance Online Publication.* April 2005, 1–9.

70 Hicklin D, Ellis L. Role of the vascular endothelial growth factor pathway in tumor growth and angiogenesis. *J Clin Oncol* 2005; 23: 1011–27.

Index